Colour Handbook of

Skin Diseases
of the
Dog and Cat

A PROBLEM-ORIENTED APPROACH TO DIAGNOSIS AND MANAGEMENT

Richard G. Harvey
BVSc, PhD, CBiol, MIBiol, DVD, Dip. ECVD, MRCVS
Royal College of Veterinary Surgeons Specialist in Veterinary Dermatology
Godiva Referrals, Coventry, UK

Patrick J. McKeever
DVM, MS, DACVD
Professor of Comparative Dermatology, College of Veterinary Medicine
The University of Minnesota, St Paul, Minnesota, USA

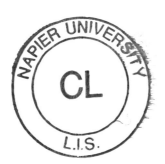

WITHDRAWN

Manson Publishing/The Veterinary Press

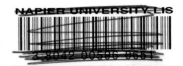

Softcover edition 2003

ISBN 1–874545–61–8

Copyright © 1998, 2003 Manson Publishing Ltd

A CIP catalogue record for this book is available from the British Library.

For full details of all Manson Publishing Ltd titles please write to:
Manson Publishing Ltd,
73 Corringham Road,
London NW11 7DL, UK.

Tel: +44 (0)20 8905 5150
Fax: +44 (0)20 8201 9233

Email: manson@man-pub.demon.co.uk
Website: www.manson-publishing.co.uk

Project manager: Paul Bennett
Text editor: Peter H. Beynon
Cover design: Patrick Daly
Colour reproduction: Tenon & Polert Colour Scanning Ltd, Hong Kong
Printed by: Grafos SA, Barcelona, Spain

Contents

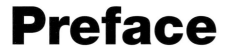

Preface

The genesis of this book lay in the authors' recognition that students and clinicians desire a problem-oriented approach to dermatology and that the dermatologic discipline has, in general, provided an etiopathologic approach. Such an approach recognizes that disease may present differently in one patient to another. Pruritus, for example, may be a major component of cheyletiellosis in some dogs and cats, whereas in others the disease is asymptomatic.

Nonetheless, the majority of dermatologic diseases have a principal component that is common to most cases and it is on this basis that the book is arranged. Some of the differential diagnoses may, at first sight, seem somewhat incongruous, until it is remembered that we have worked within the confines of a problem-oriented approach. We ask for your understanding.

Acknowledgements

The authors would like to acknowledge the support given by their families through the sacrifices they have made to allow us the time to complete this book. We are also grateful for the wonders of modern technology, without which this book would not have come to fruition. Finally we would like to thank the referring veterinarians who have trusted their dermatologic cases to us so that we could accumulate the knowledge and experience necessary to undertake this book.

Introduction

A PRACTICAL APPROACH TO THE DIAGNOSIS OF DERMATOLOGIC CASES

A dermatologic case can be viewed as a jig-saw puzzle with history, clinical findings, and diagnostic procedures being the major pieces. As with a puzzle, one piece by itself will generally not let you know what the picture is but, if you combine the pieces, the picture becomes clear. Likewise, a clinician will generally need the information in the history, the clinical findings, and the results of diagnostic procedures to see the picture or arrive at a definitive dermatologic diagnosis.

Approach, history, and signalment

Initially it is important to determine what the client's concerns are. In many chronic cases these concerns may be different from, or not relate to, the primary disease but reflect concerns due to secondary manifestations. Also it is important to determine what the client's expectations are, as they may be unrealistic since many cases cannot be cured, just controlled.

Signalment and particulars about the animal's diet and environmental surroundings are obtained next as these may give clues to contagion, zoonotic potential, and idiosyncratic managemental factors. Information pertaining to other body organs (appetite, thirst, exercize capability) is also important because the dermatologic lesions may reflect systemic disease.

Attention should then be focused on the skin by learning the initial appearance and location of lesions, subsequent changes, and the time frame of any progression. Finally, one can inquire if problems are also occurring in any people or other animals that have contact with the patient and what the response has been to at-home or veterinary prescribed therapies.

Physical examination

The skin and all body organs should be examined in a systematic manner. It is important to record the findings so that progress can be monitored objectively rather than subjectively. This methodology will also ensure that information is available should another clinician evaluate the case. It is especially important to note the distribution of lesions along with the types of lesions and whether they are primary or secondary.

Differential diagnosis

Using information obtained from the history and physical examination a differential diagnosis or list of rule outs is developed. Findings obtained on the history and physical examination are compared to key features of the diseases in the differential diagnosis so that they can be prioritized.

Diagnostic plan

Consideration of the prioritized differential diagnosis will allow formulation of a diagnostic plan, which will yield either a definitive diagnosis or allow diseases to be ruled out. This plan is reviewed with the animal's owner and the reasons for, likelihood of success, and cost of the various diagnostic procedures is explained to the client. Communication is essential as many cases take a considerable amount of time to work up and may incur considerable expense. It is important to ensure that the owners understand and accept this.

Therapy

After explaining the various treatment options, their expected success rate, cost, and possible side-effects a treatment plan is developed that is acceptable to the client. If appropriate, follow-up examinations are scheduled to assess progress and/or adjust medication doses.

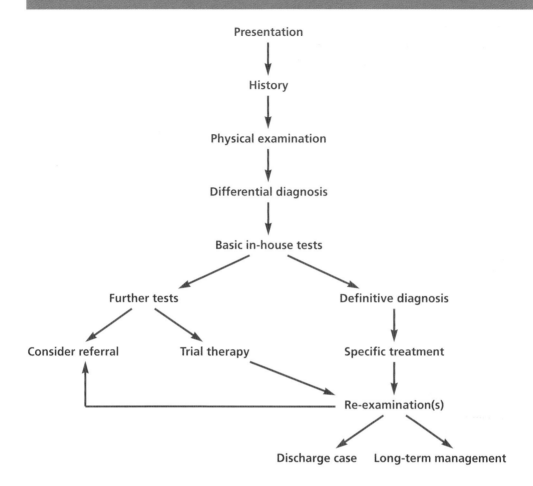

Algorithm summarizing the approach to the dermatologic case.

TERMINOLOGY USED IN THE DESCRIPTION OF DERMATOLOGIC LESIONS

Primary lesions

Primary lesions are directly associated with the disease process. They are not pathognomonic but give a valuable clue as to the type of disease process occurring.

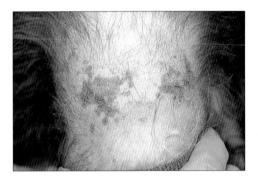

Macules are flat areas of discoloration up to 1 cm (0.4 in) in diameter whereas *patches* are larger than 1 cm in diameter. Illustration shows hemorrhagic macules and patches.

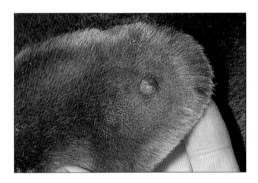

Papules are small, solid elevated lesions up to 1 cm (0.4 in) in diameter, in this case a mast cell tumor.

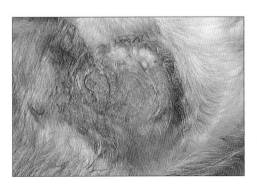

A plaque is a flat, solid elevated lesion of more than 1 cm (0.4 in) in diameter. The lesions illustrated are eosinophilic plaques on a cat.

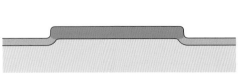

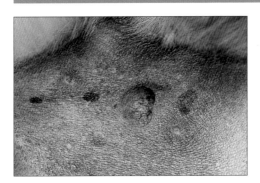

A nodule is a solid elevation of the skin greater than 1 cm (0.4 in) in diameter. The nodule illustrated is a mast cell tumor on the abdomen of a dog. A *tumor* is a large nodule, although not necessarily neoplastic.

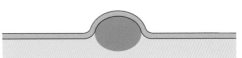

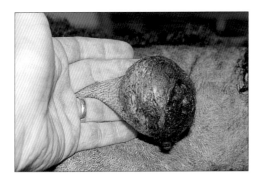

A tumor is a large growth. A lipoma on the flank of a dog is illustrated.

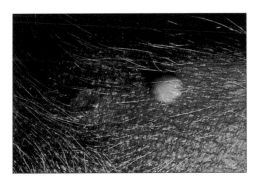

A pustule is a small circumscribed skin elevation containing purulent material.

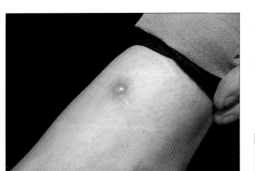

A vesicle is a circumscribed elevation of the skin up to 1 cm (0.4 in) in diameter filled with serum. The illustrated vesicle occurred on this veterinary nurse's arm within minutes of a flea bite. A bulla is a vesicular lesion greater than 1 cm (0.4 in) in diameter.

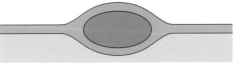

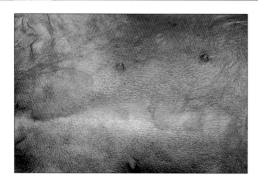

A wheal is an irregular elevated edematous skin area which often changes in size and shape. The wheals in this case were acute, transient and of unknown etiology.

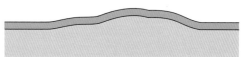

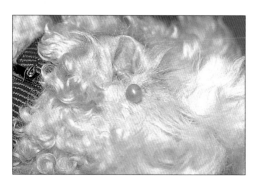

A cyst is an enclosed cavity with a membranous lining which contains liquid or semisolid matter. The illustration is of a cystic basal cell tumor on the head of a dog.

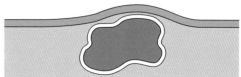

Secondary lesions

Secondary lesions are a result of trauma, time, and degree of insult to the skin. Often primary lesions evolve into secondary lesions. Thus papules become pustules which become focal encrustations, often hyperpigmented.

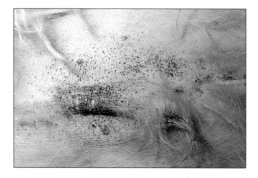

Comedones are the results of sebaceous and epidermal debris blocking a follicle. They may be seen in many disease but are often very prominent in case of hyperadrenocorticism, as in this instance.

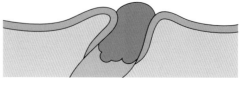

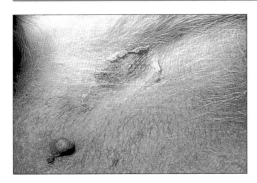

Scale results from accumulations of superficial epidermal cells that are dead and cast off from the skin. In this case there is an epidermal collarette surrounding a postinflammatory patch of hyperpigmentation. This presentation is frequently seen in cases of superficial pyoderma.

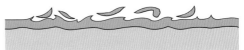

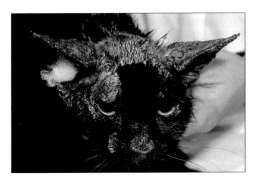

Crust is composed of cells and dried exudate of serum or blood. This cat has pemphigus foliaceus.

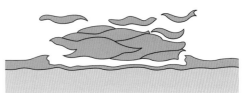

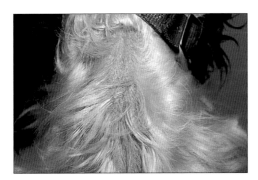

Erythema is reddening of the skin. In this Springer Spaniel the erythema is due to *Malassezia pachydermatis* infection.

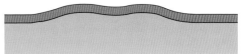

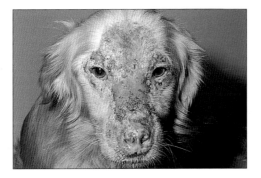

An erosion occurs following loss of the superficial part of the epidermis as on the face of this dog with discoid lupus erythematosus. Erosions heal without scar formation.

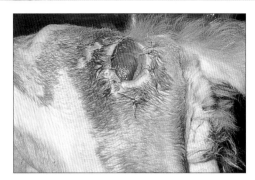

An ulcer is deeper than an erosion and occurs following loss of the epidermis and exposure of the deeper tissues of the dermis. Lesions may scar, as in this decubital ulcer overlying the bony prominence of the hip.

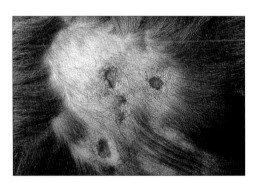

Sinus or fistula implies a draining lesion. This dog has panniculitis and there are draining fistulas on the flank. The term sinus is usually reserved for an epithelialized tract that connects a body cavity and the skin surface.

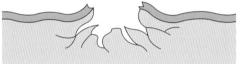

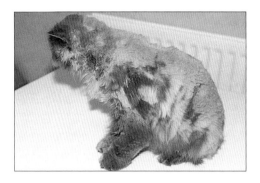

An excoriation results from self-trauma. In some cases, often cats, the damage can be extensive, as in this Persian cat with food allergy.

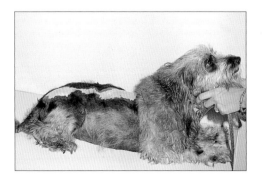

A scar results from the abnormal fibrous tissue that replaces normal tissue after an injury, such as a burn as in this case.

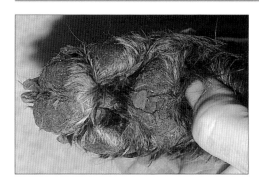

A fissure results when thickened, usually lichenified or heavily, crusted skin splits. The illustration shows the foot of a dog with necrolytic migratory erythema.

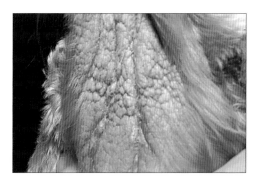

Lichenification occurs following chronic inflammation, as in this case of *M. pachydermatis* infection. There is thickening of the skin associated with accentuation of normal skin markings.

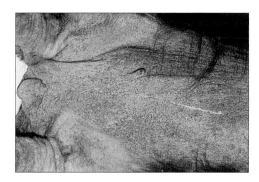

Hyperpigmentation, an increase in cutaneous pigmentation, usually occurs after chronic inflammation, as with this West Highland White Terrier with atopy. Hyperpigmentation may also be seen in cutaneous changes associated with an endocrinopathy.

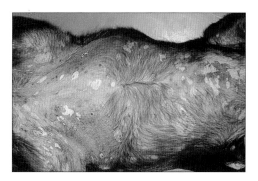

Hypopigmentation, a decrease in cutaneous pigmentation, occasionally follows inflammation, as in this case where it occurred after a superficial pyoderma. Vitiligo, a rare, non-inflammatory condition, is characterized by symmetrical hypopigmentation.

Pruritic Dermatoses

GENERAL APPROACH
1 Rule out ectoparasites, particularly fleas.
2 Do not over-diagnose allergy.
3 Remember that superficial pyoderma is pruritic.

DISEASES THAT MAY BE REFRACTORY TO STEROID THERAPY
- Sarcoptic mange
- Calcinosis cutis
- *Pelodera* dermatitis
- *Malassezia pachydermatis* dermatitis
- Allergic contact dermatitis
- Dietary intolerance
- Mycosis fungoides

PRURITIC DISEASES ASSOCIATED WITH ZOONOTIC LESIONS
- Sarcoptic mange
- Cheyletiellosis
- Flea infestation

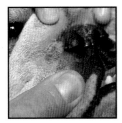
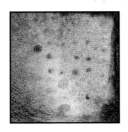
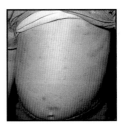
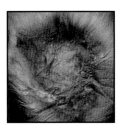

Flea Bite Hypersensitivity

DEFINITION

Flea bite hypersensitivity is a pruritic dermatosis resulting from immediate or cell-mediated hypersensitivity to various proteins in the saliva of fleas.

ETIOLOGY AND PATHOGENESIS

Fleas deposit salival proteins within the epidermis and superficial dermis during feeding. Hypersensitivity to these proteins induces local edema and a cellular infiltrate which produce the erythematous papule that may follow the bite. It is now considered that all signs resulting from infestation with fleas are a consequence of hypersensitivity and that flea bite dermatitis *per se* does not exist[1]. In the dog it has been shown that early and regular exposure to fleas results in delayed and, in some cases, less severe expression of flea bite hypersensitivity[2].

CLINICAL FEATURES

Dogs exhibit a more predictable spectrum of clinical signs than cats. There is no breed incidence, except that atopic dogs are predisposed to flea bite hypersensitivity and there is a breed incidence similar to that of atopy. The most commonly affected age group is dogs between 1 and 3 years old[3].

In dogs, pruritus is present, although the expression of this, and the owner's ability to identify it, will vary. Lesions are predominantly over the caudal back (**1**, **2**), tail, and perineum, although in some individuals the limbs, rostral trunk, and head may be affected[3]. Other changes, such as alopecia (which may be symmetrical), excoriation, hyperpigmentation, and lichenification, may be visible, although the degree of these changes will depend on the duration of the dermatosis and the degree of pruritus experienced by the animal. Acute pyotraumatic dermatitis and secondary superficial pyoderma is variably reported and is probably more common in hot, humid climates than temperate ones.

Cats rarely manifest a primary lesion, although they do manifest a wider spectrum of clinical signs associated with flea bite hypersensitivity than do dogs. Crusted papules (**3**) are the most common sign[4]. Symmetrical alopecia (**4–6**), eosinophilic plaque (**7**), and linear granuloma (**8**) may also be associated with flea bite hypersensitivity.

DIFFERENTIAL DIAGNOSES

- Pediculosis
- Sarcoptic mange
- Cheyletiellosis
- Ectopic *Otodectes cynotis* infestation
- Trombiculidiasis
- *Lynxacarus radovsky* infestation
- Superficial staphylococcal pyoderma
- Dermatophytosis

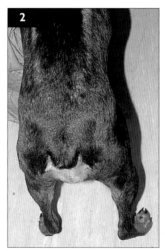
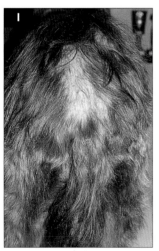
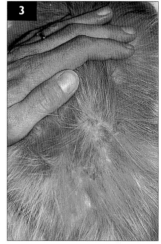

1–3 Flea bite hypersensitivity. Patchy alopecia on the dorsal lumbosacral region and tail base of a crossbred dog (**1**); Rottweiler with symmetrical alopecia and self-trauma (**2**); erythematous crusted papules on the dorsal lumbosacral region of a cat (**3**).

Flea Bite Hypersensitivity

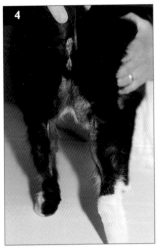

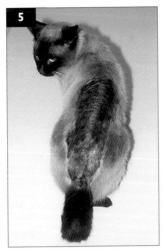

4–6 Flea bite hypersensitivity. Alopecia in the perineum and on the caudal aspects of the hindlimbs in a cat (**4**); alopecia and hyperpigmentation due to acromelanism, along the dorsal midline of a dark-pointed Siamese cat (**5**); extensive alopecia involving the entire caudal trunk and hindlimbs of a cat (**6**).

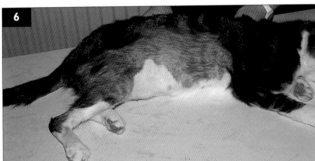

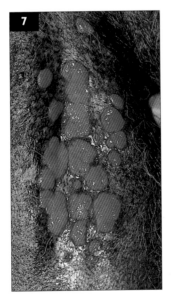

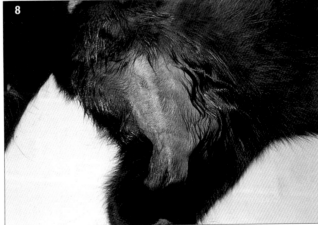

7, 8 Flea bite hypersensitivity. Cluster of eosinophilic plaques on the caudal aspect of the hindlimb of a cat (**7**); linear (collagenolytic) granuloma on the medial aspect of the hindlimb of a cat (**8**).

Flea Bite Hypersensitivity

- Atopy
- Dietary intolerance
- Pemphigus foliaceus
- Drug eruption

DIAGNOSTIC TESTS

A diagnosis of flea bite hypersensitivity requires the demonstration of:

- Compatible clinical signs.
- The presence of fleas or flea feces on the animal.
- In the dog, a positive reaction following intradermal injection of an aqueous solution of flea allergen (**9**).

In practice, a diagnosis of flea bite hypersensitivity should not be ruled out in the face of a negative reaction after the intradermal injection of flea allergen, particularly in cats[5]. Furthermore, it may prove difficult to demonstrate fleas on an affected animal – commonly, flea feces are the only sign of flea infestation. In some cases it may be necessary to examine animals in contact with an affected animal to demonstrate fleas. The presence of *Dipylidium caninum* in the animal and of erythematous papular lesions on members of the household are also findings supportive of the presence of fleas in the immediate environment.

MANAGEMENT

Adult fleas are obligate ectoparasites[5] and topical flea control is mandatory. However, the development of the life cycle from egg through to pupa occurs in the immediate domestic environment of the infested pet rather than on the host, and this requires environmental treatment[6,7]. Although the interior of houses are the preferred breeding environment, fleas may breed out of doors, particularly in warm climates, although, in reality, it appears that flea burdens in the garden are small[7]. Contact with other cats is much more likely to be the source of infection. The principal strategic problem in trying to control a domestic flea population is dealing with young adult fleas within the protective pupal case. These can yield live, viable adults for periods of 2–4 weeks after all eggs, larvae, and other adults have been killed, and repeated applications of environmental treatment may be necessary in some cases.

Environmental treatment

All environmental treatment within the home should be preceded by vacuum cleaning as this has been shown to be an effective method of removing adult fleas from the flooring[7]. It also reduces the numbers of eggs and larvae within the carpet[8] and elevates the carpet pile, thus permitting penetration of the pulicide to the base of the pile where the larvae will concentrate. A comparative study showed that the application of an insect growth regulator (IGR) to, for example, permethrin, significantly increased the efficacy of an environmental treatment protocol to control fleas with 100% reduction at 60 days being recorded[6].

There are a number of environmental products available, such as combinations of organophosphates (dichlorvos and iodofenphos), permethrin, and IGRs such as methoprene and lufenuron. These agents are variably efficient at killing all life stages, apart from the pre-emerged adult, and most preparations have good residual activity for 2 or 3 months. In some countries an inert compound containing electrostatically charged synthetic borate crystals is available, and this has been claimed to be effective for up to 6 months.

Topical treatment

Proprietary shampoos and washes are not particularly effective since they are rinsed off before they have acted on the fleas and thus have little, or no, residual activity. Flea collars with pulicidal activity (such as those containing diazinon) may be of value, particularly in cats, where their convenience is high[8]. However, flea collars alone will not provide adequate control of flea infestation and they may impart a false sense of security to the owner.

Aerosol preparations containing organophosphates (such as dichlorvos and fenitrothion) or permethrin are very popular products, although the difficulties in ensuring adequate application result in limited residual action, in the order of 8 days in one study[11]. Fenthion exhibits good knockdown and has a residual efficacy of 85–95% 2–4 weeks after application[9,10]. Microencapsulated clorpyriphos environmental spray results in adulticidal activity for 8–10 weeks. Topical application of permethrin liquid preparations is a relatively recent innovation and is claimed to be effective for periods of some 4 weeks. Topical washes with, or 'spot on' applications of, fipronil (a GABA antagonist) have a residual effect for

Flea Bite Hypersensitivity

1–2 months after application, although in cases of severe flea bite hypersensitivity, applications may be required at monthly intervals. Imidocloprid, as a 'spot on', applied in the dorsal interscapular region of dogs, or the back of the neck in cats, kills fleas on the animal and provides residual action for 4 weeks in dogs and 3 weeks in cats.

Topical application of systemic organophosphates, such as fenthion, is effective and easy to use[8], although their use is rapidly becoming outmoded by the non-organophosphate products, such as fipronil.

Systemic and other treatments

Insect growth regulators, such as methoprene (environmental application) or lufenuron (oral application) act at specific immature stages and have little effect on adult insects[12,13]. Because the affect on adult numbers is slow, in the clinical situation simultaneous administration of a topical adulticide is recommended for prompt reduction of the adult population[14].

The potential for vaccination, either against the immunogenic salivary proteins or against concealed antigens within the flea gut, is being explored and offers exciting possibilities for the future management of fleas[15,16].

Although flea control is mandatory, it may not be sufficient to result in complete control of the dermatosis. In such cases, anti-inflammatory treatment will be necessary. Systemic antihistamines, systemic glucocorticoids or essential fatty acid supplements may be indicated, either as sole treatments or in combination.

KEY POINTS

- Flea bite hypersensitivity is common.
- Flea bite hypersensitivity may be difficult to demonstrate to sceptical clients.
- If you suspect flea bite hypersensitivity, treat it and re-examine the animal after 3 or 4 weeks.
- Always use an adulticide on all the animals in the household and an environmental IGR in the home.

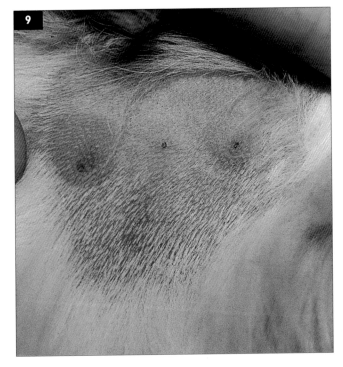

9 Positive intradermal flea test. The wheal on the left is the positive control (histamine); the central injection (negative control – saline) has produced no reaction. An aqueous solution of flea allergen was injected on the right. Note the positive reaction (a wheal).

Atopic Dermatitis

DEFINITION
Atopic dermatitis (atopy, atopic disease, allergic inhalant dermatitis) is characterized in the veterinary literature as an inherited tendency to develop IgE antibodies and resultant clinical allergy to environmental allergens[1].

ETIOLOGY AND PATHOGENESIS
The pathogenesis of atopic dermatitis is complex and new concepts on the etiology of the disease are still emerging. In humans it has been shown that atopic dermatitis is associated with elevated T-lymphocyte activation, hyperstimulatory Langerhans cells, defective cell-mediated immunity, and B-cell IgE overproduction. In addition, abnormal biochemical responsiveness and mediator release by monocytes, mast cells, and eosinophils contribute to the dermatitis[2]. Furthermore, it is possible for the cutaneous inflammation to be self-perpetuating due to continual scratching and secondary skin changes, even in the absence of allergen.

CLINICAL FEATURES
Generally, clinical signs of atopic dermatitis are first seen when animals are between 1 and 3 years of age. However, the disease has been first noted in the very young (approximately 12 weeks of age) and in the very old (approximately 16 years of age). If sensitivities develop to pollens, the condition is likely to be seasonal. However, many animals exhibit perennial disease, a reflection of the importance of allergy to house dust mites and house dust.

The breed predisposition to atopic dermatitis will vary with the local gene pool, but in the USA, UK, and Europe a number of breeds are recognized to be particularly at risk. These include Cairn Terriers, West Highland White Terriers, Scottish Terriers, Wire-haired Fox Terriers, Dalmatians, English and Irish Setters, Labrador and Golden Retrievers, German Shepherd Dogs, Newfoundlands, Boxers, Boston Terriers, English Bulldogs, Beagles, Miniature Schnauzers, and Chinese Shar-Peis[3]. There is no feline breed predisposition.

Clinically, animals are pruritic although the degree of pruritus may vary over periods of time and from individual to individual. Erythema and secondary skin changes, such as hyperpigmentation and lichenification, may be found interdigitally (**10**), in the ears (particularly on the concave aspect of the pinnae and in the vertical canal (**11**)), along the ventrum, in the perineum, on the axilla (**12–14**), on the face (particularly periocularly, but occasionally on the lips (**15**)). Alopecia may occur in any of the affected areas depending on the duration and degree of inflammation. Frequently, secondary infection with *Staphylococcus intermedius* or *Malassezia pachydermatis* will occur (**16–18**). The staphylococcal infection is usually a superficial pyoderma and typically presents as erythematous papules that may develop to pustules, but more often progress to small crusts or circular areas of alopecia with a scaling border (epidermal collarettes).

Chronic erythematous otitis externa is a frequent finding. Protracted erythema will often lead to hyperplasia of the tissues on the inside of the pinnae and the ear canals. It also predisposes to increased secretions from the glands lining the ear canals, which can act as a growth medium for bacteria and yeast, predisposing to otitis externa.

Small intradermal papules may occur between the toes and develop into cysts that break and drain a serosanguinous fluid. Interdigital granulomas may follow.

Cocker Spaniels, Springer Spaniels, West Highland White Terriers, and Scottish Terriers will often have areas of alopecia, erythema, hyperpigmentation, and greasy scale on the ventral neck, and this is frequently secondarily infected with *M. pachydermatis*.

DIFFERENTIAL DIAGNOSES
- Flea bite hypersensitivity
- Sarcoptic mange
- Dietary intolerance
- *Malassezia pachydermatis* dermatitis
- Superficial pyoderma
- Cheyletiellosis
- Pediculosis
- Contact dermatitis
- *Pelodera strongyloides* dermatitis

DIAGNOSTIC TESTS
History and clinical signs may allow for a presumptive diagnosis. Intradermal skin testing (**19**), if performed properly, will result in positive results that concur with the history in approximately 85% of cases. To prevent inaccurate test results, short-acting steroids, such as prednisone, prednisolone, or methylprednisolone, should be discontinued 3 weeks prior to testing, and repository injectable steroids should be discontinued 6–8 weeks prior to testing. Antihist-

Atopic Dermatitis

amines should be discontinued 7–10 days before testing. Control of pruritus, pending testing, may be achieved by bathing the animal every 1–3 days using emollient moisturizing shampoos, oatmeal and paroxamine-based shampoo, or alternatively a simple cleansing shampoo followed by application of a conditioner containing paroxamine, if available. Lotions or sprays containing 1% hydrocortisone may be applied to pruritic inflamed skin twice daily as long as it is not applied to the skin site used for testing.

Serologic allergy testing (RAST, ELISA, and liquid-phase immunoenzymatic assay) can be performed to determine if there are increased concentrations of allergen-specific IgE present. The problem with these procedures is the high rate of occurrence of false positives.

Almost all normal dogs, dogs with skin disease, and all dogs with atopic dermatitis will react to at least one, and sometimes many, substances[4]. One study showed that serologic allergy testing based on the RAST could not differentiate between normal dogs and dogs which had atopic dermatitis[5].

SYMPTOMATIC TREATMENT

Glucocorticoids
Methylprednisolone (0.05–0.1 mg/kg) is the preferred agent for the control of erythema and pruritus. Prednisolone and prednisone may also be used (0.1–0.2 mg/kg), but they are more likely to cause polyuria–polydipsia and polyphagia in some dogs. Induction doses should be given

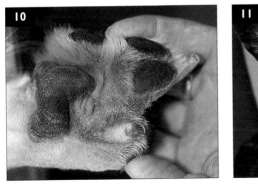

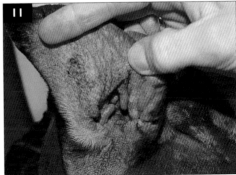

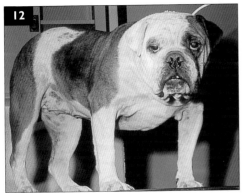

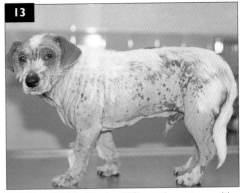

10–13   Atopy. Plantar interdigital erythema in a West Highland White Terrier (**10**); erythematous otitis externa in a Boxer (**11**); erythema in the axillae, groins, and medial aspects of the proximal limbs in an English Bulldog (**12**); extensive erythema and alopecia on the ventral trunk and proximal limbs of a Jack Russell Terrier (**13**).

Atopic Dermatitis

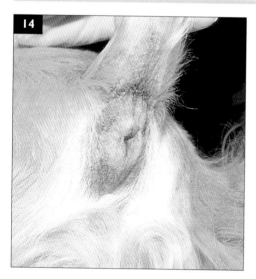

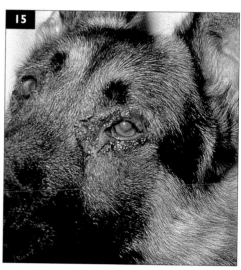

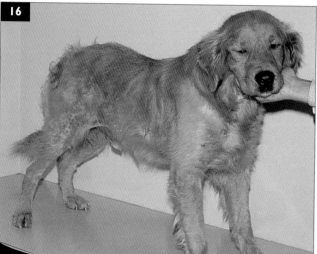

14–17 Atopy. Perineal erythema in a Cocker Spaniel (**14**); facial excoriations in a German Shepherd Dog (**15**); erythroderma (generalized erythema, scale, and alopecia) in a Retriever (**16**); erythematous papules and localized erythematous alopecia in the groins of a Labrador Retriever (**17**).

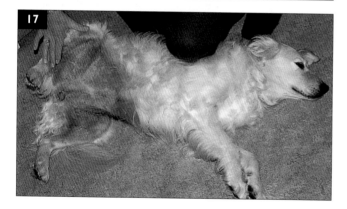

Atopic Dermatitis

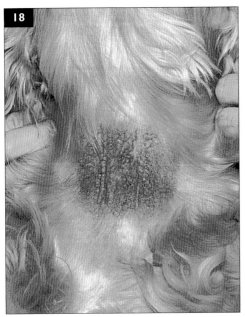

18   Atopy. Focal hyperpigmentation and erythema on the ventral neck of a Cocker Spaniel due to secondary *Malassezia pachydermatis*.

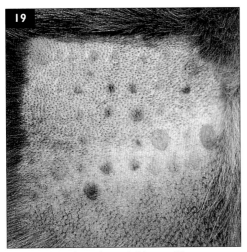

19   Positive intradermal skin test. The green dots are text highlighter and positive reactions are seen as darkly colored (edematous) swellings.

twice daily for 8 days, then once daily in the morning for 8 days, and then on alternate mornings. The dose is then decreased by 20% every 8 days to determine the least amount that will keep the animal comfortable. At this time, antihistamines or essential fatty acid supplements may be administered in an attempt to further reduce the dose (see below). The client should be forewarned that the minimal dose may change if the animal is exposed to fleas, contracts a secondary infection, is exposed to a hotter and more humid environment, or if it encounters a higher dose of the antigen. However, failure promptly to re-establish control of pruritus in a case which was previously well controlled, should prompt suspicion of secondary infection with *S. intermedius* or *M. pachydermatis*, and ever-increasing doses of glucocorticoid should not be permitted without re-examination.

Methylprednisolone acetate (0.25–1.0 mg/kg IM) or betamethasone (0.08–0.4 mg/kg) injections are generally not recommended because of the prolonged pituitary adrenal suppression. However, occasional use of these injectable steroids may be warranted if the dermatitis is extremely severe, if only 1–3 injections are needed per year to control a seasonal allergy, or if the client finds it impossible to administer oral medications to the animal.

Antihistamines

Antihistamine therapy may be additive (or even synergistic) with fatty acid supplements. Given that fatty acid supplements have a lag phase before maximal effects are seen, it may be beneficial to delay antihistamine therapy for 4 weeks.

Chlorpheniramine (0.4 mg/kg PO q 8 h), diphenhydramine (2–4 mg/kg PO q 8 h), and hydroxyzine (2 mg/kg PO q 8 h) may be useful in controlling pruritus and erythema if it is not severe. Clients are instructed to try each independently for 2 weeks to determine which works best with the fewest side-effects. Clemastine fumerarate (0.05 mg/kg PO q 8 h) and ketotifen (2–4 mg/kg PO q 8 h) may also be effective but the cost will be higher. Terfenadine, astemizole, and lortadine have not proved beneficial for the treatment of pruritus due to allergies in dogs[4].

Antibacterial agents

To control secondary bacterial infection, appropriate antibacterial agents should be given for 2–3 weeks (see Superficial Pyoderma, page 108).

Atopic Dermatitis

Shampoos

If a secondary bacterial infection is present, shampoos containing benzoyl peroxide should be used every 4–7 days, depending on the severity of lesions. Shampoos containing chlorhexidine or ethyl lactate are not as irritating as those containing benzoyl peroxide and may be more appropriate for animals which have severely inflamed skin. If yeasts are found on impression smears or skin scrapings, shampoos containing miconazole or ketoconazole should be used. Scaling should be treated with shampoos containing tar and salicylic acid, unless it is due to xeroderma (see below).

Conditioners and humectants

The use of skin and coat conditioners and humectants after bathing has been found to be beneficial – to prevent drying of the skin (xeroderma) and reduce irritation of the animal's dermatitis. Emollient moisturizing shampoos are indicated in these cases. A conditioner containing oatmeal and paroxamine has been found to be particularly beneficial.

Topical antipruritics

Focal areas of inflammation may be treated with either sprays or lotions containing 1% hydrocortisone or an ointment containing neomycin, isoflupredone acetate, and tetracaine. The latter is used when the erythema is of a more severe nature.

Fatty acid supplements

Supplements containing omega-3 and/or omega-6 fatty acids may be useful in cases where the pruritus is minimal or as adjunct therapy in more severe cases[6–12]. The response to fatty acid supplements is dose related (the more that is given, the better the effect) and there is a time lag of up to 12 weeks before maximal response is seen.

Immunotherapy

Hyposensitization has been reported to provide benefit to 50–80% of dogs with atopic dermatitis[3]. In addition, approximately 75% of atopic dogs can be controlled without the use of systemic glucocorticoids when hyposensitization is combined with other nonsteroidal treatments[3]. In the authors' experience, 60–65% of atopic dogs can be maintained on hyposensitization alone, another 15–20% can be maintained with hyposensitization plus other non-steroidal treatments, while 20–25% do not benefit from hyposensitization. It may take animals as long as 6–12 months to respond to immunotherapy and, therefore, critical clinical evaluation should not take place until this time. The percentage of dogs with an excellent response to hyposensitization appears to be greater when therapy is based on intradermal rather than serologic testing[3,13] and when hyposensitization is based on a strong intradermal reaction pattern in a 2–6-year-old animal. Chronically affected older animals with longstanding disease appear to be associated with a poorer response.

SUMMARY

The management of the atopic dog must be tailored to the individual patient. Owners should be advised that it is not possible to predict which dog will respond to which therapy. The aim should be to minimize the use of glucocorticoids and to control bacteria, yeast, fleas, and xerosis.

One suggested plan of action, which encompasses all of these aims, is:

1 Order immunotherapy.
2 Start fatty acid supplements.
3 Initiate glucocorticoid therapy if the dogs are severely affected.
4 After 4 weeks (with glucocorticoids at the lowest possible dose and fatty acids starting to exert effects), begin trial antihistamine therapy.
5 Start immunotherapy and, if possible, withdraw other therapies.
6 Aim to minimize glucocorticoid use.
7 Regular re-examinations are essential.

KEY POINTS

- Atopy is common – perhaps 5% of dogs are affected.
- Bilateral otitis externa occurs in 55% of atopic dogs.
- Recurrent superficial pyoderma and malassezial infection are common in atopic dogs.
- The pruritus is usually steroid responsive.

Adverse Reactions to Food (Dietary Intolerance)

DEFINITION
Dietary intolerance is an uncommon dermatosis caused by an abnormal response to an ingested food or additive.

ETIOLOGY AND PATHOGENESIS
The etiology of most cases of dietary intolerance is not determined, but may involve either food intolerance or food hypersensitivity. Food intolerance is any clinically abnormal response to the ingestion of a food that does not have an immunologic component, such as food poisoning, food idiosyncrasy, metabolic reactions, and dietary indiscretions[1]. Food hypersensitivity is an abnormal response to a food or food additive that is immunologically mediated. Unless a particular case is proven to be immunologically mediated, the preferred term is 'adverse reaction to food or dietary intolerance'.

Although many dietary ingredients have been documented as causing adverse reactions in the dog, the most frequently implicated are beef, cow's milk, and cereals[2-6]. Too few cases have been studied in the cat to determine the ingredients that are most likely to cause a problem[2,7,8].

CLINICAL FEATURES
The incidence of adverse reaction to food is controversial and difficult to determine as it may coexist with atopic dermatitis. About 10–15% of all cases of allergic dermatosis are reportedly attributable to adverse reactions to food[2,9].

There is no sex or breed predisposition and although age predisposition is rarely reported, two large studies found that 33% and 52% respectively of the cases with adverse reactions to food were less than 1 year of age[3,10].

Pruritus is the most prominent clinical sign in the majority of cases. In a few cases, primary lesions such as papules may be noted, but most lesions result from self-trauma and accompanying secondary infection. Thus erythema, scale, hyperpigmentation, lichenification, and alopecia may be seen[2-6](20). The location of any dermatologic lesions can be quite varied (21, 22). Unilateral or bilateral otitis externa may be a clinical feature of dogs with an adverse reaction to food and may occur in the absence of other signs of skin disease[2,6].

Pruritus, crusting, and excoriations of the head and neck are the most common clinical findings of adverse reaction to food in cats (23). Other dermatologic findings in cats may include localized or generalized scale or crusts, miliary dermatitis, symmetric or localized areas of alopecia, eosinophilic granulomas, erythema of the pinna, and otitis externa[2,5,7,8]. No age, breed, or sex predisposition has been noted in cats.

DIFFERENTIAL DIAGNOSES: DOGS
- Atopy
- Flea bite hypersensitivity
- Drug eruption
- Superficial staphylococcal folliculitis
- Ectoparasitism
- Contact dermatitis
- Defects in keratinization

DIFFERENTIAL DIAGNOSES: CATS
- Flea bite hypersensitivity
- Ectoparasitism
- Dermatophytosis
- Atopy
- Idiopathic miliary dermatitis
- Psychogenic alopecia
- Pyoderma
- Drug eruption
- Feline acne

DIAGNOSTIC TESTS
Definitive diagnosis is based on feeding a restricted diet, composed of unique ingredients to which the animal has not been previously exposed. The length of a diet trial necessary to confirm an adverse reaction to food is controversial, and in most cases a duration of 3 weeks has been recommended. However, one prospective study of 51 dogs found that only 25.5% responded in this period, while 33.3% required 4–6 weeks, 23.5% required 6–7 weeks, and 17.6% required 8–10 weeks[10]. Most authorities now recommend a duration of at least 6 weeks in order to rule out dietary intolerance. If improvement is noted, the original diet is reinstated. If the clinical signs deteriorate, the restricted diet is reimposed. The sequence of improvement, deterioration, and subsequent improvement is diagnostic. Challenge studies may be instituted at this point if the offending component is to be identified.

Although there are a number of commercial 'hypoallergenic diets' available, these should be used with caution, at least during the diagnostic phase, until clinical trials with challenge have shown them to be as efficacious as home-prepared diets. Given that 75% of proven cases have involved reactions to beef, cereal, or dairy

Adverse Reactions to Food (Dietary Intolerance)

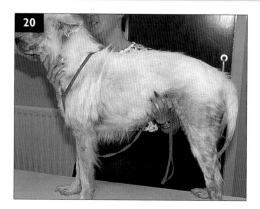

20–22 Dietary intolerance. A Samoyed with extensive alopecia, scale, and crust (**20**); a Rottweiler with a focal lesion on the forelimb (**21**); a Jack Russel Terrier with symmetrical alopecia secondary to pruritus (**22**).

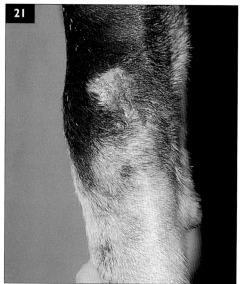

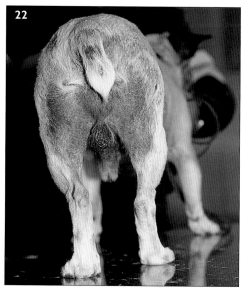

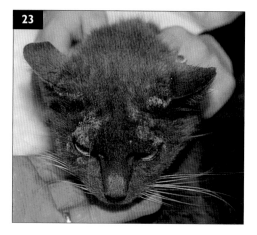

23 Dietary intolerance. Extensive alopecia, scale, and crust on the head of a domestic shorthair cat (the crusting is due to self-trauma).

Adverse Reactions to Food (Dietary Intolerance)

products[2,3,4], it is sensible to avoid these when composing a restricted diet. The authors recommend for dogs either boneless turkey or vegetables. These may be prepared and cooked in advance, divided into portions, and frozen until required. The turkey or vegetables are mixed with boiled rice and fed according to the directions given below. For cats, a diet of 100 g (3.5 oz) rice and 100 g (3.5 oz) chicken (poached in water which is added back as gravy) is adequate[8].

Other diagnostic procedures, such as intradermal skin testing, ELISA or RAST, have been shown to have a very low sensitivity, which is the ability to detect true positive reactions based on dietary provocation[9].

Vegetarian test diet for dogs
Vegetables:
1.4 kg (3 lb) carrots
1.4 kg (3 lb) peas
1.4 kg (3 lb) green beans
1.4 kg (3 lb) fresh or tinned tomatoes
285 g (10 oz) broccoli
450 g (1 lb) greens (turnip, kale, spinach)

Cook the vegetables in water according to the instructions on the packaging. Do not add seasoning. Separate into eighteen 0.6 l (20 fl oz) containers or freezer bags and place in the freezer until required.

Rice:
2 kg (4 lb 6oz) white rice

Cook the white rice in 5 cups of water according to instructions, but without butter or seasoning.

Vegetable and rice mixture:
Mix one portion of vegetables with the cooked rice and feed as directed below. Refrigerate any unused mixture.

Feeding instructions:
Feed half to three-quarters of a cup of the vegetable–rice mixture for each 4.5 kg (10 lb) body weight. For very large dogs, you may have to feed extra rice. To prevent diarrhea, slowly switch over to the vegetarian diet over an 8–10 day period of time. The dog's stools may be softer on the vegetarian diet. Compared with most commercial foods, this diet is low in protein and some dogs may lose weight while on it.

Turkey and rice diet for dogs
2.5 kg (10 cups) cooked rice
450 g (1 lb) cooked turkey
1 1/3 tsp calcium carbonate
1 tsp dicalcium phosphate
5 tbsp vegetable oil
1 tsp salt substitute (potassium chloride)
Non-flavored, additive-free multivitamin/mineral supplement

Bake or boil the turkey (dark and white meat). Cook the rice according to directions and add salt substitute to the water. Grind or finely chop the turkey and set aside. Pulverize the calcium carbonate, dicalcium phosphate, and vitamin/mineral supplement. Mix the oil, minerals, and supplements with the rice and then add the turkey. Mix well, cover, and refrigerate.

Table 1 Feeding Guidelines for Turkey and Rice Diet for Dogs	
Weight of dog	**Amount to feed daily**
1.8–5.4 kg (4–12 lb)	140–280 g (5–10 oz)
5.4–9.0 kg (12–20 lb)	280–450 g (10–16 oz)
9.0–22.5 kg (20–50 lb)	450–900 g (1–2 lb)
22.5–36.3 kg (50–80 lb)	900–1,360 g (2–3 lb)

MANAGEMENT
Feed a complete and balanced, highly digestible, limited antigen diet that does not contain the offending ingredients (as identified in the challenge studies).

KEY POINTS
- Dietary intolerance is rare.
- The pruritus may be refractory to steroid therapy.
- Recurrent otitis externa and recurrent superficial pyoderma may be associated with dietary intolerance.

Sarcoptic Mange

DEFINITION

A contagious dermatosis of dogs, and rarely cats, due to infection with the mite *Sarcoptes scabiei* var. *canis*. Sarcoptic mange is characterized by progressive, often unremitting, pruritus and self-trauma.

ETIOLOGY AND PATHOGENESIS

Most of the pruritus associated with sarcoptic mange is due to hypersensitivity to the mite (**24**) and its secretions[1]. Thus, initial infection in a naïve animal is associated with an asymptomatic period during which the mite multiplies (the lag period). This lag period may be from 3–6 weeks in duration in some animals[2]. An animal infected by the mite on subsequent occasions exhibits a very much shorter lag period. Once hypersensitivity ensues the clinical features of intense pruritus are noted.

CLINICAL FEATURES

The first signs of sarcoptic mange are usually tiny erythematous papules, greyish-yellow crust, and pruritus, first noted on the tips of the pinnae, elbows, or hocks (**25**). Adjacent skin, particularly of the ventral abdomen, is affected and, ultimately, generalized disease may ensue (**26**). Pruritus is intense and may be unremitting. Self-trauma results in a patchy alopecia and may induce severe excoriation. There may be weight loss and polylymphadenopathy. Zoonotic lesions are common (**27**).

DIFFERENTIAL DIAGNOSES

- Dietary intolerance
- *Malassezia pachydermatis* dermatitis
- *Pelodera strongyloides* dermatitis
- Flea bite hypersensitivity
- Atopic dermatitis

DIAGNOSTIC TESTS

A careful evaluation of the history and consideration of the clinical signs will often allow a tentative diagnosis of scabies. The diagnosis is confirmed by identifying the mite, or ova, in skin scrapings. This may be difficult and microscopic examination of multiple skin scrapings and concentration/flotation techniques may be necessary. The presence of a pinnal scratch reflex is highly suggestive, although not pathognomonic, of scabies.

MANAGEMENT

Miticidal treatment of the affected animal, and all in-contacts, is curative. Treatment with topical organophosphates, amitraz, or systemic ivermectin (0.2–0.3 mg/kg) on 2, and occasionally 3 occasions, at intervals of 2 weeks is usually required. Ivermectin is contraindicated in Collie breeds, Collie cross-breeds, and certain herding breeds. Fipronil dips may also be efficacious. Environmental application of a suitable miticidal is also advocated since the mites have some capacity to survive off the host for short periods[3].

KEY POINTS

- Always be alert for scabies.
- A good history, particularly early in the disease, may be enough to prompt suspicion.
- If you suspect scabies, treat it.

Sarcoptic Mange

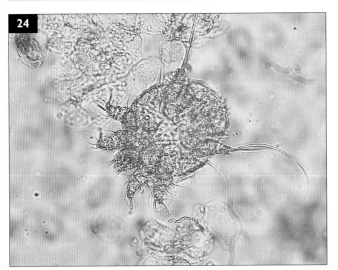

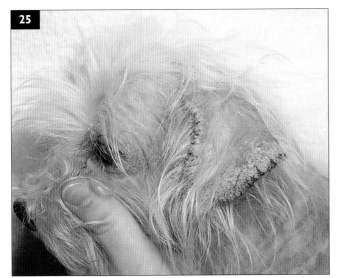

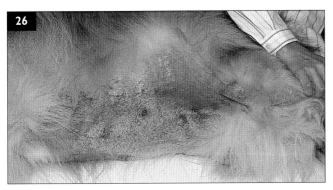

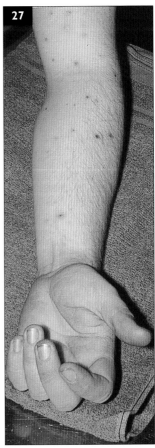

24–27 *Sarcoptes scabiei* var. *canis*. Photomicrograph of an adult mite in a skin scraping (**24**); severe self-trauma, alopecia, erythema, and crusting (particularly on the pinnal edge) of a Maltese dog (**25**); sarcoptic mange in a Rough Collie demonstrating erythema and crust (**26**); zoonotic lesions of scabies on the forearm of an owner (**27**).

Cheyletiella spp. Infestation

DEFINITION
This infestation (walking dandruff) is a scaling or crusting, variably pruritic dermatitis due to the presence of *Cheyletiella* spp. mites living on the skin surface.

ETIOLOGY AND PATHOGENESIS
Three species of mites are responsible for the majority of clinical cases in dogs, cats, and rabbits. Although none are host specific, *C. yasguri* is found more frequently in dogs, *C. blakei* in cats, and *C. parasitovorax* in rabbits[1]. The mites live on the skin surface and the eggs are attached to the hair shafts. The mites are characterized by prominent hooks at the end of accessory mouthparts (**28**). The life cycle is approximately 35 days and is completed on one host. The adult female can live off the host for a variable period, about 10–14 days[2,3]. The mites are easily transmitted from one animal to another via direct contact and this is how infestation generally occurs. Occasionally, transmission may occur by coming into contact with mites in the environment.

CLINICAL FEATURES
Diffuse scaling over the dorsum of the animal (**29**) is the characteristic feature of infestation in dogs and rabbits[1,3]. Pruritus in dogs is usually mild, but may be severe in some animals and absent in others. Although variably pruritic scaling may be a feature in cats, small (0.2–0.4 cm/ 0.08–0.16 in) crusted papules, with an erythematous base (**30**), found over the dorsum are a more common finding[4], particularly in long-haired cats. In these individuals the lesions are generally pruritic[5]. Both dogs and cats can be asymptomatic carriers. People associated with infected animals will show signs in 30–40% of cases[3]. The classic signs are small, pruritic, erythematous papules in groups of two or three, usually on the arms and trunk (the parts which come in contact with infested animals) (**31**).

DIFFERENTIAL DIAGNOSES
- Flea bite hypersensitivity
- Staphylococcal folliculitis
- Pediculosis
- Atopic dermatitis
- Dermatophytosis
- Dietary intolerance
- Demodicosis
- Poor nutrition, particularly essential fatty acid deficiency

- Ectopic *Otodectes cynotis* infestation
- Idiopathic defects in keratinization
- Psychogenic dermatitis

DIAGNOSTIC TESTS
Skin scrapings taken from scaling or crusty areas may demonstrate the mites or eggs which are attached to the hair[1,3]. Tape strips are also a useful method of demonstrating the eggs and mites. Generally, mites are easier to demonstrate in dogs than cats. Microscopic examination of scale and hair collected by grooming the coat with a fine-toothed comb is the most reliable diagnostic method in cats. Mites cannot be demonstrated in all animals and trial therapy may be necessary in some case to confirm a diagnosis.

MANAGEMENT
Selenium sulfide shampoos weekly for 4–5 weeks are curative. Weekly dips of lime sulfur or pyrethrin, diluted according the manufacturer's recommendations, can also be used to control infestations in dogs, cats, and rabbits. Three amitraz dips given at 2-week intervals would be appropriate for adult dogs. Ivermectin injections (0.2–0.3 mg/kg) repeated at 2-week intervals for 3 treatments would also be effective in cats, rabbits, and those breeds of dogs where ivermectin is not contraindicated, such as the Collie breeds, Collie cross-breeds, and certain herding breeds. Fipronil may also be effective. All associated animals should be treated concomitantly. As the mites may live in the environment for up to 10 days, it would be appropriate to thoroughly vacuum floors and furniture that the animals have access to and treat these areas with a flea premise spray.

KEY POINTS
- Cheyletiellosis may be very hard to prove – if you suspect it, treat it.
- Remember to treat the environment, in addition to all in-contact cats or dogs.

Cheyletiella spp. Infestation

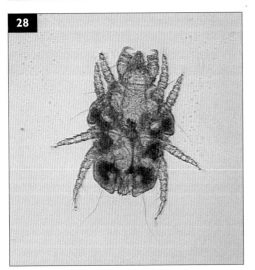

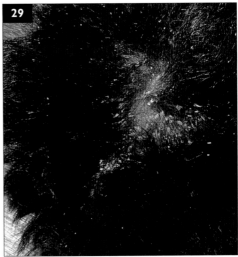

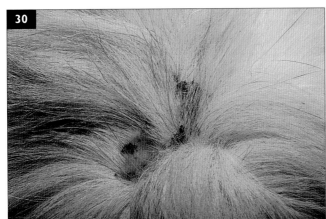

28–31 Cheyletiellosis. Adult *Cheyletiella yasguri* (**28**); typical signs of scale on the dorsal trunk of a dog (**29**); crusted erythematous papules on the dorsal trunk of a cat (**30**); zoonotic lesions on the abdomen of a man in contact with an infested pet (**31**).

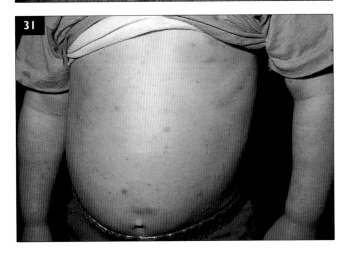

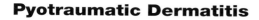

Pyotraumatic Dermatitis

DEFINITION
Pyotraumatic dermatitis (acute moist dermatitis, hot spot) is a localized area of acute inflammation and exudation in skin that is traumatized by licking, scratching, or rubbing.

ETIOLOGY AND PATHOGENESIS
There is no single etiology, but rather multiple factors that predispose to the development of pyotraumatic dermatitis. Some of these factors include: acute focal inflammation resulting from allergic conditions, such as atopic dermatitis, allergic contact dermatitis, flea bite and other parasite hypersensitivities; skin maceration due to continued wetting or accumulation of moisture under a thick coat; trauma due to abrasions, foreign bodies in the coat, or irritation from clipper blades; and a primary irritant contacting the skin. Serum exudation from the inflammatory process creates a favorable climate for bacterial overgrowth and surface pyoderma.

CLINICAL FEATURES
Lesions are noted more frequently during hot, humid weather. Animals are presented because they are persistently licking or scratching a particular area which can vary in size. The areas most commonly involved are the dorsal and dorsolateral lumbosacral region and the periaural region[1]. Affected skin is erythematous, moist and, in a majority of cases, exudative (32–34). The typical lesion will evidence alopecia or thinning of the hair. However, hair may still cover the lesion if it is detected early or if it is in a location that is difficult to lick or scratch. Excoriations are occasionally present due to licking or scratching.

DIFFERENTIAL DIAGNOSES
- Calcinosis cutis
- Superficial burn
- Irritant contact dermatitis
- Flea bite hypersensitivity
- Atopic dermatitis
- Deep folliculitis and furunculosis

DIAGNOSTIC TESTS
Diagnosis is generally made on the clinical appearance of lesions and a history of predisposing factors. Impression smears may be appropriate for determination of the number and type of bacteria, and a skin biopsy would be appropriate if calcinosis cutis was suspected.

MANAGEMENT
If the lesions are painful or the animal is fractious, sedation may be necessary for initial treatment. Any remaining hair should be clipped from affected areas and the lesions cleaned with a shampoo containing chlorhexidine or ethyl lactate and thoroughly rinsed with clean water. The lesion can then be treated with a drying solution of 2% aluminum acetate (Domeboro solution) for 3–5 minutes to decrease exudation. After cleaning and drying, an antibiotic–steroid cream or ointment can be applied. Application of the drying solution and antibiotic corticosteroid preparation can be continued at home by the owner 2–3 times a day. If the lesion is extensive or severe, systemic corticosteroids at anti-inflammatory doses can be used for 3–7 days, or as necessary, to reduce the inflammation and shorten the time necessary for resolution of the lesion. Most lesions resolve in 3–7 days but may recur if predisposing factors are not corrected.

Some individuals of certain breeds, particularly Labrador Retrievers and St. Bernards[2], may be affected by deeper infection and may require systemic antibacterial therapy (see Deep Pyoderma, page 124).

KEY POINTS
- Do not underestimate the capacity of this disease to cause problems.
- Treat aggressively and make regular reexaminations.

Pyotraumatic Dermatitis

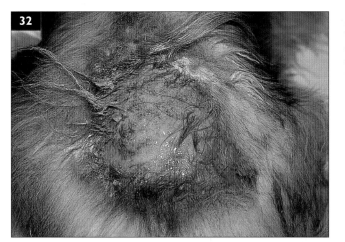

32 Pyotraumatic dermatitis. A well-demarcated moist, erythematous, alopecic patch on the dorsal lumbosacral region of a Collie cross.

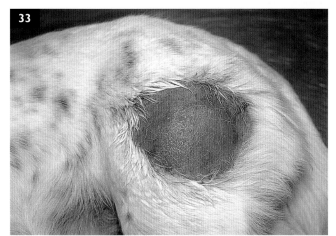

33, 34 Pyotraumatic dermatitis.

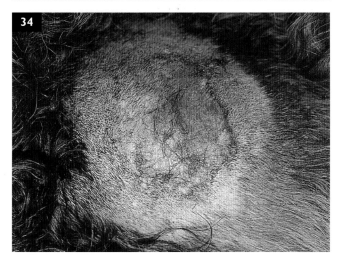

Malassezia pachydermatis Dermatitis

DEFINITION

A pruritic, often glucocorticoid resistant, dermatitis associated with the presence of the lipophilic, non-mycelial yeast *Malassezia pachydermatis*.

ETIOLOGY AND PATHOGENESIS

Malassezia pachydermatis (**35**) is considered a normal inhabitant and opportunist pathogen of the canine external ear canal, although it may also be found in the rectum, anal sacs, and vagina. Low numbers of yeast may be found on the inflamed skin that is associated with a number of conditions, such as atopy or defects in keratinization. Increased prevalence of *M. pachydermatis* dermatitis is also associated with previous antibacterial therapy and combinations of antibacterial and glucocorticoid therapy[1]. The presence of the yeast has been associated with erythematous, hyperpigmented dermatitis, although the status of the organism, as a primary agent, is not known.

CLINICAL FEATURES

Malassezia pachydermatis dermatitis in dogs is a highly pruritic dermatosis, often refractory to systemic glucocorticoids[2,3]. In dogs the disease is associated with erythema (**36**), variable but often a yellowish/grey greasy scale, hyperpigmentation, self-trauma, and alopecia (**37**, **38**). In cats, otitis externa, acne, and generalized exfoliative dermatitis have been attributed to a related organism, *M. sympodialis*.

DIFFERENTIAL DIAGNOSES

- Idiopathic defects in keratinization
- Demodicosis
- Atopic dermatitis
- Dietary intolerance
- Sarcoptic mange
- Superficial pyoderma

DIAGNOSTIC TESTS

The presence of the yeast is established on the basis of impression smears or tape strip cytology, culture, and histopathologic examination of biopsy material[4]. *Malassezia pachydermatis* has an elongated, oval shape and exhibits unipolar budding.

MANAGEMENT

Although it may appear to act as a primary pathogen, an underlying disease should always be suspected and exhaustive tests may be necessary to rule out the differential diagnoses. Elimination of the yeast from the skin surface may be achieved, at least in the short term, by systemic ketoconazole (10 mg/kg q 12 h) for 10–14 days or topical shampoos containing miconazole or ketoconazole. In a few cases, complete resolution of the dermatosis occurs and no further treatment is necessary. Most commonly, the yeast is found to be only partially responsible for the clinical signs, and in these instances the underlying disease must be identified and managed and the yeast numbers controlled by regular shampoo therapy.

KEY POINTS

- The pruritus associated with *M. pachydermatis* may be refractory to steroid therapy.
- Most, although not all, cases are associated with underlying disease.

Malassezia pachydermatis Dermatitis

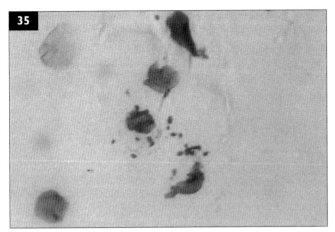

35–38   *Malassezia pachydermatis*. Photomicrograph of yeast organisms on and around squames (**35**); interdigital erythema and hyperpigmentation in a Cocker Spaniel (**36**); erythema, alopecia, and hyperpigmentation in the groins and ventral abdomen of a West Highland White Terrier (**37**); symmetrical patches of erythema, alopecia, and hyperpigmentation in a Basset Hound (**38**).

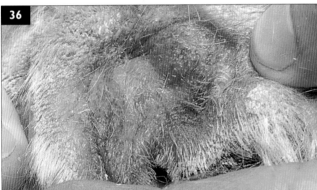

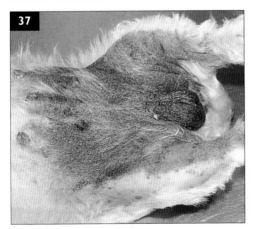

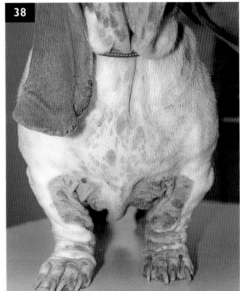

Intertrigo

DEFINITION
Intertrigo, or skin fold dermatitis, is an inflammatory condition occurring in skin that has intimate contact with adjacent skin.

ETIOLOGY AND PATHOGENESIS
Lip, facial, vulvar, body, and tail fold dermatitis result from inflammation which occurs when skin is closely opposed to skin. There is local abrasion, inflammation, and an accumulation of surface secretions, which result in maceration and secondary infection.

CLINICAL FEATURES
Lip fold dermatitis (**39**) results from the overlapping of redundant skin of the lower lip. The redundant skin forms a crevice which entraps food particles and saliva, producing an ideal environment for bacterial growth. The resultant surface infection is characterized by a foul odor, which most clients associate erroneously with dental disease. Affected skin is erythematous, at times ulcerated, and occasionally covered by a small amount of exudate.

Facial fold dermatitis (**41, 42**) occurs more frequently in brachycephalic breeds, such as Pekingese, English Bulldogs, and Pugs. The interiginous areas between folds of skin over the bridge of the nose and under the eyes become macerated and inflamed due to epiphora or accumulation of sebaceous or apocrine secretions. A secondary bacterial infection may occur.

Vulvar fold dermatitis is more common in obese animals which have a small vulva deep within a perivulval fold. Accumulation of urine and vaginal secretions causes irritation and maceration of adjacent skin, resulting in severe inflammation, secondary bacterial infection, and occasional ulceration. Affected animals exhibit increased licking of the vulvar area and this is generally the primary concern of clients.

Tail fold dermatitis (**40**) occurs more often in English Bulldogs, Boston Terriers, and Pugs. The dermatitis results from pressure and friction of corkscrew tails on the skin of the perineum as well as maceration which may occur under skin that folds over the tail.

Body fold dermatitis occurs in those animals which have redundant skin thrown up into folds, such as Basset Hounds and Chinese Shar-Peis. Folds are most frequently found on the limbs and trunk. As in other folds, the accumulation of surface secretions results in inflammation and secondary infection.

DIFFERENTIAL DIAGNOSES
- *Malassezia pachydermatis* infection
- Atopic dermatitis
- Demodicosis
- Mucocutaneous candidiasis
- Epitheliotropic lymphoma

DIAGNOSTIC TESTS
Clinical findings confirm a diagnosis, but impression smears should be taken from affected areas to determine the presence of bacteria or yeast. Skin scrapes should be taken to rule out *Demodex canis*, and impression smears or tape strips should be examined to rule out *M. pachydermatis* and *Candida* spp. Cutaneous lymphoma is rare and only diagnosed by histopathologic examination of biopsy material.

MANAGEMENT
Soiled hair that is excessive should be clipped and affected areas cleaned with shampoos containing chlorhexidine or ethyl lactate, or with benzoyl peroxide gel. If lesions appear moist, they can be treated 2–3 times a day for 5 minutes with a drying solution containing aluminum acetate (Burrow's solution). After cleaning and/or drying, an antibiotic–steroid cream or ointment can be applied. If deep bacterial infection appears to be present, treatment with systemic antibiotics would be indicated.

Owners should be forewarned that medical treatment will only control the condition and that surgical intervention is necessary for a cure. Cheiloplasty and episioplasty are appropriate procedures for lip and vulvar fold dermatitis respectively. Tail amputation and removal of redundant skin is the preferred approach for tail fold dermatitis. Facial and body folds may also be removed surgically, but they may be considered desirable traits in some show animals and this therefore necessitates a careful discussion of the procedure with the clients prior to surgery.

KEY POINT
- Although intertrigo is often self-evident, do not overlook the role of infection.

Intertrigo

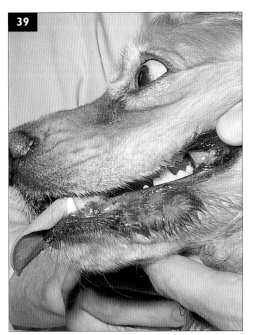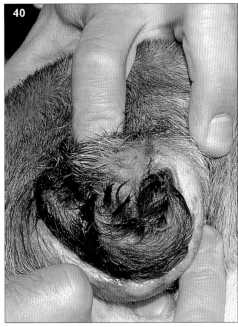

39, 40   Skin fold dermatitis. An extensive patch of erythema and erosion in the lip fold of a Cocker Spaniel (**39**); erythema and alopecia around the base of the tail in a Bulldog (**40**).

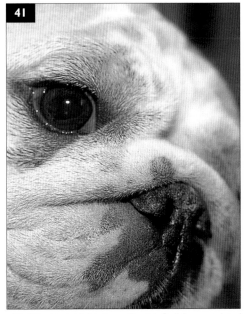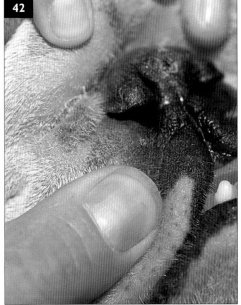

41, 42   Facial folds in an English Bulldog need to be separated to reveal fold pyoderma.

Pediculosis

DEFINITION
Pediculosis is the infestation of the skin and hair with lice.

ETIOLOGY AND PATHOGENESIS
Lice are wingless, dorsoventrally flattened insects that are host specific and spend their entire life cycle on the host. Pet infestations are more common in Europe than North America[1]. Biting lice (Mallophaga) would include *Trichodectes canis* (**43**), which is the most common louse in dogs; *Heterodoxus spineger*, which may infest dogs in warmer climates; and *Felicola subrostratus*, which is the most common louse in cats. Sucking lice (Anoplura) have narrow heads, mouthparts designed for piercing and sucking, and claws designed to cling to the hair of the host. *Linognathus setosus* (**44**) is the sucking louse of dogs. Cats do not have a species of sucking louse that infests them.

The entire life cycle is completed on the host within 3 weeks[1]. Operculate eggs (nits) (**45**) are deposited on hairs and hatch into nymphs, which undergo several moults prior to becoming adults. Transmission occurs by direct contact or by grooming with contaminated brushes or combs.

CLINICAL FEATURES
The clinical appearance of pediculosis can be quite variable and can include asymptomatic carriers; seborrhea sicca with mild pruritus; rough, dry hair coat; alopecia, papules, and crusts with mild to moderate pruritus; and severe inflammation, alopecia, excoriations, and crusting with extensive pruritus. Occasional cases of pediculosis may appear as miliary dermatitis in cats and may mimic flea bite hypersensitivity in dogs. Heavy infestations with sucking lice (**46**) may result in anemia.

DIFFERENTIAL DIAGNOSES
- Cheyletiellosis
- Dermatophytosis (cats)
- Sarcoptic mange
- Atopic dermatitis
- Keratinization disorders
- Dietary intolerance
- *Neotrombicula* spp. infestation
- Flea bite hypersensitivity

DIAGNOSTIC TESTS
Diagnosis is based on finding the lice or the nits on the skin or hair.

MANAGEMENT
Two treatments at 14-day intervals using either pyrethrin sprays, shampoos, or dips will be effective in most cases. One ivermectin injection (0.2 mg/kg SC) has been reported to be effective for pediculosis[2]. Ivermectin is contra-indicated in Collie breeds, Collie cross-breeds, and certain other herding breeds. A single treatment with fipronil has also been shown to be effective in *T. canis* infection[3].

KEY POINT
- Although easily treated, this condition may not be suspected by clinicians as diagnosis may be difficult.

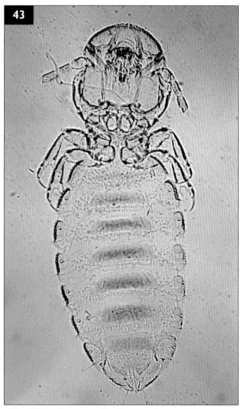

43 *Trichodectes canis*. (Photomicrograph courtesy of M. Geary.)

Pediculosis

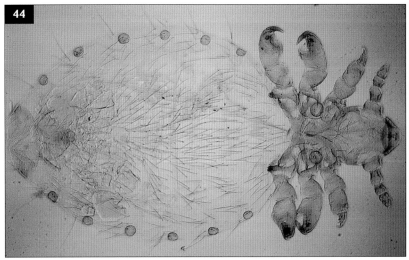

44   *Linognathus setosus.* (Photomicrograph courtesy of M. Geary.)

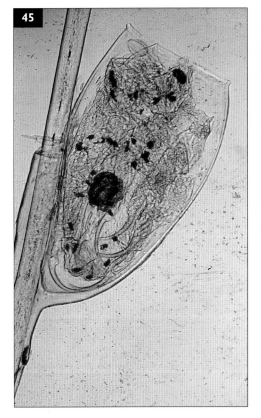

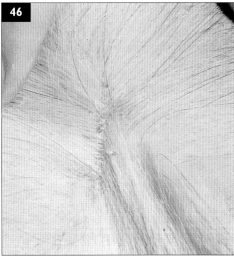

45, **46**   Pediculosis. An empty ova (nit) on the hair shaft (**45**); lice on the skin surface of a heavily infested pup (**46**).

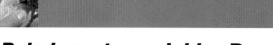

Pelodera strongyloides Dermatitis

DEFINITION
Pelodera strongyloides, or rhabditic, dermatitis is an erythematous pruritic dermatitis caused by cutaneous infestation with the larvae of *P. strongyloides*.

ETIOLOGY AND PATHOGENESIS
Pelodera strongyloides is a free-living nematode that has a direct life cycle[1]. It is found in damp soil or moist, decaying organic matter, such as straw, leaves, hay, and rice hulls. Larvae may invade skin which comes into contact with the contaminated soil or organic material and initiate cutaneous inflammation.

CLINICAL FEATURES
Lesions associated with this infestation occur in areas of skin that come into contact with the ground or bedding, but their appearance will vary markedly between cases. Focal or diffuse alopecia may be present with or without erythema (**47, 48**). Papules, pustules, and crusts may be present in some cases. In chronic cases the skin may become lichenified and hyperpigmented. Pruritus can vary from minimal to intense.

DIFFERENTIAL DIAGNOSES
- Sarcoptic mange
- Atopic dermatitis
- Contact irritant dermatitis
- Demodicosis
- Ancylostomiasis
- Dirofilariasis
- Dermatophytosis
- Bacterial folliculitis

DIAGNOSTIC TESTS
Skin scrapings should be performed to demonstrate the small, motile nematode larvae (563–625 μm in length (**49**))[2]. In some cases the larvae are easy to demonstrate and in others it can be very difficult.

MANAGEMENT
The primary goal of management is to change the animal's environment so that it is not coming into contact with soil or bedding harboring the larvae. Old, damp straw, hay, or other organic material should be removed from doghouses, kennels, or yards. After cleaning the inside of doghouses and the surfaces of runs, they can be sprayed with malathion (28 g of 57–59% malathion per 4.5 liters of water). New bedding consisting of wood chips, old blankets, or shredded paper can then be placed. Animals should be bathed using a mild shampoo. Systemic antibacterial therapy (see Superficial Pyoderma, page 108) would be appropriate if secondary bacterial infection is present.

Systemic glucocorticoids, such as methylprednisolone (0.05–0.1 mg/kg PO q 12 h) or prednisolone and prednisone (0.1–0.2 mg/kg PO q 12 h) can be used for 3–10 days, or as necessary, to control severe pruritus. Once the environment is cleaned, the lesions should be self-limiting. Giving affected animals 1–3 weekly parasiticidal dips using medications appropriate for scabies has been previously advocated[1,2]. However, the efficacy of this is not known as there have been no studies performed to show whether these treatments shorten the course of clinical disease or not.

KEY POINT
- The pruritus associated with *P. strongyloides* may be refractory to steroid therapy.

Pelodera strongyloides Dermatitis

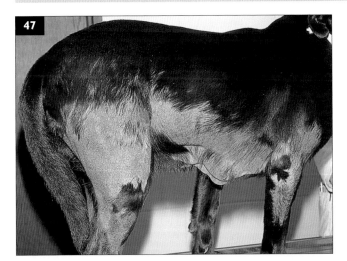

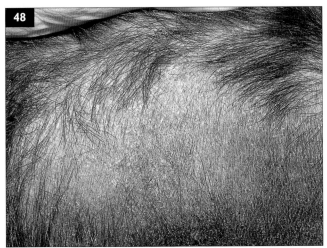

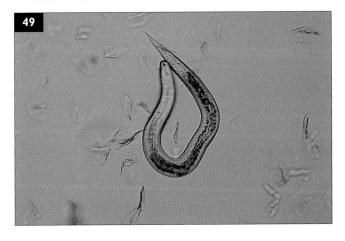

47–49 *Pelodera* dermatitis. Extensive alopecia, crusting, lichenification, and hyperpigmentation on the dependent aspects of the body (**47**); alopecia and hyperpigmentation (**48**); a photomicrograph of the nematode, *P. strongyloides*, found in skin scrapings (**49**).

Harvest Mite Infection

DEFINITION
A seasonal dermatosis associated with infestation of the parasitic larvae of harvest mites (chiggers) such as *Neotrombicula autumnalis* and *Eutrombicula alfredugesi*.

ETIOLOGY AND PATHOGENESIS
Adult harvest mites are free-living and non-parasitic. Eggs are laid in batches on vegetation in the late summer. The parasitic larvae (**50**) infest the host in groups of up to several hundred, often clustering on the head, ears, feet, or ventrum. The larvae feed for a few days and then leave. Since infestation may be non-pruritic in some cases, it is probable that those individuals displaying pruritus are manifesting a hypersensitivity to the mite or its products.

CLINICAL FEATURES
The infestation is a seasonal threat to the free-ranging dog or cat. The mite is more commonly found on lighter, well-drained ground than on heavy clay and in areas of rough vegetation rather than parkland or gardens. Infested animals may be asymptomatic. Those displaying signs are pruritic. Examination of the affected area reveals clusters of orange-red larvae (**51**), sometimes associated with a papular or papulocrustous dermatitis[1]. Most commonly the mites are found in the interdigital regions, on the ventral abdomen, or in the folds at the base of the pinnae.

DIFFERENTIAL DIAGNOSES
• Atopy
• Contact allergic or irritant dermatitis

DIAGNOSTIC TESTS
Careful examination of the affected areas will reveal tiny, orange-red patches which are clusters of larvae. In some cases the mites have left the host before it is presented to the veterinarian, and in these cases local knowledge of the disease is important as summer seasonal pedal pruritus may suggest atopy.

MANAGEMENT
Since the larvae are a seasonal threat and are associated with rough vegetation, the logical approach is to restrict access during periods of risk. In reality this is usually not practical. It is possible that some of the dips with a residual action against ticks, such as amitraz or fipronil[2,3], may be useful in preventing harvest mite infestation.

If mites are found on an affected animal, they are easily removed with a topical ectoparasitic aerosol, wash, or dip. The pruritus usually abates quickly, but in some cases a short course of prednisolone (0.5–1.1 mg/kg PO q 12–24 h) may be necessary.

KEY POINT
• Trombiculidiasis causes summer seasonal pedal (and possibly otic) pruitus. So does atopy. Be careful.

Harvest Mite Infection

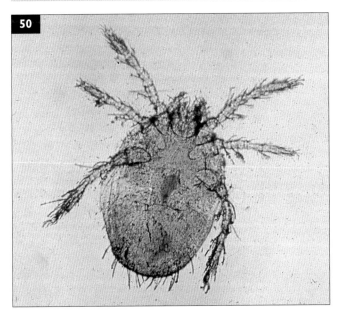

50   Six legged, orange-red colored larva of *Neotrombicula autumnalis*, the harvest mite or chigger.

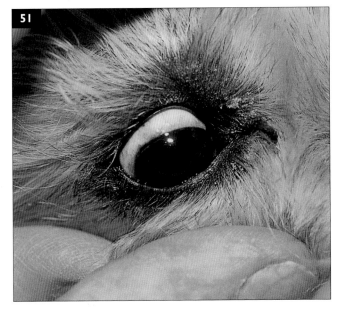

51   Trombiculidiasis. A cluster of trombiculid mites at the medial canthus of a cross-bred dog.

Allergic and Irritant Contact Dermatitis

DEFINITION

Allergic and irritant contact dermatitis are rare, predominantly ventral, pruritic dermatoses characterized by erythematous papules.

ETIOLOGY AND PATHOGENESIS

Allergic contact dermatitis is a Coombs type 4 (cell-mediated) hypersensitivity to small, low molecular weight chemicals (haptens) which are present in the animal's environment. Irritant contact dermatitis results from inflammation within the skin following exposure to noxious substances in the animal's environment. First exposure to any foreign substance (potential allergen or otherwise) results in initiation of a stereotyped response[1] during which the hapten is phagocytosed by Langerhans cells and presented to the immune system. On continued, or subsequent, exposures to the substance, the immune system is activated resulting in inflammation, epidermal necrosis, and a predominantly neutrophilic infiltrate[2]. Although allergic and irritant contact dermatitis are induced by completely different mechanisms, the histopathologic and immunocytologic findings are similar, which suggests that common immunologic pathways are involved in both processes[1]. From a clinical standpoint it is difficult to distinguish allergic contact dermatitis from irritant contact dermatitis, particularly if the dermatosis is acute. It is appropriate, therefore, to consider these diseases together.

CLINICAL FEATURES

The refractory period for allergic contact dermatitis is reported to be rarely less than 2 years[3] and, therefore, one would not expect it to appear in animals less than this age. However, the inquisitive nature of puppies and, perhaps, their juvenile pelage, might predispose them to exposure to irritants; thus irritant contact dermatitis might be expected to occur in young animals. German Shepherd Dogs comprised 50% of the case load in one series of confirmed allergic contact dermatitis[4].

Most cases of allergic contact dermatitis are perennial, although seasonal examples will be met, typically to vegetative allergens. Acute irritant dermatitis may result in erythema (**52**), edema, vesiculation, and even erosion or ulceration, of the epidermis[5]. The primary lesions of allergic contact dermatitis are erythematous macules, papules (**53**) and, occasionally, vesicles[4]. Secondary lesions tend to mask these primary lesions, except perhaps at the periphery of the affected areas where there is usually a well-defined margin between affected and normal skin (**54**).

The distribution of the lesions will reflect the areas exposed to irritants. Although initially confined to sparsely haired regions, prolonged contact will result in extension to adjacent areas and, with time, the chin, ventral aspect of the pinna, neck, medial aspects of the limbs, and the entire ventrum will be affected[6]. Generalized reactions may be seen in cases of sensitization to shampoos[3]. Chronic otitis externa may result from sensitivity to topical neomycin.

DIFFERENTIAL DIAGNOSES

- Atopy
- Dietary intolerance
- Sarcoptic mange
- Superficial pyoderma
- *Malassezia pachydermatis* dermatitis
- *Pelodera strongyloides* dermatitis

DIAGNOSTIC TESTS

A tentative diagnosis is based on history, clinical signs, and rule outs. The histopathologic picture of biopsy samples from some cases of acute irritant contact dermatitis may be characterized by intraepidermal spongiosis or vesiculation accompanied by necrosis of keratinocytes, but most histopathologic samples are non-diagnostic[4]. Exclusion trials and closed patch testing may be necessary if definitive diagnosis is necessary for management.

If the environment is suitable, exclusion trials are useful tests. The animal is restricted to one uncarpeted room, for example, or kept off grass. If the dermatitis goes into remission, provocative exposure may allow identification of the allergen. Closed patch testing may be indicated if exclusion trials are unrewarding (**55**), but this is a specialist procedure and referral is advised. Briefly, the animal is hospitalized, the thoracic wall close-clipped, and samples from a standard panel of chemicals (such as The European Standard Battery of Allergens) are placed into Finn chambers (small nickel cups) which are taped to the clipped skin. In addition, samples from the household, such as carpet fibres or vegetation, can be placed into adjacent chambers. An Elizabethan collar and foot bandages are used to prevent the animal removing the Finn chambers. The sites are inspected at 48 hours and erythematous indurated sites classed as positive. Punch biopsies can be taken from positive sites to confirm the reaction.

MANAGEMENT

If the allergen or irritant can be identified, and if exposure can be restricted, then the prognosis is

Allergic and Irritant Contact Dermatitis

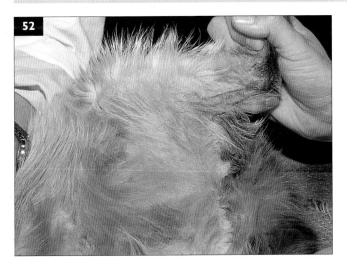

52 Irritant contact dermatitis. Erythema and alopecia following exposure to irritant oil.

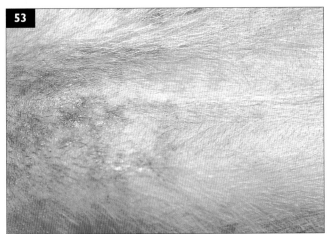

53, 54 Allergic contact dermatitis. Primary lesions (erythematous papules) on the ventral midline of a Labrador Retriever (**53**); well-demarcated erythema and alopecia in the groin and ventral abdomen of a Labrador Retriever (**54**).

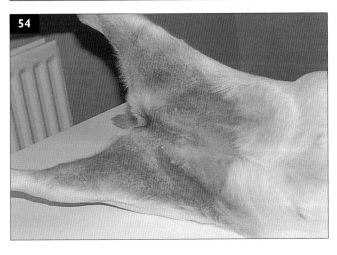

Allergic and Irritant Contact Dermatitis

good. Failure to identify the cause or prevent access results in reliance on symptomatic therapy, usually with systemic glucocorticoids. In some individuals, complete control may be very hard to achieve without the side-effects of glucocorticoid therapy becoming apparent.

KEY POINTS
- Allergic contact dermatitis is rare.
- The pruritus may be refractory to steroid therapy.

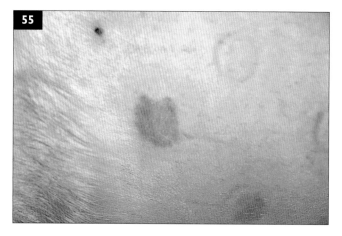

55 Positive closed patch test read after 48 hours. Circular impressions of the Finn chambers are apparent and the edematous, erythematous patches are readily visible.

Notoedric Mange

DEFINITION
A contagious dermatosis of cats due to infection with the mite *Notoedres cati*. Notoedric mange is characterized by intense, often unremitting, pruritus and self-trauma.

ETIOLOGY AND DIAGNOSIS
Infection with the mite results in severe pruritus, presumably due to a hypersensitivity, as is the case with canine scabies, although the biology and life cycle of the mite are less well understood[1].

CLINICAL FEATURES
There is no breed, age, or sex predisposition. Affected cats exhibit intense pruritus on the head and pinnae. The initial lesions are an erythematous, papular dermatitis, but a greyish crust soon becomes apparent, affecting the anterior edges of the pinnae in particular (56). There is local lymphadenopathy.

DIFFERENTIAL DIAGNOSES
- Dietary intolerance
- Otodectic acariasis
- Atopic dermatitis
- Dermatophytosis

DIAGNOSTIC TESTS
Microscopic examination of skin scrapings will usually reveal adult mites, eggs, or immature larvae.

MANAGEMENT
Ivermectin (0.2–0.3 mg/kg) repeated after 10 days is curative. Topical application of malathion or lime sulfur is also effective.

KEY POINT
- Notoedric mange may be confined to localized areas of a country or to small groups of cats.

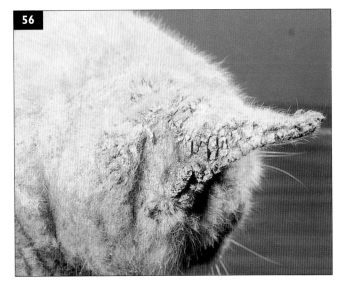

56

56 Notoedric mange. Accumulation of greyish crust on the rostral aspect of the pinna.

Epitheliotropic Lymphoma

(Cutaneous T Cell Lymphoma, Mycosis Fungoides)

DEFINITION
A rare, cutaneous neoplasm of dogs and cats characterized by epidermotropic T lymphocytic infiltration of the skin.

ETIOLOGY AND PATHOGENESIS
Certain T lymphocytes express membrane receptors which ensure that they repeatedly migrate through the dermis and epidermis. Epitheliotropic lymphoma results when one, or several, clones of these cells become malignant, although the stimulus for this neoplastic transformation is not known[1,2]. The neoplastic lymphocytes infiltrate the upper dermis and epidermis resulting in thickening, hyperkeratosis, plaque, and ulceration.

CLINICAL FEATURES
Epitheliotropic lymphoma is a disease of the older dog and cat and there is no breed or sex predisposition. The most common presentation in both dogs and cats is of a pruritic hyperkeratosis which is non-responsive to systemic glucocorticoids[1,3,4]. The disease typically progresses to an erythroderma on which plaques of silvery-white scale develop. Nodules or ulcerations of the skin may develop late in the course of the disease (57, 58). More rarely, epitheliotropic lymphoma presents as symmetrical raised lesions or solitary, often perioral, ulcerated plaque or tumor[3,5].

DIFFERENTIAL DIAGNOSES
- Atopic dermatitis
- Dietary intolerance
- Sarcoptic mange
- *Malassezia pachydermatis*
- Other causes of secondary defects in keratinization should be considered

DIAGNOSTIC TESTS
The diagnosis of mycosis fungoides is made on the basis of histopathologic examination of biopsy samples.

MANAGEMENT
Epitheliotropic lymphoma is often refractory to treatment. Partly this reflects the benign nature of the initial signs and the time which elapses before diagnosis is made. Topical nitrogen mustard, retinoids, and radiotherapy have been reported as inducing clinical improvement in some cases, but none of these are readily available and none have induced even medium-term remission[2,3,6]. Euthanasia is the only practical and humane option in most instances.

KEY POINTS
- The pruritis associated with epitheliotropic lymphoma may be refractory to steroid therapy.
- The initial signs may be so mild that suspicion is not aroused.

Epitheliotropic Lymphoma

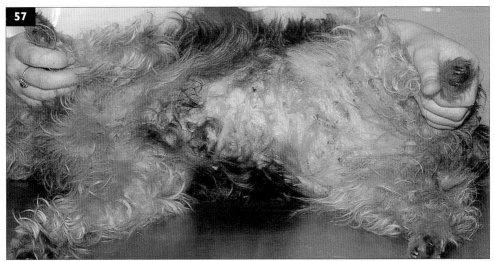

57 Epitheliotropic lymphoma. Erythroderma, nodules, and crusting on the ventral abdomen of a Yorkshire Terrier.

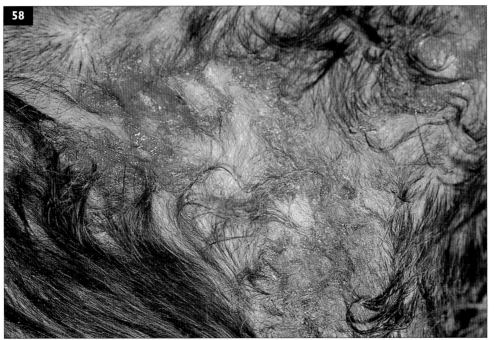

58 Erythematous, ulcerated plaques of mycosis fungoides.

Psychogenic Dermatoses

DEFINITION
Psychodermatoses result from continued, local or multifocal self-trauma, which is a consequence of an obsessive–compulsive, behavioral or self-mutilation disorder.

ETIOLOGY AND PATHOGENESIS
The origin of most psychodermatoses is unknown. In some cases the lesions may result from local inoculation or continued attention to local underlying tissue damage[1], whereas in other cases, evidence of sensory nerve axonopathy has been reported[2]. However, in most cases an underlying physical cause is not detected and lesions have been reported to result from boredom, lack of environmental stimulation, separation anxiety, and 'psychic stressors' such as an addition to the household or changes in work practice of a member of the household[1,3]. More recently, it has been suggested that the majority of cases (and particularly the refractory cases) are a manifestation of an obsessive–compulsive disorder, which would not be expected to respond to behavioral therapy[4]. Self-mutilation syndromes may also represent stereotypic behavior, itself a reflection of endorphin induction[5].

Whatever the cause, the animal exhibits continued, or chronic relapsing, attention to one or several areas of the body, typically the distal limb (acral lick dermatitis, self-mutilation) or flank (flank sucking), distal tail (tail chasing) or trunk (feline psychogenic alopecia). The consequences of this continued trauma are, progressively, saliva staining, focal alopecia, local thickening, hyperpigmentation, erosion, and ulceration. Secondary infection is uncommon.

CLINICAL FEATURES
There is a breed predisposition among dogs and German Shepherd Dogs, Doberman Pinschers, Irish Setters, Labrador and Golden Retrievers, Great Danes, and St. Bernards are overrepresented[3]. The most common manifestation is a local, well-circumscribed, hyperpigmented, alopecic plaque on the rostral aspect of the distal limb. Occasionally, multiple lesions will be present. Severe self-trauma will result in erosion (59) and, sometimes, ulceration but this is uncommon. There is no local lymphadenopathy. Digital compression fails to express either serosanguinous fluid or pus.

Flank sucking results in salivary wetting of a localized area of one (usually) flank, and is almost exclusively confined to Doberman Pinschers[3]. An underlying dermatitis is not common[3]. Tail chasing and biting rarely results in dermatitis since the tail is not usually 'caught'. Self-mutilation is very rare and is extremely distressing to the owner, as affected animals may inflict such serious damage to their distal limbs that autoamputation results.

Psychodermatoses in cats may affect both cross-bred 'domestic' cats and pedigree breeds. Both psychogenic alopecia and psychogenic dermatitis may result, depending on the degree of attention to which the skin is subjected. The lesions are most commonly found along the dorsal midline or are symmetrical (60), arranged in the groins and ventral abdomen (61). Hair loss may be extensive but it is not usually associated with dermatitis. Occasionally, cats will, however, persistently damage the skin, and erosion followed by ulceration will result.

DIFFERENTIAL DIAGNOSES
Dogs
- Localized folliculitis/furunculosis
- Demodicosis
- Fungal granuloma
- Cutaneous neoplasia
- Reaction to referred pain from an underlying osteo- or osteoarthritic condition

Cats
- Flea bite hypersensitivity
- Atopic dermatitis
- Dietary intolerance
- Demodicosis
- Telogen defluxion secondary to internal disease

DIAGNOSTIC TESTS
The diagnosis of a pychodermatosis is essentially one of exclusion. Flank sucking, tail chasing, and self-mutilation may be suspected from the history, although hypersensitivities, ectoparasitic dermatoses, anal sacculitis, and (in the case of self-mutilation) digital neoplasia should be considered.

Localized lesions of acral lick granuloma are the most difficult to diagnose definitively. Localized folliculitis/furunculosis is the most common cause of a solitary lesion on the forelimb of a dog. Digital pressure may express pus from the lesion, in which case it should be submitted for bacteriologic culture and sensitivity and followed by 4–6 weeks of appropriate antibacterial therapy (see Deep Pyoderma,

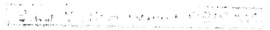

Psychogenic Dermatoses

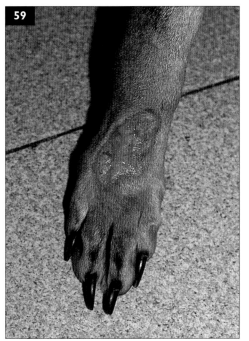

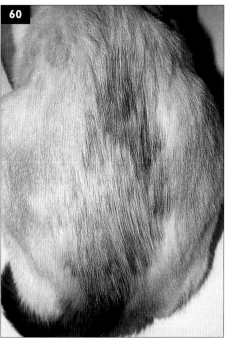

59 Acral lick granuloma. An erythematous, eroded, well-demarcated plaque on the distal aspect of the forelimb of a Doberman Pinscher.

60 Symmetrical alopecia on the lumbo-sacral region of a Siamese cat. Note the acromelanism.

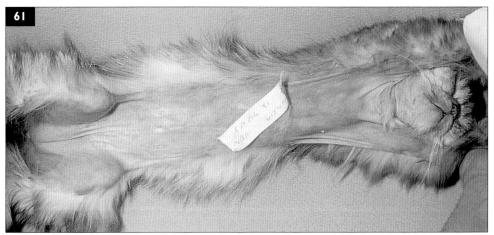

61 Psychogenic alopecia. Extensive, symmetrical alopecia on the ventral body surfaces of a Persian cat.

Psychogenic Dermatoses

page 124). A biopsy should be performed if doubt remains since it rules out most of the other differential diagnoses and will identify changes consistent with acral lick granuloma. Radiographic examination to search for underlying orthopedic conditions may be indicated in some cases. Animals with multiple lesions on several limbs are more likely to have a psychodermatosis.

The principle differential diagnosis of self-induced symmetrical alopecia in the cat is flea bite hypersensitivity, and every effort must be made to demonstrate that fleas are not the cause of the problem. Demodicosis and dermatophytosis may be ruled out by microscopic examination of skin scrapings and fungal culture, respectively. Underlying internal disease may be eliminated from the differential diagnosis by appropriate laboratory tests and by examination of the distal ends of plucked hairs – they will be gently tapering in cases of telogen defluxion, but obviously broken and fractured if self-epilation is the cause of the alopecia.

MANAGEMENT

Once the diagnosis of a psychodermatosis is made, the aim should be to try and identify any behavioral component of the condition. For example, changes in the work pattern of the household, changes in the family structure, or the addition of a new pet, either in the household or within the immediate neighborhood, may produce sufficient stress to precipitate the disorder[1]. Attention seeking, confinement and, rarely, boredom may be discovered to be the inciting cause[3,4], and specific actions to rectify the animal's environment may be successful. The use of amitryptaline (1–2 mg/kg q 12 h for dogs and 5–10 mg/kg q 12 h for cats) may allow the owner to reduce the degree of the animal's anxiety whilst attending to the underlying cause. Unfortunately, many cases of simple acral lick granulomas and most cases of multiple acral lick lesions, flank sucking, and self-mutilation are refractory to this approach, perhaps suggesting an obsessive–compulsive disorder[4], and pharmacological control must be attempted.

Recently, two groups of compounds have been reported to be beneficial in the management of psychodermatoses. Tricyclic antidepressants such as amitryptaline (the dose is given above) and doxepin (3–5 mg/kg q 12 h to a maximum of 150 mg/animal q 12 h) may be tried[4]. Clomipramine (1–3 mg/kg q 12 h) and fluoxetine (1 mg/kg q 24 h) in particular have proven successful[4] and warrant further investigation. Narcotic antagonists, such as naltrexone, have been shown to alleviate the signs of stereotypic licking and chewing in both dogs and cats[5–7]. However, these agents are expensive and difficult to obtain.

KEY POINTS
- Acral nodules are often infected.
- Solitary nodules, on the forelimbs in particular, may respond completely to antibacterial therapy.
- Behavioral causes are uncommon.

Ancylostomiasis (Hookworm Dermatitis)

DEFINITION
Hookworm dermatitis is a condition character-ized by erythematous papular lesions that occur following cutaneous penetration by the larvae of hookworms.

ETIOLOGY AND PATHOGENESIS
The dermatitis develops from the cutaneous penetration of the third stage larvae of *Uncinaria stenocephala* or *Ancylostoma* spp. located in the soil that the animal contacts[1]. Skin lesions are more often associated with *Uncinaria* spp. infestation than with *Ancylostoma* spp. Larvae enter the skin primarily at areas of desquamation but occasionally they may enter via hair follicles[2]. In contrast to *Ancylostoma* spp., *Uncinaria* spp. rarely completes its life cycle by percutaneous penetration[2,3].

CLINICAL FEATURES
The condition is more frequently noted in hook-worm-infested dogs which are housed on dirt runs with poor sanitation. Lesions are primarily located on the feet, but may be seen on any area of skin that touches the ground. Erythematous papules constitute primary lesions, but chronically affected skin often becomes diffusely erythematous and thickened and may exhibit alopecia (**62**). The epithelium of the footpads becomes roughened due to the development of keratinized papillae. Chronically affected footpads may eventually become soft and spongy, especially at the pad margins[4]. Nails may grow faster, become ridged, twisted on their long axis, thicker at the base, and in severe cases break off. Arthritis of the distal interphalangeal joints may be a sequela[4]. Pruritus is usually mild but can vary in intensity[2,4].

DIFFERENTIAL DIAGNOSES
- Atopic dermatitis
- Demodicosis
- Contact dermatitis
- *Pelodera strongyloides* dermatitis
- Bacterial pododermatitis
- Trauma

DIAGNOSTIC TESTS
Diagnosis is based on a history of being housed on dirt runs or kennels, poor sanitation, as well as the clinical findings. A positive fecal examination for hookworm eggs provides supporting evidence but does not confirm a diagnosis. Generally, larvae cannot be demonstrated on microscopic examination of skin scrapings.

MANAGEMENT
All affected and associated dogs should be given appropriate anthelmintic treatment and a prophylactic program should be started. Frequent removal of feces from the runs and kennels, as well as improved sanitation, should be initiated. If feasible, dirt runs or kennels should be relocated so that animals are removed from the parasitized environment. Sodium borate ($0.5 \ kg/m^2$) may be used to destroy larvae on the ground, although owners should be made aware that this treatment will kill vegetation[1].

KEY POINT
- Ancylostomiasis is unusual, although it may occur in certain groups of dogs, e.g. racing Greyhounds.

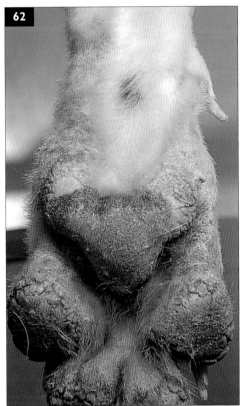

62   Hookworm dermatitis. Note the extensive erythema and scale formation in this chronic case.

Schnauzer Comedo Syndrome

DEFINITION
A follicular keratinization disorder of Miniature Schnauzers characterized by comedo formation along the dorsal midline.

ETIOLOGY AND PATHOGENESIS
The syndrome has been reported to occur because of an inherited developmental defect of the hair follicles leading to abnormal keratinization, comedo formation, follicular plugging and dilation and, in some cases, a secondary bacterial folliculitis[1-3].

CLINICAL FEATURES
Lesions develop in young-adult Miniature Schnauzers who are predisposed to the defect. They extend laterally from the dorsal midline and are located from the neck to the sacrum. In many cases, lesions are more prominent on the lumbar sacral region (**63**). In early or mild cases the lesions may not be visualized, but only noticed by the palpation of small papules over the dorsum. With progression, papular comedones become obvious and thinning of the hair occurs in the affected areas (**64**). A secondary bacterial folliculitis may develop and this will often be accompanied by pruritus and pain. Small crusts may develop in association with the infection.

DIFFERENTIAL DIAGNOSES
- Demodicosis
- Bacterial folliculitis
- Dermatophytosis
- Flea bite hypersensitivity

DIAGNOSTIC TESTS
History and clinical signs provide a tentative diagnosis and histopathologic examination of biopsy samples will allow confirmation.

MANAGEMENT
Mild cases with few lesions require no treatment. The majority of the more severe cases can be controlled with benzoyl peroxide shampoos. Initially, the frequency of shampooing should be twice weekly. This may be reduced to weekly or biweekly, as appropriate, for control. If a secondary bacterial folliculitis is present, systemic antibiotic therapy for 2 weeks would be indicated (see Superficial Pyoderma, page 108). Cases refractory to topical therapy may be treated with isotretinoin (1–2 mg/kg PO q 24 h)[2]. Response is generally noted in 3–4 weeks, after which the dose may be reduced to every 2–3 days as necessary for control.

KEY POINT
- Do not make the mistake of forgetting to eliminate all possible differential diagnoses.

Schnauzer Comedo Syndrome

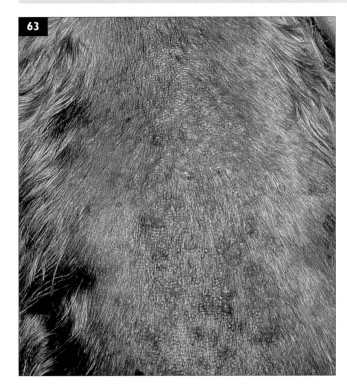

63 Schnauzer comedo syndrome. Erythema. Comedones and crust on the dorsal lumbar sacral region.

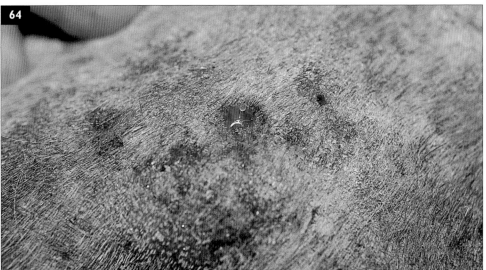

64 Schnauzer comedo syndrome demonstrating secondary infection and furunculosis.

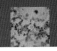

Nodular Dermatoses

GENERAL APPROACH

1 Not all nodules are neoplastic.
2 Biopsy all nodules – prognosis depends on a definitive diagnosis.
3 Cytologic evaluation of nodules before surgery should be part of routine management. Thus if cytology suggests mast cell neoplasia, a surgical margin of at least 2 cm (0.8 in) on *all* sides (that is, left, right, top, bottom, *and* underneath) should be left.

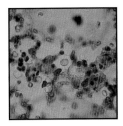
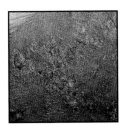
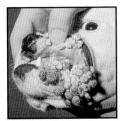
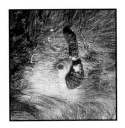

Epidermal and Follicular Inclusion Cysts

DEFINITION
Epidermal and follicular inclusion cysts are non-neoplastic swellings with an epithelial lining.

ETIOLOGY AND PATHOGENESIS
Epidermal inclusion cysts may result from the traumatic implantation of keratinaceous material of epidermal origin into the dermis. Follicular inclusion cysts may result from traumatic occlusion of the follicular canal, resulting in the accumulation of pilosebaceous material[1].

CLINICAL FEATURES
These lesions are common in the dog and uncommon in the cat. There is no breed, age, or sex predisposition. Epidermal inclusions cysts are well demarcated, soft, painless swellings up to 5 cm (2 in) in diameter (**65**), which may occur anywhere on the body, although the dorsal and lateral trunk are the most common sites[1]. Occasionally, a patent pore connects the interior of the cyst to the skin surface. The contents may rupture to the surface and are softly granular or paste-like in nature, often yellowish-grey in color. Follicular inclusion cysts are more common on the limbs and head[1] and are smaller and harder than epidermal inclusion cysts, often only 2–5 mm (0.1–0.2 in) in diameter.

DIFFERENTIAL DIAGNOSIS
- Abscess
- Hematoma
- Cutaneous neoplasia

DIAGNOSTIC TESTS
Clinical examination, aspiration cytology, and sectioning of excised lesions will allow for diagnosis. Histopathologic examination of excised samples will confirm the clinical diagnosis.

MANAGEMENT
Surgical excision is curative, although affected animals tend to produce new lesions in due course. Owners should be advised to refrain from squeezing the cysts since this results in the expression of more material into the dermis, only to provoke further reaction.

KEY POINT
- Do not be tempted to squeeze these out – dermal inflammation will follow and recurrence is certain.

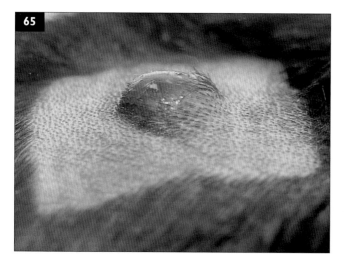

65 Epidermal inclusion cyst. A large, well-demarcated plaque-like lesion on the dorsal trunk of a cross-bred dog.

Papillomatosis

DEFINITION
Cutaneous papillomas (warts) are a thickening of the epidermis supported by finger-like projections of the dermis resulting in multiple fronds.

ETIOLOGY AND PATHOGENESIS
Most lesions are induced by a DNA papovavirus, but idiopathic, non-viral squamous papillomas can occur[1-3]. The lesions of viral papillomas may be transmitted by either direct or indirect contact, with an incubation that varies from 2–6 months[3].

CLINICAL FEATURES
Cutaneous viral papillomatosis is common and occurs primarily in young dogs. Lesions occur as single or multiple white-to-flesh-colored, pedunculated or cauliflower-like masses (**66**), which can range in size from 2–3 mm (0.01 in) in diameter to 3 cm (1.2 in)[3]. They are generally located on the oral mucosae but may also be found on the tongue, palate, pharynx, epiglottis, lips, conjunctiva, cornea, eyelids, and skin[2-4]. A less common form is the inverted cutaneous papilloma, which occurs most frequently on the ventral abdomen and groin, and appears as a 1–2 cm (0.4–0.4 in) raised lesion with a central pore. Frond-like projections extend into the center of crater-like lesions[1]. Cutaneous horn may occasionally be a presenting sign of either of these two types of papillomas[2]. Viral papillomas are usually benign and will regress over a period varying from weeks to months. However, in rare instances, malignant transformation into squamous cell carcinomas has been documented[5].

Idiopathic, non-viral papillomas are uncommon and occur mainly in older animals. Lesions tend to be small (1–5 mm/0.04–0.2 in) in diameter, appear pedunculated or verrucose, and are located mainly on the head, eyelids, and feet[2,3].

DIFFERENTIAL DIAGNOSES
- Sebaceous gland adenoma
- Infundibular keratinizing acanthoma

DIAGNOSTIC TESTS
Diagnosis may be based on history and clinical appearance of lesions. Excision and histopathologic examination should be considered if they are unusual in appearance.

MANAGEMENT
Treatment may not be necessary as canine viral papillomas usually undergo regression within 3 months, and the affected animals develop an immunity to further infection. Large masses of regressing lesions may give off a foul odor. If the lesions are numerous and large so that they interfere with mastication, they may be treated via cryosurgery (two freeze-thaw cycles) or electrosurgery. Autogenous or commercially produced vaccines have not been documented to be of value, and squamous cell carcinomas occasionally will arise at injection sites[6].

KEY POINT
- A common condition and rarely needs more than identification.

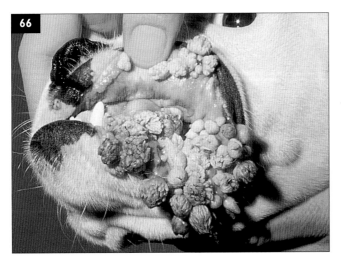

66 Papillomatosis. Multiple, verrucose papillomas on the oral mucosa of a young dog.

Mast Cell Neoplasia

DEFINITION
Mast cell tumors are relatively common and potentially very malignant tumors derived from dermal mast cells.

ETIOLOGY AND PATHOGENESIS
The etiology of mast cell neoplasia is not known. The cells are normal constituents of the canine and feline dermis[1,2]. In some cases, particularly where there are multiple neoplasms, there may be significant release of vasoactive mediators, such as histamine or heparin, resulting in paraneoplastic activity[1,2]. This may range from local erythema and edema to peptic ulceration and coagulopathies.

CLINICAL FEATURES
Mast cell tumors are most common in older dogs[1,3]. There is no sex predisposition but some breeds are predisposed, such as Boxers, Labrador Retrievers, and Staffordshire Bull Terriers[1,2,3]. The most common presentation in cats is of a solitary dermal nodule, although multiple lesions may be encountered[4,5]. A syndrome of benign mastocytoma, presenting as multiple, cutaneous papules and nodules has been reported in Siamese kittens[6]. In dogs the tumors usually begin as single or multiple dermal nodules (**67, 68**), but their clinical appearance and subsequent behavior varies and is very unpredictable. Size may vary from 1–10 cm (0.4–4.0 in); they may be soft or firm and are well-circumscribed[3]. Broadly speaking, dermal mast cell tumors are either rather slow growing, solitary nodules or rapidly growing, often poorly defined, nodules with a tendency to early metastasis[7].

DIFFERENTIAL DIAGNOSIS
- Histiocytoma
- Bacterial or fungal granuloma
- Foreign body granuloma
- Other cutaneous neoplasms

DIAGNOSTIC TESTS
Clinical suspicion may be confirmed by examination of stained needle aspirate samples[3,7]. Examination of appropriately stained samples gives information sufficient to ensure that wide (2–3 cm/0.8–1.2 in) margins are excised but does not give sufficient information to allow grading of the tumor. All excised neoplasms should be submitted for histopathologic examination. Unfortunately it has so far proved difficult to predict biologic behavior, or even optimum treatment modality (other than surgery), with histopathologic classification of mast cell morphology[7,8].

MANAGEMENT
All canine mast cell tumors should be considered potentially malignant and, for discrete lesions, wide local excision is the best treatment[3,4]. A wide surgical margin of 2–3 cm (0.8–1.2 in) *on all surfaces* is advised, even for apparently well-demarcated lesions. In some areas of the body (the distal limb, for example), this degree of excision may necessitate sliding or other types of surgical graft. There is little evidence that excision of solitary nodules should be followed up with chemotherapy.

A staged management regime for canine mast cell tumors has been proposed[3,8,9] and the following table is based on these references:

Stage 1: One tumor confined to the dermis with no regional lymph node involvement
- Wide surgical excision with cimetidine (5 mg/kg PO q 6 h) if there is histamine release.

Stage 2: One tumor confined to the dermis with regional lymph node involvement
- Surgical excision plus radiotherapy.
- Cimetidine if there is histamine release.

Stage 3: Multiple tumors, or large infiltrating tumors, with or without regional lymph node involvement
- Surgical excision may be helpful but chemotherapy mandatory. Prednisolone (40 mg/m^2 PO q 24 h for 7 days, then 20 mg/m^2 PO alternate days) and vincristine (0.5 mg/m^2 IV once weekly).
- Cimetidine if there is histamine release.

Stage 4: Any tumor with distant metastases
- Prednisolone (40 mg/m^2 PO q 24 h for 7 days, then 20 mg/m^2 PO alternate days) and vincristine (0.5 mg/m^2 IV once weekly).
- Cimetidine if there is histamine release.

Intralesional triamcinolone (1 mg/cm tumor diameter) has been suggested as an appropriate adjunct in stage 3 and 4 mast cell tumors[10]. There has also been considerable interest in the use of intralesional, and post-surgical infiltration of surgical site, with deionized water[11].

KEY POINTS
- Potentially a highly malignant neoplasm.
- Wide excision on *all* aspects gives the best chance of cure.
- Radiotherapy for recurrent lesions is recommended.

Mast Cell Neoplasia

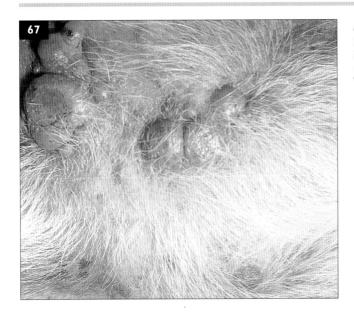

67 Mast cell neoplasia. Multiple erythematous nodules in the groins of a dog. (Illustration courtesy of G.T. Wilkinson.)

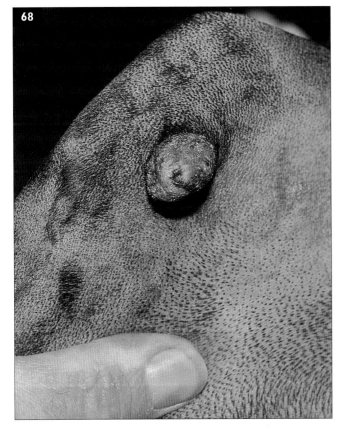

68 Mast cell neoplasia. Solitary, ulcerating nodule on the stifle of a dog.

Basal Cell Tumor

DEFINITION
Basal cell tumors are benign neoplasms which arise from the basal keratinocytes of the epidermis.

ETIOLOGY AND PATHOGENESIS
It is possible that basal cell tumors result from neoplastic change within epidermal stem cells[1]. The stimulus which results in a normally cycling cell changing to a cell with neoplastic potential is not known.

CLINICAL FEATURES
There is no sex predisposition. Most basal cell tumors occur in older dogs and cats, typically on the head and dorsal trunk[2–4]. Poodles and Cocker Spaniels are predisposed[5]. Basal cell tumors are among the most common cutaneous neoplasms in the cat; slightly less common in the dog[2–5]. The neoplasms are well encapsulated, occasionally cystic, and freely movable (**69**). They tend to be small and in the cat most are less than 2.5 cm (1 in) in diameter (**70**)[2,4].

DIFFERENTIAL DIAGNOSES
- Bacterial or fungal granuloma
- Foreign body granuloma
- Follicular cyst
- Other cutaneous neoplasms

DIAGNOSTIC TESTS
Although the cytologic appearance of basal cell tumors may be characteristic[6], the definitive diagnosis is best made by histopathologic examination of biopsy or excision samples.

MANAGEMENT
Surgical excision is the most effective form of treatment[1].

KEY POINT
- Very common tumor.

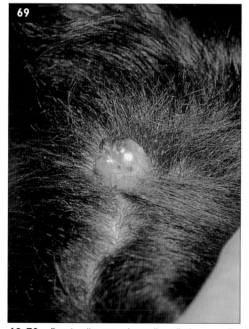
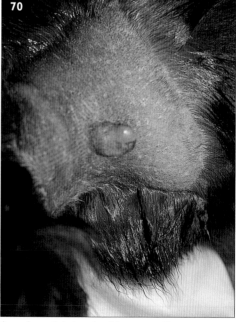

69, 70   Basal cell tumor. A small, well-circumscribed, alopecic nodule basal cell tumor on the trunk of a dog (**69**); a cystic, well-circumscribed basal cell tumor on the lateral neck of a domestic shorthair cat (**70**).

Collagenous Nevi

DEFINITION

A collagenous nevus is a circumscribed developmental defect of the skin, characterized by collagenous hyperplasia.

ETIOLOGY AND PATHOGENESIS

The mechanisms of nevus formation have not been determined[1].

CLINICAL FEATURES

Collagenous nevi generally appear as firm, well-circumscribed, slowly enlarging nodules of the skin and subcutis, that vary in size from 0.5–5 cm (0.2–2 in) in diameter[2]. Lesions are usually multiple (71) and are located more frequently on the head, neck, and proximal extremities. Middle-aged animals are more likely to be affected, but lesions have also been reported in younger animals[2]. Slowly enlarging lesions localized to one area of the body have been reported[2].

DIFFERENTIAL DIAGNOSES

- Other cutaneous neoplasms
- Bacterial and fungal granuloma
- Sterile nodular granuloma and pyogranuloma
- Deep mycotic infections

DIAGNOSTIC TESTS

Histopathologic examination of biopsy or excision samples is diagnostic.

MANAGEMENT

Surgical excision of the nodules is the treatment of choice in most cases. Reoccurrence occurs rapidly, at an accelerated rate, in those animals exhibiting large lesions localized to one area of the body[2].

KEY POINT

- Unpredictable, essentially benign lesions.

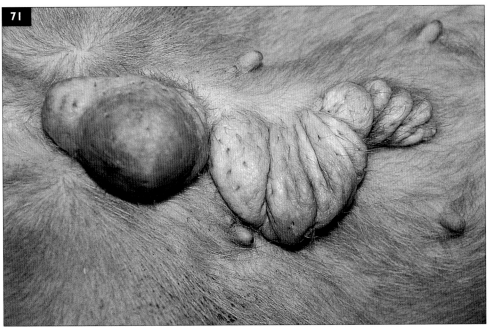

71 Multiple, flaccid collagenous nevi in the ventral midline of a dog.

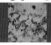

Melanocytic Neoplasia

DEFINITION
Melanocytic neoplasms are variably malignant tumors which arise from melanocytes within the skin. They are relatively uncommon in the dog and rare in the cat.

ETIOLOGY AND PATHOGENESIS
In humans, melanocytic neoplasms may be induced by actinic radiation[1]. It has not been determined whether this is so in dogs and cats. The canine tumors are usually benign when they arise on the head and trunk, but malignant when they are intraoral or on the distal limb[2,3]. The reason for this regional pattern of behavior is not known. Feline melanocytic neoplasms are usually malignant, particularly those arising on the eyelid[4].

CLINICAL FEATURES
Melanomas occur with increased frequency in Airedales, Scottish Terriers, Boston Terriers, and Cocker Spaniels; males may be predisposed[4]. The benign tumors, which are dermal in origin, may occur anywhere on the head, trunk, or proximal limb[5], and are well-circumscribed, domed, hairless, and between 0.5–2 cm (0.2–0.8 in) diameter[4]. Melonomas which arise on the distal limb (72) are similar in presentation, although with a tendency to ulcerate and to invade the nail bed[3], and may be malignant. Feline melanomas usually occur on the head, particularly the pinnae[4].

DIFFERENTIAL DIAGNOSES
- Melanocytic nevi
- Squamous cell carcinoma
- Bacterial and fungal granuloma
- Foreign body granuloma
- Other cutaneous neoplasia

DIAGNOSTIC TESTS
Aspiration cytology may help to suggest a diagnosis of melanoma, although care must be taken to differentiate them from mast cell tumors[6]. However, given the tendency for pedal and digital lesions to behave in a malignant manner, the decision to perform radical excision, in cases where significant surgery is indicated, should be based on histopathologic criteria, not cytologic. Clinical staging with local lymph node excision, thoracic radiography, and blood panels should follow suspicion of malignant melanoma, given its tendency to metastasize[6].

MANAGEMENT
Truncal melanomas are typically benign and excision with a 1 cm (0.4 in) margin is curative in most cases[6]. Benign melanotic tumors arising on the distal limb usually require amputation of the digit to achieve adequate excision with no long-term complications[3,6,7]. The management of malignant lesions should also involve local excision and, perhaps, local amputation, although the owners should be cautioned that most dogs will die of the effects of distant metastasis, typically to the lungs by way of the local lymph nodes[3].

KEY POINTS
- Be prepared to be aggressive in the management of digital masses.
- Treat non-responding digital erythema or ulceration with suspicion.

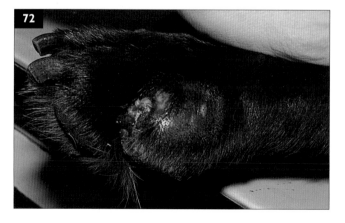

72 Melanoma. Malignant lesion, heavily pigmented, on the foot of a Labrador Retriever.

Hyperandrogenism

DEFINITION
Hyperandrogenism results from chronic stimulation of androgen dependent tissue by excess serum concentration of androgenic hormones.

ETIOLOGY AND PATHOGENESIS
Most cases of hyperandrogenism result from excessive androgen synthesis by testicular neoplasms, particularly interstitial cell tumors, although it may occur in male dogs in the absence of testicular neoplasia[1-3]. Rarely, the syndrome occurs in neutered animals, a consequence of adrenal androgen synthesis[2]. The androgen dependent tissues are the tail gland and the prostate gland in the male, and perianal gland tissue in both males and females. Under androgen influence these tissues exhibit hyperplasia and, sometimes, adenomatous change. Androgens also stimulate epidermal hyperproliferation, enhance sebum secretion, and retard the initiation of anagen[2].

CLINICAL FEATURES
Hyperandrogenism is most commonly seen in elderly, entire male dogs[2,3]. There is hyperplasia of the tail gland, perianal gland hyperplasia, and prostatomegaly[3] (73, 74). Testicular neoplasia may be detected[1,2]. Spayed bitches and males are predisposed to perianal gland neoplasia compared with entire bitches[4]. Cocker Spaniels of both sexes are predisposed to perianal gland neoplasia[4], and male English Bulldogs, Samoyeds, and Beagles are predisposed to perianal gland adenomas[4]. In some cases there may also be a greasy seborrhea, precipitated by the cutaneous effects of prolonged androgen excess[2]. In bitches there is perianal gland hyperplasia and, in some cases, exhibition of masculine behavior, such as mounting[2].

DIFFERENTIAL DIAGNOSIS
* Perianal gland adenocarcinoma

DIAGNOSTIC TESTS
The triad of tail gland hyperplasia, perianal gland hyperplasia, and prostatomegaly in an elderly male dog is diagnostic. Serum testosterone concentrations may be elevated[3].

MANAGEMENT
The adenomatous changes and hyperplasia are androgen dependent and castration is the treatment of choice[2-4]. If the condition occurs in a bitch, then adrenal gland neoplasia or hyperplasia should be investigated.

KEY POINT
* Common, especially in elderly, entire males.

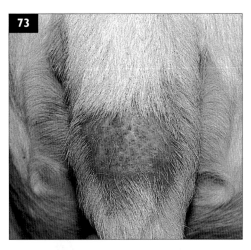

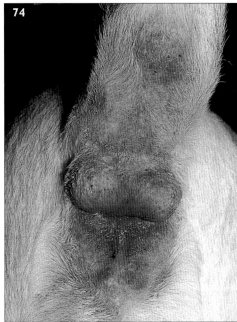

73, 74 Hyperandrogenism in an adult male Staffordshire Bull Terrier. There is a nodular alopecic swelling of the tail gland (**73**); hyperplasia of the perianal tissues (**74**).

Panniculitis

DEFINITION
Panniculitis is inflammation of the subcutaneous fat, which may result from several different etiologies.

ETIOLOGY AND PATHOGENESIS
Lipocytes (fat cells) can be damaged by many factors, but the end-product of these various etiologies is the release of free lipid into the extracellular space. These lipids undergo hydrolysis to fatty acids, which can incite further inflammation and granulomatous reactions[1,2].
- Post-injection panniculitis occurs infrequently in the cat and rarely in the dog. It may be underdiagnosed because clinical signs may not be obvious, or may seem inconsequential. This condition has been associated with various vaccines[3] and injection of other medications, including antibiotics. It is postulated that the reaction results from a combination of foreign body and hypersensitivity reactions[3].
- Traumatic panniculitis occurs when blunt trauma, chronic pressure, or decreased blood supply induces focal ischemia[1].
- Infectious panniculitis occurs when bacteria or deep mycotic agents become established in the panniculus.
- Immune-mediated panniculitis occurs with immune-mediated vascular diseases, such as systemic lupus erythematosus, the reactions occurring due to hypersensitivity to drugs, infectious agents, or visceral malignancy[1,2,4]. Erythema nodosum-like panniculitis is a septal panniculitis associated with vascular damage due to systemic hypersensitivity reactions.
- Nutritional panniculitis occurs as feline pansteatitis, which results from a severe, absolute or relative, deficiency of vitamin E, often a result of a diet rich in oily fish[5].
- Idiopathic panniculitis encompasses all of the sterile inflammatory diseases of the panniculus that have unknown etiologies. Examples would be idiopathic sterile nodular panniculitis and sterile pedal panniculitis of the German Shepherd Dog[6,7].

CLINICAL FEATURES
Lesions usually occur as solitary nodules[1]. The lesions are variably firm and painful and, in one survey, 35% of nodules were accompanied by fistulous draining tracts[1]. They are most commonly located over the ventrolateral neck, chest, and abdomen[1,2]. There is no age or sex predisposition, but Dachshunds are more frequently affected than other breeds of dogs. Animals with sterile nodular panniculitis are more likely to have multiple lesions (**75, 76**). The larger lesions of these animals, as well as lesions in animals with erythema nodosum-like panniculitis, tend to ulcerate and drain an oily, clear to yellowish-brown liquid[1,2,4].

Sterile pedal panniculitis of the German Shepherd Dog appears as well-demarcated fistulous tracts that have slightly swollen erythematous borders[7,8]. They are most frequently located dorsal to the midline of the tarsal or carpal pad, but lesions have also been associated with other pads. The fistulous tracts drain a small amount of serous to milky, viscid fluid.

Feline pansteatitis is manifested by multiple nodules of varying firmness occurring in the subcutis and abdominal mesenteric fat[5]. Fistulation is rare. Systemic signs, such as fever, malaise, and pain, may precede or occur in conjunction with the development of nodules.

DIFFERENTIAL DIAGNOSES
- Abscess
- Cutaneous bacterial or fungal granuloma
- Deep bacterial folliculitis and furunculosis
- Cutaneous mycobacterial infection
- Deep mycotic infections
- Cutaneous cysts
- *Cuterebra* spp. infestation
- Cutaneous neoplasia
- Foreign body reactions

DIAGNOSTIC TESTS
Excision, or wedge biopsy, with samples submitted for both histopathologic examination and culture and sensitivity is the minimal data base for diagnosis.

MANAGEMENT
Panniculitis secondary to systemic disease should resolve when appropriate treatment is instituted. Solitary lesions may be removed surgically. If the panniculitis is due to bacterial or fungal infections, appropriate treatment for the specific agent should be instituted based on *in vitro* culture and sensitivity testing. Cats with pansteatitis should be fed a nutritionally balanced diet and, at least until in remission, should be given vitamin E (10 IU/kg) daily. Animals with idiopathic panniculitis respond well to systemic glucocorticoids[1,2]. Methylprednisolone (0.3–1.0 mg/kg) or prednisolone (2.0 mg/kg) may be given daily until lesions resolve (usually 3–6 weeks); after this the dose is tapered. Many animals will enter

Panniculitis

long-term or permanent remissions. If lesions return, prolonged alternate day steroid therapy may be necessary for control. Daily supplementation with vitamin E (300 IU) may have a steroid-sparing action in some cases[8].

KEY POINT
- Huge differential. All lesions characterized by sinus and not known to be abscessation should be biopsied.

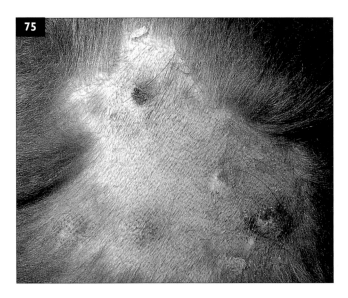

75 Panniculitis. Several erythematous nodules on the lateral trunk of a dog.

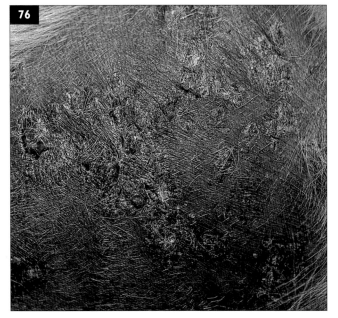

76 Hyperpigmented plaques and sinus formation associated with panniculitis.

Cryptococcosis

DEFINITION
Cryptococcosis is a deep mycotic disease resulting from infection with *Cryptococcus neoformans.*

ETIOLOGY AND PATHOGENESIS
Cryptococcus neoformans is a saprophytic, small (1–7 μm), budding yeast with a world-wide distribution. It is characterized by a mucoid, polysaccharide capsule that can vary in size from 1–30 μm. The capsule helps to prevent desiccation of the organism and also enables the yeast to escape detection from the immune system of the mammalian host[1]. Although the organism has been isolated from several sources (including soil), it is most frequently associated with pigeon droppings. Based on circumstantial evidence, the most likely route of infection is through inhalation of airborne organisms[1,2]. They may be deposited in the upper respiratory tract resulting in nasal granulomas, or proceed to the alveoli and induce pulmonary granulomas. Extension of infection from the respiratory tract occurs by local invasion through the cribiform plates to the CNS, or by hematogenous and lymphatic spread[1,3]. Cutaneous infection via traumatic inoculation has also been proposed[4]. Concurrent diseases which are immunosuppressive, such as FeLV or FIV infection in cats and ehrlichiosis in dogs, have been associated with cryptococcal infections. However, underlying diseases are often not detected in companion animals with cryptococcosis.

CLINICAL FEATURES
Cats
Cryptococcosis is the most frequently diagnosed deep mycotic infection in cats. There is no sex predisposition and affected animals range in age from 1–13 years (median 5 years)[2,3]. Signs of upper respiratory disease occur in 55% of the cases and include a mucopurulent, serous or hemorrhagic, unilateral or bilateral chronic nasal discharge. Flesh-colored, polyp-like masses in the nostrils or a firm, hard subcutaneous swelling over the bridge of the nose (**77**) will be found in 70% of the cases with a nasal discharge. Skin lesions are present in 40% of the cases and usually consist of papules or nodules (**78**) that may be either fluctuant or firm and range from 1–10 mm (0.04–0.4 in) in diameter. Larger lesions often ulcerate, leaving a raw surface with a serous exudate[2,4]. Neurologic signs occur in

25% of the cases and may include depression, amaurotic blindness, ataxia, circling, paresis, paralysis, and seizures[1,3]. Ocular involvement may also be present. Regional lymphadenopathy, low-grade fever, malaise, anorexia, or weight loss may occasionally occur[1].

Dogs
Cryptococcosis is less frequently diagnosed in the dog than in the cat. Clinical signs related to ocular and CNS lesions are the most common abnormalities[3]. Skin lesions consisting of papules, nodules, ulcers, abscesses, and draining tracts occur in 25% of the cases and often involve the nose, tongue, gums, lips, hard palate, or nailbeds[3].

DIFFERENTIAL DIAGNOSES
- Deep pyoderma and bacterial abcessation
- Other deep mycotic infections
- Cutaneous neoplasia

DIAGNOSTIC TESTS
Cytologic examination of nasal exudate, skin exudate, or CSF and tissue aspirates generally reveals pleomorphic (round to elliptical, 2–20 μm in diameter) organisms which are characterized by a capsule of variable thickness which forms a clear or refractile halo (**79**). The LCAT is a serological method for detecting capsular polysaccharide antigen in serum, urine, and CSF. Titers parallel the severity of infection, and may be used to monitor response to therapy[1]. Histopathologic examination of excision or biopsy samples is diagnostic.

MANAGEMENT
Fluconazole (50 mg/cat PO q 12 h for 2–4 months) is the recommended therapy[5]. Therapy should be continued for 1–2 months beyond clinical resolution of lesions or until the LCAT titers are negative. Itraconazole (5 mg/kg PO q 12 h) or ketoconazole (10 mg/kg PO q 24 h) has also been reported to be effective[4–6].

KEY POINT
- *Always* obtain a histopathologic report on nodules biopsied, or excised, from cats. Many cutaneous nodules in the cat are malignant but some will be cyptococcosis and will be treatable.

Cryptococcosis

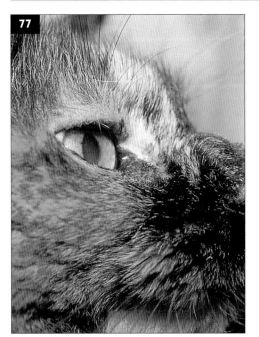

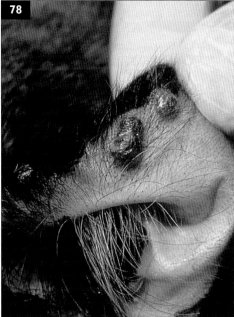

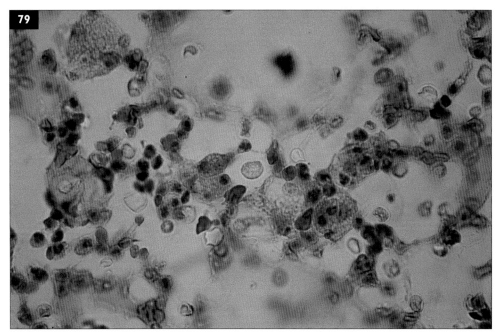

77–79   Cryptococcosis. A nodular lesion on the face of a domestic shorthair cat with cryptococcosis (**77**); papules and nodules on the pinna of a domestic shorthair cat with cryptococcosis (**78**); a photomicrograph of *Cryptococcus* spp. demonstrating the refractile, clearly defined capsule around the yeast (**79**).

Infundibular Keratinizing Acanthoma

DEFINITION
Infundibular keratinizing acanthomas (keratoacanthomas or intracutaneous cornifying epitheliomas) are benign nodular neoplasms of the skin of dogs[1].

ETIOLOGY AND PATHOGENESIS
The neoplasm evolves from the epithelium of the infundibulum or isthumus of the hair follicle[2,3]. The central portion of the tumor is filled with keratin.

CLINICAL FEATURES
The incidence of infundibular keratinizing acanthomas is higher in pure-bred dogs and the Norwegian Elkhound is particularly predisposed[3]. Animals are generally less than 5 years of age when lesions first appear, and males may have an increased incidence[3]. Neoplasms generally appear as well-circumscribed dermal or subcutaneous masses ranging is size from 0.5–4.0 cm (0.2–1.6 in) in diameter with a pore that opens to the skin surface (**80**). Digital pressure on the mass may cause the expulsion of white to gray keratin debris through the pore. A keratinized plug may protrude from the pore in some cases and, if large, it may appear as a cutaneous horn. Occasionally, neoplasms will be found entirely in the dermis or subcutaneous tissue with no communication to the skin surface. Lesions may appear inflamed if the wall becomes disrupted, allowing keratin into the surrounding tissue, where it evokes a foreign body reaction[2]. Lesions are usually solitary, but may be generalized in the Norwegian Elkhound and have been reported to be multiple in Keeshounds, German Shepherd Dogs, and Old English Sheepdogs[1].

DIFFERENTIAL DIAGNOSES
- Follicular and other cysts
- Cutaneous horn
- Foreign body reaction
- Sterile nodular panniculitis
- Deep mycotic infection
- *Cuterebra* spp. infestation
- Sterile nodular granuloma or pyogranuloma
- Bacterial granuloma
- Other cutaneous neoplasms

DIAGNOSTIC TESTS
Excision biopsy with subsequent histolopathologic examination.

MANAGEMENT
Surgical excision is the treatment of choice for solitary lesions. Surgical removal of multiple lesions is often not satisfactory as new lesions will still continue to develop. Retinoids, such as isotretinoin (2 mg/kg PO q 24 h) and etretinate (1.0–1.2 mg/kg PO q 24 h), have been helpful in the treatment of multiple lesions in some dogs[4,5]. These drugs tend to prevent development of new lesions and result in regression of small lesions, but often have little effect on larger lesions. Larger lesions may be pretreated with cryotherapy prior to retinoid therapy as this will often improve overall results. Clinical side-effects of retinoids include conjunctivitis, hyperactivity, pruritus, pedal and mucocutaneous junction erythema, stiffness, vomiting, diarrhea, and keratoconjunctivitis[5]. Laboratory abnormalities include hypertriglyceridemia, hypercholesterolemia, and increased levels of alanine aminotransferase, aspartate aminotransferase, and alkaline phosphatase[5]. Pretreatment measurement of tear production, hemogram, chemistry profile, and urinalysis is recommended and should be repeated after 1–2 months. Further monitoring is then performed as necessary. Generally, the clinical and laboratory side-effects are self-limiting with discontinuation or decrease in dose of the drug. In addition, it is extremely important to remember that all retinoids are potent teratogens.

KEY POINTS
- An unusual tumor, rarely seen in practice.

Infundibular Keratinizing Acanthoma

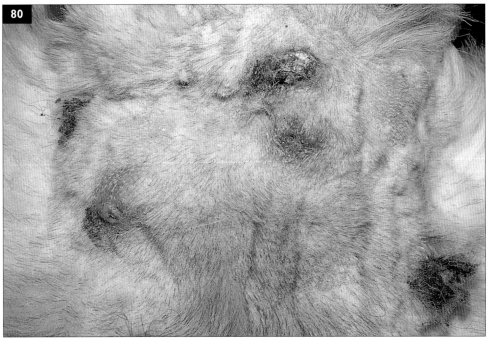

80   Keratoacanthoma. Crusted nodules in the groin of a dog.

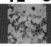

Systemic Histiocytosis and Other Histiocytoses

DEFINITION
Systemic histiocytosis is a rare condition characterized by progressive infiltration of the skin and internal organs with abnormal histiocytes. Other, rather poorly characterized histiocytic conditions, such as histiocytosis and malignant histiocytosis, are also recognized

ETIOLOGY AND PATHOGENESIS
The etiology of systemic histiocytosis is not known, although it is not consistent with neoplasia[1]. The disease may reflect uncontrolled proliferation of histiocytes in response to an unknown stimulus[2]. Male Bernese Mountain Dogs are predisposed[1], and a polygenic mode of inheritance has been proposed in this breed. Other breeds may be affected[3]. The gradual infiltration of internal organs by abnormal histiocytes results in signs of systemic disease in addition to the cutaneous lesions.

CLINICAL FEATURES
Dermatologic lesions are most apparent[1], with poorly defined alopecic papules, nodules, and plaques (**81, 82**), which may become ulcerated or encrusted[1,2]. Cutaneous lesions are particularly found on the head, pinnae, sheath, and scrotum, with the neck, trunk, and limbs much less frequently affected[1]. The clinical course of the disease is characterized by episodes of weight loss and depression interspersed with periods of remission.

DIFFERENTIAL DIAGNOSES
- Bacterial or fungal granuloma
- Cutaneous neoplasia
- Canine Langerhans cell tumor
- Foreign body granuloma
- Idiopathic sterile granuloma and pyo-granuloma syndrome
- Malignant histiocytosis

DIAGNOSTIC TESTS
The breed predisposition and waxing and waning nature of the disease are suggestive of systemic histiocytosis, but histopathologic examination of biopsy samples is necessary for definitive diagnosis. This is particularly important when attempting to differentiate cutaneous histiocytosis (predominantly young animals and only dermal lesions) and malignant histiocytosis (aggressive systemic disease in older dogs), since the former is a benign dermatosis.

MANAGEMENT
The disease has a progressive course. The periods of clinical remission make assessment of treatment difficult. Systemic antibacterial agents, glucocorticoids, and cytotoxic agents have not proved useful[1,2].

KEY POINT
- These are a group of poorly defined conditions. Biopsy and histopathologic examination is critical for prognosis.

Systemic Histiocytosis and Other Histiocytoses

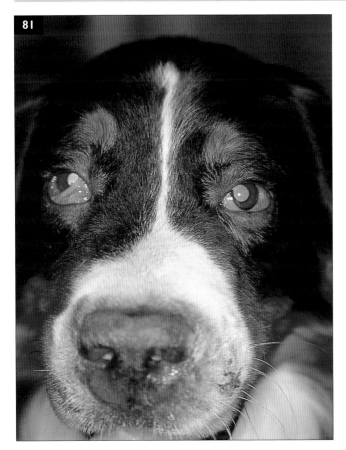

81 Systemic histiocytosis. Poorly defined crusted papules and nodules adjacent to the planum nasale in a Bernese Mountain Dog.

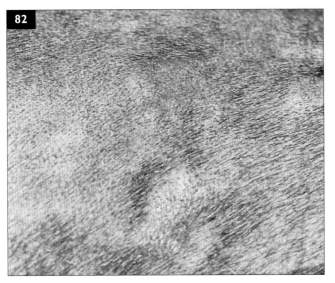

82 Cutaneous histiocytosis. Three poorly defined erythematous nodules. (Illustration courtesy of D.W. Scott)

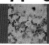

Cuterebra spp. Infestation

DEFINITION
A nodular lesion of the skin due to the presence of *Cuterebra* spp. larvae.

ETIOLOGY AND PATHOGENESIS
Adult *Cuterebra* spp. flies are large, resemble a bumble bee, and neither feed nor bite. Females lay their eggs along rabbit runs and near rodent burrows. If a host brushes up against these eggs, they hatch instantaneously and the first-stage larvae crawl into the host's fur[1,2]. From here they enter the host through natural body openings. Migration occurs to the skin where the third stage becomes clinically noticeable in the subcutaneous tissue[1,2]. Larvae may also undergo aberrant migrations in the brain, pharynx, nostrils, and eyelids[2-4].

CLINICAL FEATURES
Lesions are generally noted in late summer or autumn as 1–2 cm (0.4–0.8 in) nodules located over the head, neck, and trunk (**83**). A fistula develops from which the larva eventually escapes.

DIFFERENTIAL DIAGNOSES
- Dracunculiasis
- Cutaneous neoplasia
- Bacterial or fungal granuloma
- Deep mycotic infections
- Panniculitis
- Foreign body granuloma
- Infected wound

DIAGNOSTIC TESTS
Opening a fistula reveals the 2.5–4.5 cm (1.0–1.8 in) dark brown to black, heavily-spined larva.

MANAGEMENT
Removal of the larva through the enlarged fistula. If not removed intact, parts of the larva left in the cavity may result in allergic or irritant reactions[1].

KEY POINT
- A rare dermatosis.

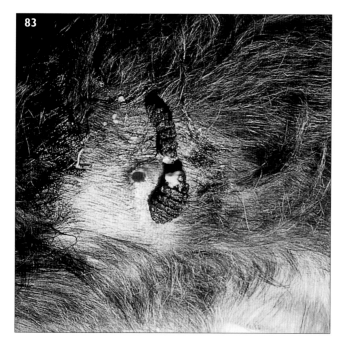

83 Cuterebriasis. A fistulated nodule in the groin of a puppy with the extracted larva adjacent to the lesion.

Dracunculiasis

DEFINITION
Dracunculiasis is a nodular dermatosis produced by the development of *Dracunculus* spp. adults in the subcutaneous tissue.

ETIOLOGY AND PATHOGENESIS
Dracunculus medinensis (guinea worm) has been reported in humans, dogs, cats, horses, cattle, and other animals in Africa and Asia[1,2]. *Dracunculus insignis* is a parasite of dogs, raccoons, mink, fox, otter, and skunks of North America[2]. The intermediate hosts are small crustacean copepods which inhabit bodies of fresh water world wide[2]. The copepods ingest first-stage larvae that have been released into water. In the copepods the larvae molt twice over a 12–14 day interval to become the infective third-stage larvae. Animals become infected when drinking water that contains these copepods. Third-stage larvae are released in the process of gastric digestion and migrate to the subcutaneous tissue where adults develop in 8–12 months.

CLINICAL FEATURES
Animals are presented with single or multiple nodules that either develop draining fistulae or ul-cerate. Urticaria, pruritus, pain, inflammation and, occasionally, pyrexia may be noted[1]. Lesions are generally located on the limbs, head, or abdomen.

DIFFERENTIAL DIAGNOSES
- *Cuterebra* spp. infestation
- Infected wound
- Foreign body
- Cutaneous neoplasia
- Deep mycotic infection
- Panniculitis

DIAGNOSTIC TESTS
Impression smears of discharge from the fistulae or ulcers may reveal the rhabdiform first-stage larvae, which are between 500 and 760 μm in length. Enlarging and exploring the fistulae may allow demonstration of the adult worms (**84**).

MANAGEMENT
The treatment of choice is surgical excision and removal of the adult worm.

KEY POINT
- May be relatively common in some regions but is generally rare.

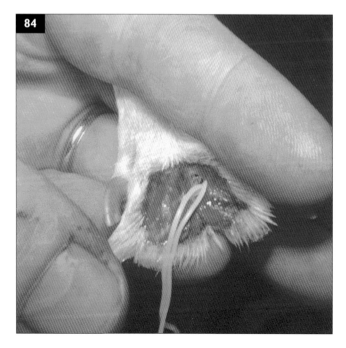

84 Dracunculiasis. A lesion in the interdigital region of a dog with the adult worm clearly visible.

Blastomycosis

DEFINITION
Blastomycosis occurs as a consequence of infection by *Blastomyces dermatidis*.

ETIOLOGY AND PATHOGENESIS
Cutaneous lesions usually occur as a consequence of hematologic spread after inhalation of spores[1,2]. Thus most cases have internal granulomas in addition to cutaneous lesions. However, primary cutaneous infection may occur after inoculation of wounds[1,2]. Large, adult, entire male hunting and sporting dogs are predisposed to blastomycosis[3], presumably because of the risk of traumatic inoculation.

CLINICAL FEATURES
Most clinical signs are slow to develop with little signs of pain, except perhaps lameness. The clinical signs will vary according to the degree of systemic involvement and the organs affected. Wide dissemination to lymph nodes, skin, oral and nasal mucosae, GI tract, bones, and CNS may be seen in a small number of animals[1,2], and these might be expected to show weight loss, anorexia, and lethargy in addition to signs referable to specific organ involvement. The cutaneous signs include subcutaneous nodules and masses, draining tracts, and recurrent abscessation (**85**)[1,2].

DIFFERENTIAL DIAGNOSES
- Penetrating foreign body
- Demodicosis
- Panniculitis
- Feline leprosy and atypical mycobacterial infection
- Nocardiosis
- Subcutaneous mycoses
- Cuterebriasis or dracunculiasis
- Cutaneous neoplasia

DIAGNOSTIC TESTS
The diagnosis of the condition is usually made by cytologic examination of exudates and aspirates which reveal 5–20 µm refractile double-walled, broad-based budding yeast (**86**), by histopathologic examination of excised tissues, and by serologic methods[1,2], although diagnosis by serologic means alone is not recommended.

MANAGEMENT
Systemic mycoses require systemic medication and treatment may be necessary for several months. Amphotericin B, alone or in combination with 5-fluorocytosine or with ketoconazole, has been recommended[1,2,4]. Amphotericin B is nephrotoxic and 5-fluorocytosine is a bone marrow depressant, and clinicians considering the use of these agents should read the detailed references. Currently, the treatment of choice is itraconazole (10 mg/kg PO q 24 h). The treatment should be continued 30 days beyond clinical and radiologic resolution of the lesions.

KEY POINT
- If you diagnose this disease, be sure to ensure that there are no systemic lesions – do not treat it as just a skin disease.

Blastomycosis

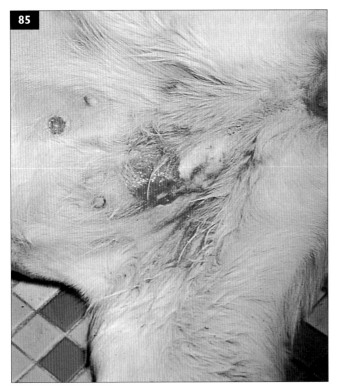

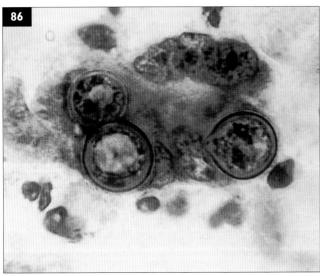

85, 86 Blastomycosis. A discharging sinus and nodular lesion in the groin of a Labrador Retriever due to blastomycosis (**85**); a photomicrograph demonstrating the refractile, spheroid shape of *Blastomyces* spp. (**86**).

Phaeohyphomycosis

DEFINITION
Phaeohyphomycoses are infections caused by de-matiaceus (darkly pigmented) fungi[1].

ETIOLOGY AND PATHOGENESIS
Phaeohyphomycoses are ubiquitous sapro-phytes. Examples of dematiaceus fungi re-ported to cause dermatologic disease in ani-mals (usually cats) include *Alternaria alter-nata*[2], *Curvularia* spp.[3], *Drechslera spicifera*[4], and *Exophiala spinifera*[3]. Subcutaneous infec-tion results from traumatic implantation and local infection. Dissemination from the site of inoculation is rare[3]. Granulomatous inflam-mation ensues and nodules, ulcerative or fis-tulous lesions, may develop[2,4].

CLINICAL FEATURES
Animals present with painless swellings or dis-charging tracts, typically on the feet (**87**), al-though the head and trunk may be affected. There may be local lymphadenopathy, but ani-mals are not usually pyrexic. The lesions are re-fractory to systemic antibacterial therapy.

DIFFERENTIAL DIAGNOSES
- Abscess following a bite wound
- Staphylococcal furunculosis
- Cutaneous neoplasia
- Sterile nodule pyogranuloma
- Arthropod-bite granuloma
- Blastomycosis
- Nocardiosis

DIAGNOSTIC TESTS
Microscopic examination of 10% potassium hy-droxide preparations from exudate or affected tissue will reveal darkly pigmented, septate hy-phae (**88**), some of which display occasional bulbous distensions[5]. Fungal culture on appro-priate media will allow definitive diagnosis. Histopathologic examination of affected tissue will reveal a granulomatous response and may allow identification of hyphae, but definitive di-agnosis is not possible.

MANAGEMENT
Surgical excision of affected tissue is curative[5]. In areas where excision may be difficult, for ex-ample, the nasal region, systemic antifungal agents, such as ketoconazole, flucytosine, or amphotericin B, may be prescribed, although medical treatment has met with variable suc-cess[2,6]. *Drechslera spicifera* infection in a cat has been treated successfully by one of the authors (PJM) using itraconazole (10 mg/kg PO q 24 h) for 8 weeks.

KEY POINT
- An ubiquitous but rare infection.

Phaeohyphomycosis

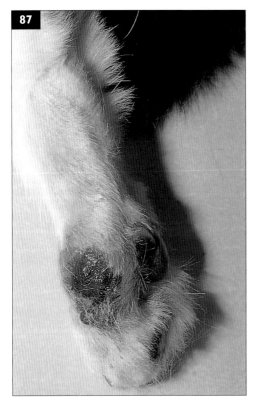

87, 88 Phaeohyphomycosis. A crusted nodule on the distal limb of a domestic shorthair cat (**87**); a photomicrograph demonstrating the dark-staining branching hyphae (**88**).

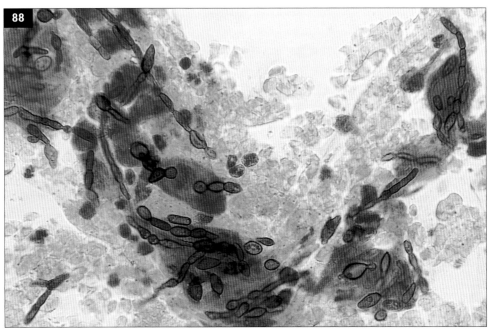

Ulcerative Dermatoses

GENERAL APPROACH TO ULCERATIVE DERMATOSES
1 Ulceration may be caused by infectious agents – avoid the use of steroids.
2 Ulceration may represent neoplasia – biopsy if you are uncertain.
3 Immune-mediated disease is uncommon.

ZOONOTIC RISKS FROM ULCERATIVE LESIONS INCLUDE
• Feline cowpox infection
• Sporotrichosis

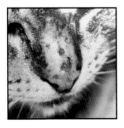
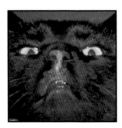
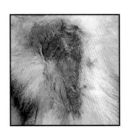
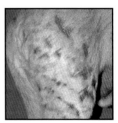

Feline Eosinophilic Granuloma Complex

DEFINITION
The eosinophilic granuloma complex comprises a group of conditions united by etiology and some histopathologic features.

ETIOLOGY AND PATHOGENESIS
The etiology of these dermatoses is unknown. Local, uncontrolled recruitment of eosinophils is thought to result in the release of potent inflammatory agents which, if allowed to accumulate, may initiate the local inflammation and collagen necrosis which is characteristic of some of these dermatoses[1]. Hypersensitivities, insect bites and stings, and bacterial infections may be associated with the occurrence of these lesions, and would account for the eosinophilia[2-4]. However, manifestations of the eosinophilic granuloma complex have been reported in specific, pathogen-free cats in which atopy and dietary hypersensitivity were ruled out[5] and no underlying cause established.

CLINICAL FEATURES
The eosinophilic granuloma complex can be classified on a number of characteristics but, on clinical presentation, three major variants are currently recognised. Cats may exhibit one or several manifestations of the complex at the same time. Some cats suffer a single episode, others exhibit recurrent lesions, while a few present with refractory lesions.

Eosinophilic plaques
These are well-circumscribed, ulcerated, moist lesions typically found on the ventral abdomen, medial thighs, or caudal trunk. There is no breed or sex incidence, although young cats may be predisposed. Adjacent lesions may coalesce, presenting as very large, plaque-like areas which appear highly pruritic (**89**).

Indolent ulcers
These are usually found on the upper lips (**90**), although they may occur on the trunk. Females are predisposed, but there is no age or breed predilection. The lesions are well-demarcated, erosive, firm, crateriform, and non-pruritic.

Collagenolytic granulomas
These are typically seen on young, female cats. Elongated, cord-like, greyish-pink, non-pruritic lesions may be seen, particularly along the caudal aspect of the hindlimb (**91**). Nodular variants may be seen on the head, pinnae, or rostral aspect of the mandible ('fat chin') (**92**).

Mosquito bite hypersensitivity
A seasonal pyrexic syndrome characterised by erosive papules on the nose and pinnae, erosive granulomas on the trunk, and hyperkeratotic footpads, which appeared to be due to mosquito bites, has been described[2,5] (**93**).

DIFFERENTIAL DIAGNOSES
- Trauma
- Cutaneous neoplasia
- Rodent or cat bites
- Feline cowpox infection
- Dietary intolerance
- Atopy

DIAGNOSTIC TESTS
Clinical history and examination will narrow the differentials. Skin scrapes and fungal cultures should be performed. Histopathologic examination of biopsy samples is usually diagnostic.

MANAGEMENT
Many cases of eosinophilic plaque are so acute that symptomatic treatment with systemic prednisolone (2 mg/kg PO q 12 h) is indicated to induce remission. Some cases appear to require adjunctive systemic antibacterial treatment, such as potentiated sulfonamides or cephalexin, to induce remission, and a few appear to respond to antibacterial agents alone[3]. Attempts to identify an underlying cause may be undertaken in cats exhibiting recurrent eosinophilic plaque or in chronic, minimally pruritic cases, such as indolent ulcer or collagenolytic granuloma. Dietary screening for food intolerance, intradermal skin testing, and screening for insect bite may all be necessary if a definitive diagnosis is required.

If a definitive diagnosis is made, then specific management may be instituted[6]. Unfortunately, many cases remain idiopathic and require symptomatic therapy.

KEY POINT
- Clinically well-recognized but poorly understood.
- Most cases require symptomatic treatment.

Feline Eosinophilic Granuloma Complex

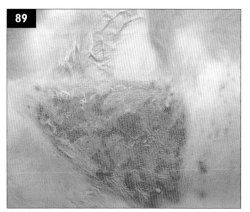

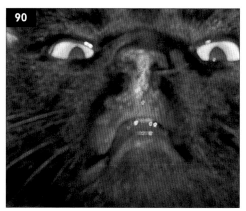

89   Eosinophilic plaque on the ventral abdomen of a cat.

90   Indolent (rodent) ulcer on the upper lip of a shorthair cat.

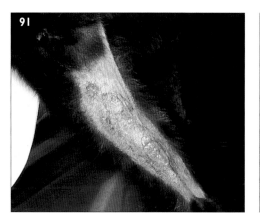

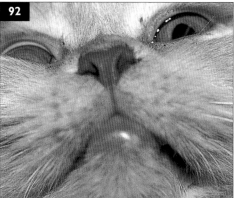

91, 92   Collagenolytic (eosinophilic) granulomas. The linear form (**91**) and the localized form on the mandible of a cat (**92**).

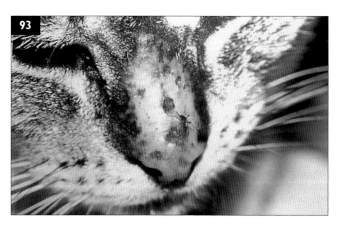

93   Feline mosquito bite hypersensitivity. (Illustration courtesy of Dr K. Mason)

German Shepherd Dog Pyoderma

DEFINITION
German Shepherd Dog pyoderma (GSP) is an idiopathic, chronic, recurrent deep pyoderma of pure-bred and cross-bred German Shepherd Dogs.

ETIOLOGY AND PATHOGENESIS
GSP is thought to be a distinct condition separate from pyoderma occurring secondary to flea bite hypersensitivity, atopic dermatitis, adverse reaction to food, demodicosis, or hypothyroidism[1-3]. *Staphylococcus intermedius* is the most commonly isolated organism. Although immunologic abnormalities have been suggested as predisposing factors, chemotaxis and killing capacities of neutrophilic leukocytes, and complement levels are normal. No specific immunoglobulin or complement deposits have been found in affected skin, and changes in serum immunoglobulin levels are non-specific[2]. Affected animals are also not hypersensitive to staphylococcal antigens[3]. However, the skin of affected dogs contains decreased numbers of T lymphocytes, and imbalance between CD4 and CD8 peripheral blood lymphocyte subpopulations has been demonstrated. Furthermore, analysis of B cell populations has shown a decrease in the level of CD21 cells, suggesting that the immunologic imbalance may be associated with defective helper cells[4].

CLINICAL FEATURES
GSP occurs most commonly in middle-aged (5–7-year-old) animals, but may be seen in animals of any age. There appears to be no sex predisposition. Lesions generally start over the lateral thighs (**94, 95**) and dorsal lumbosacral areas, but any area of the body may be affected. Typical lesions include the development of erythematous to violaceous papules, pustules, epidermal collarettes, furuncles, erosions, ulcers, crusts, and sinuses (**96**), which drain a hemopurulent material. Varying degrees of alopecia and hyperpigmentation may be noted and the peripheral lymph nodes are generally enlarged. Lesions may be pruritic and/or painful.

DIFFERENTIAL DIAGNOSES
- Demodicosis
- Pyoderma secondary to other diseases
- Cutaneous infections secondary to systemic mycosis
- Cutaneous infections of subcutaneous or opportunistic fungi or algae
- Opportunistic mycobacterial infection
- Pythiosis
- Neoplasia

DIAGNOSTIC TESTS
History and clinical findings are not pathognomonic. Microscopic examination of multiple skin scrapings is mandatory. Histopathologic examination of biopsy samples is diagnostic of deep pyoderma but may not rule out underlying diseases such as endocrinopathy. Bacterial culture and sensitivity testing is mandatory.

MANAGEMENT
Affected animals fall into one of two groups: those which respond completely to a single (albeit prolonged) course of systemic antibacterial agents, and those which require chronic therapy to maintain remission.

It is not possible to predict into which group an individual might fall. Therefore all cases should be subject to the same approach:

1 Submit swabs for bacterial culture and sensitivity testing.
2 Start therapy with bacteriocidal antibacterial agents, such as trimethroprim potentiated sulfonamide (30 mg/kg PO q 12 h) or cephalexin (25 mg/kg PO q 12 h) pending laboratory results.
3 Reassess after 3 weeks in the light of laboratory results (assuming resistance is not predicted).
4 Adjust the therapy if the clinical response is poor and laboratory results suggest resistance.
5 Continue therapy until *all* lesions have resolved (anticipate 4–12 weeks) and add a further 2 weeks.
6 Stop therapy.
7 Assess for relapse.
8 Those that relapse require reassessment for internal disease and further antibacterial treatment. Further relapse may indicate the need for long-term alternate day therapy (full dose antibacterial treatment but every 48 hours) or 2 days therapy per week, or 7 days on, 7 days off treatment.

KEY POINTS
- Poorly understood.
- About 50% of cases will require long-term antibacterial therapy.

German Shepherd Dog Pyoderma

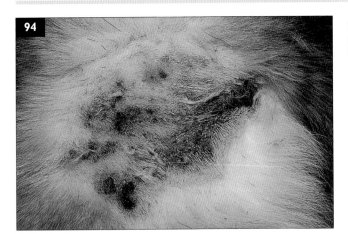

94, 95 Pyoderma ulcers and sinus formation in the groin of a German Shepherd Dog.

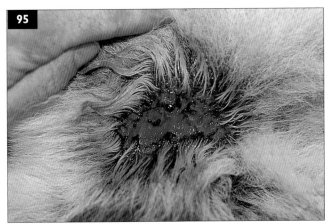

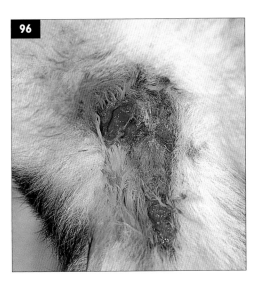

96 Deep pyoderma. A close up of the lateral elbow in a German Shepherd Dog demonstrating a poorly defined, crusted area of ulceration.

Calcinosis Cutis

DEFINITION
Calcinosis cutis results from dystrophic mineralization of the dermal and adnexal elastin and collagen fibres, and is virtually pathognomonic for hyperadrenocorticism[1].

ETIOLOGY AND PATHOGENESIS
Calcinosis cutis has not been reported in the cat. The mechanism which results in the deposition of soluble calcium and phosphate ions onto the collagen and elastin matrix is not known. A chronic, granulomatous, inflammatory response is commonly induced by the mineralization[1]. Calcinosis cutis is more commonly associated with iatrogenic hyperadrenocorticism rather than the naturally occurring disease[2]. The reason for this is not known. Calcinosis cutis occurs in a variable proportion of cases, from 1.7–40%[3,4], presumably reflecting the various proportion of iatrogenic to naturally occurring disease in case series.

CLINICAL FEATURES
Calcinosis cutis usually is found on the dorsum or in the axillae or groins[4]. Dogs typically present with erosive, crusted, ulcerated, and gritty-feeling patches of erythema and erythematous or crusted papules (**97, 98**). Close examination may reveal a pale accumulation of mineral within intact lesions. The affected areas are often secondarily infected, particularly if mineral is being slowly eliminated through the skin, and these cases are usually extremely pruritic, failing to respond to both systemic antibacterial or glucocorticoid therapy.

DIFFERENTIAL DIAGNOSES
- Pyotraumatic dermatosis
- Superficial pyoderma
- Other causes of dystrophic or metastatic calcification
- Irritant dermatitis
- Cutaneous neoplasia

DIAGNOSTIC TESTS
The degree of pruritus is often the first indication that these lesions are not simply pyoderma. Many, but not all, dogs will have other signs suggestive of internal disease, such as pu/pd, muscle wasting, and exercise intolerance, which will raise suspicion of hyperadrenocorticism. Close examination of the lesions, and palpating them, will often allow an appreciation of mineralization. This is even more apparent when skin scrapes and biopsy samples are taken. Histopathologic examination of biopsy samples may be necessary to provide a definitive diagnosis. Once calcinosis cutis is identified, then a search for the underlying cause should be made.

MANAGEMENT
Identify and attend to the underlying cause of the mineralization. Complete resolution is to be anticipated provided the underlying problem is treatable.

KEY POINT
- The pruritus associated with this dermatosis may be refractory to steroid therapy.

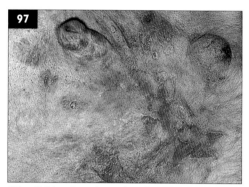

97 Calcinosis cutis causing ulceration, crusting, and papules in the groin and medial thighs of a dog with iatrogenic hyperadrenocorticism.

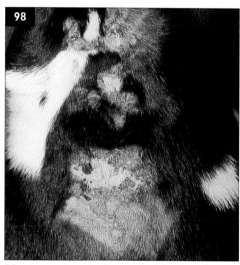

98 Large, alopecic plaque of calcinosis cutis on the dorsal neck of a French Bulldog.

Decubital Ulcers

DEFINITION
Decubital ulcers (pressure sores) occur mainly over bony prominences because of continual localized pressure to the skin.

ETIOLOGY AND PATHOGENESIS
Animals which are recumbent due to neurologic deficits or musculoskeletal problems are predisposed. Compression of the skin and subcutaneous tissue collapses blood vessels, resulting in ischemia, necrosis, and subsequent ulceration. Laceration, friction, burns from heating pads, irritation from urine or fecal material, malnutrition secondary to inadequate diet, anemia, or hypoproteinemia may also be contributing factors[1].

CLINICAL FEATURES
The initial clinical finding is hyperemia. Tissue necrosis and ulceration follow if the pressure is not relieved. Lesions most frequently occur in skin overlying the scapular acromion, lateral epicondyle of the humerus, tuber ischii, tuber coxae, trochanter major of the femur, lateral condyle of the tibia (99) and the lateral sides of the fifth digits of the forelimbs and hindlimbs. Secondary bacterial infection can lead to undermining of the skin beyond the ulcer edges. Osteomyelitis can develop in bone underlying the ulcer.

DIFFERENTIAL DIAGNOSES
• Cutaneous neoplasia
• Pyoderma
• Deep mycotic infection

DIAGNOSTIC TESTS
Diagnosis is based on clinical findings and histopathologic examination of biopsy samples.

MANAGEMENT
Ideally, decubital ulcers should be prevented by turning the recumbent animal frequently (every 2 hours) and providing soft bedding, such as a water mattress. Providing adequate nutrition and keeping the skin clean, via twice daily bathing or whirlpool baths, is also important, particularly in the long-term hospitalized patient. Particular attention should be paid to protecting the skin from contact with urine by using a cage rack and applying petrolatum to areas of skin that urine is likely to contact[2]. Once ulcers have developed, they may be managed by either non-surgical or surgical means. Non-surgical management consists of wound lavage and topical antibacterial therapy[2].

Doughnut bandages can be placed over the ulcer to avoid direct pressure on the wound. Surgical treatment is accomplished by débridement of necrotic and infected tissue, and wound closure to heal by primary intention[1]. The preventive measures previously mentioned must be strictly adhered to following surgery.

KEY POINT
• Be aware that decubital ulcers can occur in hospitalized patients.

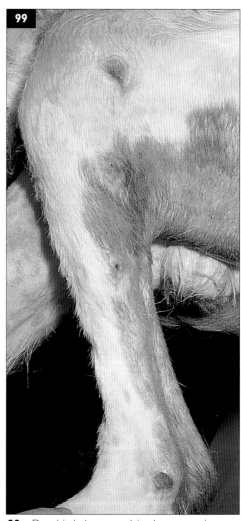

99 Decubital ulcers overlying bony prominences on the lateral stifle and hock.

Squamous Cell Carcinoma

DEFINITION
A relatively common, malignant neoplasm of dogs and cats arising from the epidermal squames.

ETIOLOGY AND PATHOGENESIS
There is little doubt that long-term exposure to high levels of actinic radiation is a major factor in the development of squamous cell carcinoma, particularly in lightly pigmented skin[1,2]. Ultraviolet B radiation has the capacity to be oncogenic and locally immunosuppressive, reducing the effectiveness of local immune surveillance[1-3]. Undoubtedly, there are other factors involved in the etiology of cases not directly attributable to actinic radiation. Squamous cell carcinomas arise in the epidermis, are locally invasive, and have a low metastatic potential[4].

CLINICAL FEATURES
Squamous cell carcinomas are relatively common in both dogs and cats, and tend to occur in older animals. Dalmatians, Bull Terriers, and Boxers and white-haired cats are predisposed[5,6]. In dogs the tumors tend to occur on the trunk and limbs (**100**), rather than on the head[4,5], whereas in cats the head, and most especially the pinnae (**101**), are predisposed sites[6,7]. Clinically, the tumors have two presentations in the dog: proliferative, vegetative, often ulcerated on the surface; and, less commonly, an erosive ulcerating form[4] (**102**). Those that occur on the foot have a much more aggressive nature and tend to metastasize early[4,7] (**103**). Black Standard Poodles are also predisposed to develop squamous cell carcinomas of the digits, at the junction of the skin and nail. More than one toe on several feet may be involved.

DIFFERENTIAL DIAGNOSES
- Traumatic injury
- Localized pyoderma
- Dermatophytosis
- Subcutaneous fungal infections
- Other cutaneous neoplasms

DIAGNOSTIC TESTS
Impression smears are of little value due to the presence of a surface inflammatory exudate[8]. A scraped sample can be stained and may reveal changes sufficient to make a tentative diagnosis of squamous cell carcinoma[8], but histologic examination of biopsy tissue or excision samples is necessary to obtain a definitive diagnosis and to grade the tumor.

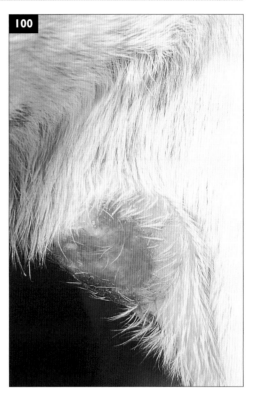

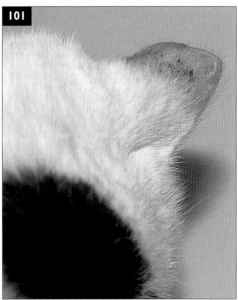

100, 101 Squamous cell carcinoma on the precrural fold of a dog (**100**) and the pinna of a cat (**101**).

Squamous Cell Carcinoma

MANAGEMENT

Surgical excision of isolated lesions is usually curative[4] except for the digital lesions, which show a tendency to metastasize to the local lymph node and then to the lung fields[4,7]. Problems may be encountered in performing adequate surgical resection of nasal and facial lesions, particularly in cats. A photodynamic therapy has recently been described which appears to offer good prospects for poor surgical candidates[9].

KEY POINT

- Non-responsive ulceration should be biopsed.

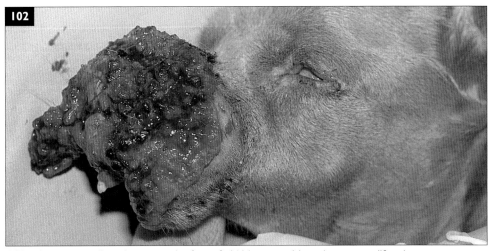

102   Squamous cell carcinoma on the face of a Weimaraner. Note the very proliferative nature of this neoplasm.

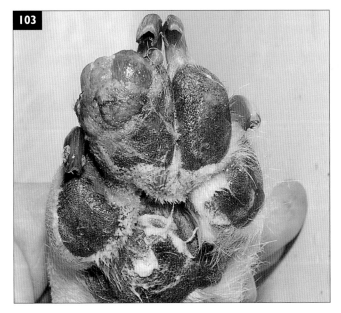

103   Ulcerated nodule of squamous cell carcinoma on the foot.

Epidermal Metabolic Necrosis

(Diabetic Dermatopathy, Hepatocutaneous Syndrome, Necrolytic Migratory Erythema, Superficial Necrolytic Dermatitis)

DEFINITION

Epidermal metabolic necrosis is an uncommon skin disorder associated with metabolic diseases such as vascular hepatopathy, diabetes mellitus, and glucagon-secreting pancreatic tumor (glucagonoma).

ETIOLOGY AND PATHOGENESIS

The syndrome in humans is generally associated with hyperglucagonemia resulting from a glucagon-secreting pancreatic islet cell tumor[1–3]. Although cases of epidermal metabolic necrosis due to glucagon-producing pancreatic tumors have been reported in the dog, the majority of cases do not have a pancreatic neoplasm. Abnormalities of the liver characterized by a moderate to severe vacuolation of hepatocytes, parenchymal collapse, and nodular regeneration are present in most cases[1,2]. These findings support an underlying metabolic/hormonal dysfunction rather than primary liver disease[1]. The exact pathomechanisms leading to the liver changes are not known. One theory is that increased plasma glucagon does play a role, even though levels are normal in most dogs in which they have been evaluated[1]. Explanations for this include a lack of sensitivity or specificity of the assay, poor correlation of peripheral plasma glucagon concentrations with increased pancreatic glucagon secretion, or due to a non-immunoreactive enteric form of glucagon[1]. A coexisting hyperglycemia and diabetes mellitus is noted in a significant number of dogs. As these findings tend to occur after the development of liver and cutaneous disease, they are not thought to be involved in the pathogenesis[1]. Most dogs have a marked decrease in the concentrations of plasma amino acids, which may lead to protein depletion of the epidermis resulting in necrolysis[1].

CLINICAL FEATURES

Epidermal metabolic necrosis is a disease of older dogs, and cutaneous changes generally precede the recognition of systemic illness. No breed or sex predisposition has been noted[1–3]. Some dogs may have a history of weight loss[2]. Hyperkeratosis, crusting, and cracking of the digital pads is the most consistent clinical finding[1,2]. Erythema, erosion, ulceration, and crusting (**104–106**) occur on the muzzle, mucocutaneous junctions, ears, pressure points (elbows, hocks, hips, and stifles), genitalia, abdomen, and axillae[1–3]. Ulcerations of the oral cavity can occur in some cases[1,2].

DIFFERENTIAL DIAGNOSES

- Pemphigus foliaceus
- Systemic lupus erythematosus
- Zinc responsive dermatosis
- Superficial bacterial or fungal infections
- Epitheliotropic lymphoma

DIAGNOSTIC TESTS

Microscopic examination of skin biopsies from erythematous plaques with mild-to-moderate adherent crusts show intracellular edema in the mid-epidermis[4]. Plasma amino acids may be low; serum alkaline phosphatase and serum alanine aminotransferase may be high. Blood glucose may be high and plasma glucagon may be elevated (if a glucagonoma is present), otherwise results are variable. Liver biopsy usually reveals evidence of chronic liver disease.

MANAGEMENT

If a glucagonoma is diagnosed, surgical removal would be the treatment of choice. Epidermal metabolic necrosis due to other causes is associated with serious internal disease and the prognosis is poor with most dogs dying or being euthanased within 5 months after the development of cutaneous lesions[2]. Administration of egg yolks as a dietary supplementation has been reported to result in partial to complete remission of cutaneous lesions in some dogs[1].

KEY POINT

- History and clinical signs are usually enough to suggest the diagnosis, but histopathologic examination of biopsy sample is mandatory.

Epidermal Metabolic Necrosis

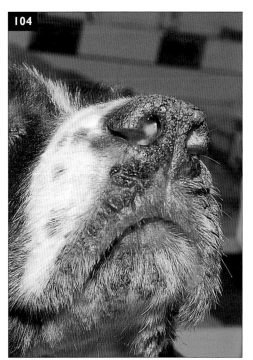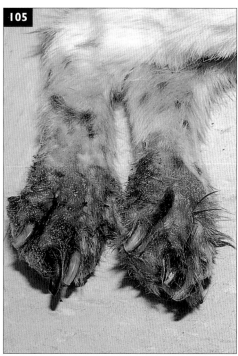

104, 105 Epidermal metabolic necrosis. Erythema, erosions, crust, and alopecia on the face (**104**) and distal limbs (**105**) of a Springer Spaniel. (Illustrations courtesy of S. Torres.)

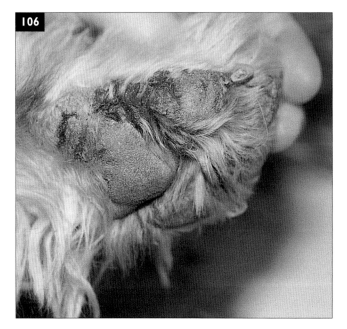

106 Epidermal metabolic necrosis. Pedal lesions characterized by severe crusting of the footpads.

Discoid Lupus Erythematosus

DEFINITION
Discoid lupus erythematosus is an uncommon dermatosis in which localized, photoaggravated skin lesions occur.

ETIOLOGY AND PATHOGENESIS
The etiology of discoid lupus erythematosus is unclear. It has been proposed that, in genetically predisposed, susceptible individuals, actinic radiation induces an inflammatory cascade which damages dermal and epidermal components, provoking a localized, chronic, immune-mediated reaction[1]. The inflammation results in erythema, scale, crusting, and depigmentation[2].

CLINICAL FEATURES
There is no age predilection, but females and some breeds, such as Shetland Sheepdogs, Rough Collies, German Shepherd Dogs, and Siberian Huskies, are predisposed[3,4]. Discoid lupus erythematosus is very rare in cats[5]. The most common site for lesions is the nose and planum nasale[2,3] (107, 108). The lips, periorbital regions, and pinnae are also affected in some cases[2,3]. Interestingly, the pinnae are more commonly affected in cats[5]. Rarely, the sheath and digits exhibit lesions[3]. Lesions are usually alopecic and erythematous and display varying degrees of depigmentation. In active lesions there may be a fine scale and even small, adherent crusts

DIFFERENTIAL DIAGNOSES
• Actinic dermatitis
• Dermatophytosis
• Nasal pyoderma
• Demodicosis
• Pemphigus complex
• Drug eruption
• Systemic lupus erythematosus
• Uveodermatologic syndrome

DIAGNOSTIC TESTS
Clinical history and examination will demonstrate that the lesions are localized and that there are no systemic signs[3]. The cardinal observation in narrowing the huge differential diagnosis is whether the lesion affects the planum nasale or not. *It is very unusual for dermatoses other than immune-mediated diseases to affect the planum nasale*: they may affect haired skin adjacent but they do not cross the border. Histopathologic examination of biopsy samples is usually diagnostic[3,4] and immunofluorescence is rarely necessary. Antinuclear antibody tests are nearly always negative[3,4].

MANAGEMENT
Systemic prednisolone will induce remission, and low dose alternate day prednisolone will keep most animals in remission[3,4]. Topical sun-blocking creams and sun avoidance will help to keep the dose as low as possible. Some cases may be kept in remission with topical hydrocortisone cream, or more powerful topical glucocorticoids, and sun blocker alone. Megadoses of vitamin E (400–800 IU daily) were reported as useful in a proportion of cases, although it does have a 1–2 month lag phase[3]. Recently, the combination of tetracycline and niacinamide (250 mg of each drug PO q 8 h in dogs under 10 kg and 500 mg of each PO q 8 h in dogs over 10 kg) was reported as a useful alternative to systemic prednisolone[6].

KEY POINTS
• The most common immune-mediated dermatosis.
• Try to avoid inducing Cushingoid changes for what is usually a localized problem.

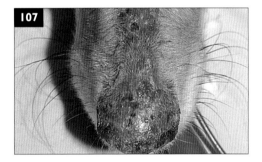

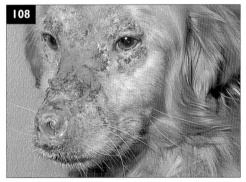

107, 108 Discoid lupus erythematosus. Lesions on the rostral face (**107**); more extensive lesions on the face (**108**).

Feline Cowpox Infection

DEFINITION
Feline cowpox infection is due to infection with a virus of the Orthopox genus, indistinguishable from cowpox virus.

ETIOLOGY AND PATHOGENESIS
It is currently believed that the virus exists within a reservoir population of small, wild mammals[1]. Cats are infected, presumably by bite wounds, and there is local multiplication at the site of inoculation. Viremia then occurs with multiple, generalized papulocrustous lesions appearing over the subsequent 7–10 days. These lesions gradually resolve and the cats usually make a complete recovery.

CLINICAL FEATURES
There is no breed, age, or sex predisposition, but hunting cats are most likely to be affected[1]. There is a sharp increase in cases in the late summer and autumn period. The primary lesion, a papulovesicle, is usually on the head or forelimb and may become secondarily infected. Multiple, usually more than ten, secondary lesions follow, most occurring on the head and trunk[1,2]. These secondary lesions begin as small, firm papules which enlarge to become flattened, crusted, alopecic areas between 0.5 and 2.0 cm (0.2 and 0.8 in) in diameter (109). Occasionally, the secondary lesions are erythematous and exudative in nature[1,2]. The lesions heal in about 4 weeks and gradually become haired again. Unless treated with systemic glucocorticoids, the cats make a complete recovery and are rarely ill[3]. Those treated with immunosuppressive agents, or cats with FeLV or FIV infection, tend to get more severe secondary lesions accompanied by bacterial infection and, occasionally, respiratory disease[1,3,4].

DIFFERENTIAL DIAGNOSES
- Cat bite abscess
- Flea bite hypersensitivity
- Dermatophytosis
- Superficial pyoderma

DIAGNOSTIC TESTS
Clinical history and local knowledge may suggest the diagnosis, but definitive diagnosis depends on histopathologic examination of biopsy samples, serology, electron microscopy, or virus isolation[3,5].

MANAGEMENT
Once the lesions are identified, then broad-spectrum antibacterial cover may be indicated. Supportive care may be required by the occasional cat, but most make a steady recovery provided that glucocorticoids are not administered.

KEY POINTS
- Do not give steroids to these cats.
- Potentially zoonotic.

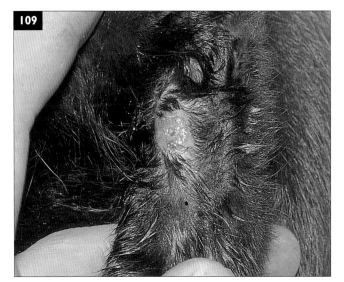

109 Erythematous erosion due to feline cowpox infection.

Drug Eruption

DEFINITION
Drug eruption is a rare diagnosis in which pleomorphic cutaneous lesions, with or without systemic signs, occur as a result of exposure to a chemical compound.

ETIOLOGY AND PATHOGENESIS
Cutaneous drug eruptions may reflect immunologic or non-immunologic reactions[1]. The animal may become sensitized to, or react to, a medication, preservative, or even the dye within a tablet. Reaction may occur to systemic or topical medications. Most drug eruptions result in extensive lesions and are unpredictable in nature. Rarely, a repeatable, localized reaction may be noted (fixed drug eruption)[2].

CLINICAL FEATURES
There is no breed, age, or sex predisposition to cutaneous drug eruption, although Doberman Pinschers appear predisposed to sulfonamide induced polyarthritis[4]. Certain drugs, particularly penicillins and sulfonamides[3], appear to be commonly implicated, (perhaps reflecting simply the volume of use), but it should be remembered that any drug has the capacity to induce a drug eruption. Clinical signs vary from urticaria and angioedema, erythematous macules (**110**) and papules or crusted vesicles (**111**) to exfoliative dermatitis or total epidermal necrosis[1,5-7](**112**).

DIFFERENTIAL DIAGNOSES
• Superficial bacterial infections
• Irritant or contact dermatitis
• Pemphigus group
• Systemic lupus erythematosus
• Cutaneous neoplasia

DIAGNOSTIC TESTS
Drug eruption may be tentatively diagnosed on the basis of known exposure to the drug, compatible clinical signs, the presence of compatible histologic features on examination of biopsy samples, lack of reaction to any concurrently administered drugs, and a resolution of the signs after withdrawal of the drug[1]. Definitive diagnosis is only possible with provocative exposure and this is inadvisable, since readministration may precipitate systemic or generalized signs.

MANAGEMENT
Removal of the offending agent and appropriate supportive therapy is sufficient in cases exhibiting only moderate signs of reaction. Some cases, such as those with extensive open skin lesions or toxic epidermal necrolysis, will require aggressive fluid therapy and anti-shock regimes. Areas with necrotic skin should be treated with topical silver sulfadiazine ointment. The value of systemic glucocorticoids is controversial[1], since most of the damage is irreversible and ongoing at the point of diagnosis. Clinicians should also bear in mind that drug reactions can occur to steroid medications. The patient's records should be flagged to indicate sensitivity to relevant drugs.

KEY POINTS
• Drug eruption is probably underrecognized.
• Do not rechallenge to confirm your diagnosis.

Drug Eruption

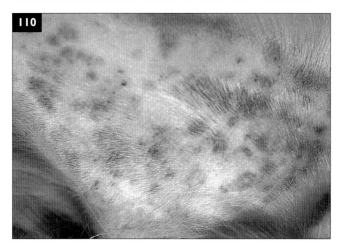

110 Erythematous cutaneous macules and patches following Imodium treatment.

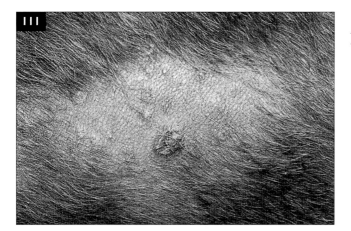

111 Fixed drug eruption on the lateral flank of an Airedale Terrier.

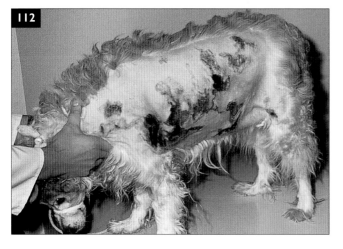

112 Toxic epidermal necrolysis secondary to drug eruption.

Nocardiosis

DEFINITION
Nocardiosis is a pyogranulomatous infection due to *Nocardia* spp. organisms.

ETIOLOGY AND PATHOGENESIS
Nocardia spp. are saprophytic aerobic bacteria that enter the body through soil contamination of wounds, inhalation, or ingestion[1,2]. Plant awns may also serve as a means to introduce the organism into tissues. Immunosuppression may predispose animals to infection. Species isolated from lesions of dogs and cats include *N. asteroides*, *N. brasileinsis*, and *N. caviae*[1]. All have a world-wide distribution, except *N. brasileinsis*, which is confined to Mexico, Central America, and South America[1]. *Nocardia asteroides* is the species most often associated with lesions in the dog and cat

CLINICAL FEATURES
Cutaneous infection typically occurs after a wound is contaminated with soil. Draining fistulous tracts, ulcers, abscesses, and subcutaneous nodules are the most common clinical findings (**113, 114**). Additional signs of fever, weakness, lethargy, pyothorax, and dyspnea may develop. Discharge from tracts, ulcers, and abscesses can vary from serosanguineous to sanguinopurulent, and is often described as 'tomato sauce colored'. *Nocardia* spp. may also produce oral lesions.

DIFFERENTIAL DIAGNOSES
- Deep pyoderma
- Pyoderma secondary to other diseases
- Cutaneous infections of systemic fungi
- Cutaneous infections of opportunistic fungi or algae
- Opportunistic mycobacterium infection
- Penetrating foreign bodies

DIAGNOSTIC TESTS
A tentative diagnosis can be made by finding gram-positive, partially acid-fast, branching, filamentous rods on either impression smears or histopathologic examination of biopsy material. Definitive diagnosis is made by culture, which may be difficult[1]. Laboratories to which the samples are submitted should be notified that *Nocardia* spp. have been included in the differential diagnosis, since specialized culture is required.

MANAGEMENT
Drainage should be established for all lesions. The *in vitro* susceptibility of *Nocardia* spp. does not necessarily predict *in vivo* efficacy[1]. Sulfadi-

azine (80 mg/kg PO q 8 h) is effective for a majority of cases. Alternatives include minocycline (5–25 mg/kg PO q 12 h), erythromycin (10 mg/kg PO q 8 h), clindamycin (11 mg/kg PO q 12 h), and ampicillin (20–40 mg/kg PO q 6 h). Amikacin (8–12 mg/kg IM or SC q 8 h) is also highly effective[1]. Treatment will generally take at least 6 weeks and should be continued 1 month beyond clinical cure. Owners should be warned that some cases will not respond and that relapses may occur.

KEY POINT
- Cats with non-responsive abscessation should be checked for FeLV infection and samples should be submitted for culture and sensitivity testing (both aerobic and anaerobic).

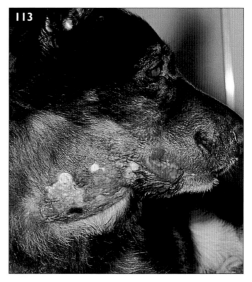

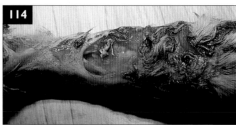

113, 114 Nocardiosis. Lesions on the ventral face and neck of a dog (**113**) and on the forelimb of a cat (**114**).

Plasma Cell Pododermatitis of Cats

DEFINITION
Plasma cell pododermatitis is a rare disorder of cats associated with plasma cell infiltration into one or more footpads[1].

ETIOLOGY AND PATHOGENESIS
The cause of the disease is not known, although the presence of elevated serum globulin concentrations, lymphocytosis, plasma cell involvement, and dermoepidermal immune complex deposition suggest an immune-mediated disorder[2,3]. The gradual accumulation of plasma cells and granulation tissue results in soft, poorly defined swelling of the affected pad. Ulceration and secondary infection of the protruding tissue usually follows.

CLINICAL FEATURES
There is no breed, age, or sex incidence. Usually only a single pad is affected, typically the central metacarpal or metacarpal pad[1]. Occasionally, a digital pad or several pads may be affected[1,2]. Initially, there is a soft, painless swelling of the affected pad (**115**), accompanied by hyperkeratotic, interlacing striae. A pale blue or violet discoloration may be apparent. If the pad ulcerates, a mound of hemorrhagic granulation tissue protrudes. There may be local lymphadenopathy but discomfort and pain are rare. Secondary infection may ensue in some cases[1] and, rarely, hemorrhage may be significant[2].

DIFFERENTIAL DIAGNOSES
The clinical presentation is almost unique. Other causes to consider include:

- Bacterial or fungal granuloma
- Collagenolytic granuloma
- Squamous cell carcinoma
- Feline herpes virus or calicivirus respiratory infection

DIAGNOSTIC TESTS
Stained impression smears may reveal plasma cells. Histopathologic examination of biopsy material is diagnostic.

MANAGEMENT
A number of therapeutic regimes have been reported, such as systemic antibacterial agents, glucocorticoids, surgical excision, bandaging, and chrysotherapy[1-3]. No one method appears superior to another, and many cases appear to resolve spontaneously.

KEY POINT
- Almost pathognomonic appearance.

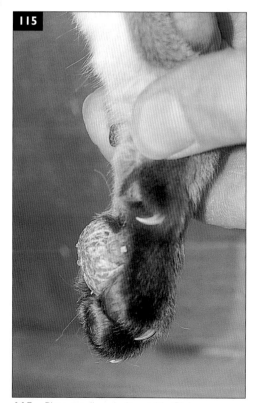

115 Plasma cell pododermatitis. Globose central pad immediately prior to ulceration.

Pemphigus Vulgaris

DEFINITION
Pemphigus vulgaris is a rare, vesicular and ulcerative condition affecting the skin and oral mucosa.

ETIOLOGY AND PATHOGENESIS
The pemphigus vulgaris antibody (IgG) binds to the intracellular portion of calcium-dependent intercellular adhesion molecules[1,2]. The binding of autoantibody is thought to interfere with cell morphology and cell-to-cell binding, and the result is loss of cohesion between the keratinocytes and acantholysis. Primary lesions are vesicles which rapidly rupture to become ulcers.

CLINICAL FEATURES
There is no breed, age, or sex predisposition[3]. Most cases present with mucocutaneous and oral ulceration and exhibit systemic signs, such as pyrexia, depression, and anorexia[3,4]. The cutaneous lesions comprise erosions and ulceration (116, 117), particularly in the axillae and groins and on the nail beds[3,4]. Lesions in cats are concentrated in the oral cavity and on the head. Systemic signs are less common[3].

DIFFERENTIAL DIAGNOSES
- Bullous pemphigoid
- Drug eruption
- Systemic lupus erythematosus
- Cutaneous neoplasia

DIAGNOSTIC TESTS
Clinical examination and history may suggest drug eruption or polysystemic disease, such as systemic lupus erythematosus. Examination of stained impression smears from fresh lesions may demonstrate acanthocytes and the Nikolsky sign may be detected. Neither of these occur in bullous pemphigoid. Histopathologic examination of biopsy samples is usually diagnostic[4], although immunohistochemical methods may be needed in a small proportion of cases.

MANAGEMENT
The aim of treatment is to induce remission as quickly as possible. High doses of prednisolone (2–4 mg/kg PO q 12 h) are the cornerstone of most therapeutic protocols[3,6]. However, the high incidence of severe side-effects[6] means that if improvement in clinical condition cannot be quickly achieved, within 7–14 days, other adjunctive agents should be used in an attempt to reduce the dose of prednisolone. Typically, azathioprine (2.2 mg/kg PO q 48 h) or, possibly, chrysotherapy (aurothioglucose 1.0 mg/kg IM weekly or auranofin 0.05–0.2 mg/kg PO q 12 h) are used[6–8]. Once remission is attained, the drug doses are slowly tapered to the minimum required to maintain remission[6].

Animals treated with azathioprine (and gold salts) require regular blood samples to monitor bone marrow status. Azathioprine should not be used in cats. Some animals require such high doses of glucocorticoid to maintain remission that severe (untreatable) side-effects are unavoidable. Euthanasia is often the only option in these instances.

KEY POINT
- A potentially devastating disease. Treat it aggressively.

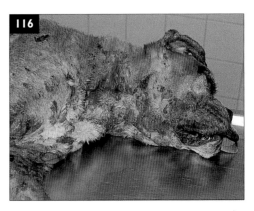

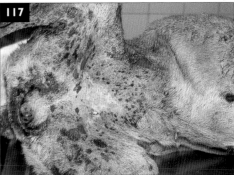

116, 117 Pemphigus vulgaris. Erosions, ulcers, and crusts on the ventral aspects of the neck (116) and the abdomen (117) in a Boxer.

Feline Cutaneous Herpesvirus and Feline Cutaneous Calicivirus Infection

DEFINITION
A rare dermatosis of cats associated with cutaneous infection with feline herpesvirus or feline calicivirus.

ETIOLOGY AND PATHOGENESIS
Feline herpesvirus (feline viral rhinotracheitis virus) and feline calicivirus usually cause upper respiratory tract infection and oral ulceration, respectively, in cats[1]. On rare occasions, cats with active, or recent, feline herpesvirus or calicivirus infection develop cutaneous lesions from which virus particles may be isolated[1-3]. Whether the virus is inoculated during grooming, acts as a secondary invader after ulceration occurs, or arrives by hematogenous spread is not known[1,3]. However, the virus does multiply within the local epithelium, and is not merely a contaminant[1,3].

CLINICAL FEATURES
Affected cats are often actively infected with either feline herpesvirus or calicivirus, and may exhibit oral ulceration in addition to evidence of upper respiratory tract infection[1-3]. Furthermore, poor body condition, surgical stress, or systemic administration of glucocorticoids is often associated with cutaneous viral infections[1-3]. Lesions usually occur on the distal limbs (118) or head, particularly in the periocular regions, although they may be generalized[1-3]. The most common cutaneous lesions are poorly defined, moist ulcers[1-3], although, occasionally, discrete crusted lesions will be noted[1]. There may be local lymphadenopathy.

DIFFERENTIAL DIAGNOSES
- Irritant contact dermatitis
- Cat bite abscessation
- Feline poxvirus infection

DIAGNOSTIC TESTS
Correlation of oral or upper respiratory tract viral infection with cutaneous ulceration will raise suspicion of cutaneous viral infection. Chemical, managemental, or surgical stress should be considered as possible causes. The animals should be checked for FeLV and FIV infection. Histopathologic examination of affected tissue may be helpful. Isolation of the viruses from affected tissue, particularly if it is disinfected before sampling[1], may help to confirm active viral infection rather than simple contamination.

MANAGEMENT
Affected cats should not be given systemic glucocorticoids. Systemic broad-spectrum antibacterial drugs should be administered and a high-quality diet fed. Topical administration of 5-iodo-2'-doxyuridine solution may be helpful in cases of feline herpesvirus infection[1].

KEY POINT
- Do not give steroids to cats with skin ulcers.

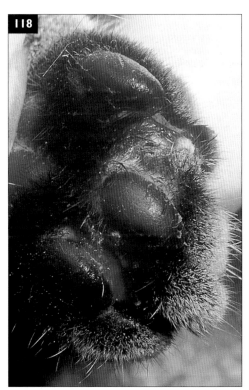

118 Interdigital erosions due to feline calicivirus infection.

Systemic Lupus Erythematosus

DEFINITION
Systemic lupus erythematosus (SLE) is a rare, multisystemic autoimmune disease.

ETIOLOGY AND PATHOGENESIS
Although the immunologic mechanisms have been elucidated, their initiating cause remains obscure. Genetic factors, viruses, hormones, drugs, and environmental conditions, such as exposure to sunlight, have all been implicated in the pathogenesis of SLE[1,2].

In most cases the primary immunologic events leading to the development of SLE are associated with defective suppressor-cell function. The result is a polyclonal gammopathy and the unrestrained production of autoantibodies. These autoantibodies may be cell or tissue specific and directed against erythrocytes, platelets, and leukocytes, or they may be directed against ubiquitous nuclear antigens that are cell/tissue non-specific.

These non-specific autoantibodies are known as antinuclear antibodies (ANA) and combine with free DNA to form DNA–antiDNA immune complexes. These immune complexes may be deposited in glomeruli causing a membranous glomerulonephritis, deposited in arteriolar walls resulting in local fibrinoid necrosis and fibrosis, or deposited in synovia where they provoke arthritis[1]. The presence of the cell/tissue specific and the cell/tissue non-specific autoantibodies, which in any patient may be found either separately or in combination, leads to the diverse clinical presentations of SLE.

CLINICAL FEATURES
In dogs, SLE occurs in middle-aged animals (mean, 5.8 years; range 2–12 years). Rough Collies, Shetland Sheepdogs, Beagles, Afghan Hounds, German Shepherd Dogs, Old English Sheepdogs, Poodles, and Irish Setters comprise the majority of the patient population[1]. There is no sex predisposition, although entire females greatly outnumber neutered females in the affected population. Clinical signs may appear suddenly or gradually, and will often wax and wane[3] making diagnosis difficult. Lameness, due to either a polyarthritis or polymyositis, occurs in 75% of cases and is the most common clinical feature[3]. Fever of unknown origin, proteinuria from glomerulonephritis, hemolytic anemia, skin lesions, thrombocytopenia, neutropenia, myocarditis, thyroiditis, splenomegaly, lymphadenopathy, and CNS disorders have also been reported in association with SLE[1–4].

Skin changes occur in about 50% of cases[1]. They may be localized or generalized and involve the face, ears, limbs, body, mucocutaneous junctions, and oral cavity. Lesions are varied and unpredictable and include alopecia, erythema, ulceration, crusting, scarring, leukoderma, cellulitis, panniculitis, and furunculosis[1–4] (**119, 120**).

SLE is rare in cats and generally presents as an antiglobulin-positive anemia. Other clinical manifestations include fever, skin lesions (alopecia, erythema, scaling, crusting, and scarring which most often involves the face, pinnae, and paws), thrombocytopenia, and renal failure[1,2,5].

DIFFERENTIAL DIAGNOSES (SKIN LESIONS)
- Dermatophytosis
- Demodicosis
- Discoid lupus erythematosus
- Epitheliotropic lymphoma
- Erythema multiforme
- Dermatomyositis
- Necrolytic migratory erythema
- Leishmaniasis
- Toxic epidermal necrolysis
- Pemphigus vulgaris
- Pemphigus foliaceus
- Bullous pemphigoid

DIAGNOSTIC TESTS
The diagnosis of SLE is challenging because of the unpredictable clinical signs and lack of a specific diagnostic test. Diagnosis has to be based on history and clinical findings plus supporting laboratory findings.

ANA test
This is an indirect immunofluorescent test that documents the presence of serum antibodies with specificity for nuclear antigens. It is the most specific and sensitive test for SLE. However, some normal dogs, many normal cats, dogs undergoing treatment with certain drugs (griseofulvin, penicillin, sulfonamides, tetracyclines, phenytoin, and procainamide), and dogs with other diseases may have detectable ANA[1,2].

Histopathologic examination of skin biopsy
This may reveal characteristic findings, such as an interface dermatitis with basal cell vacuolation, and necrosis of basal cells with the formation of colloid or Civatte bodies. Lesions may also involve the hair follicle outer root sheaths. Lichenoid inflammation of the dermis may also be present[4].

Systemic Lupus Erythematosus

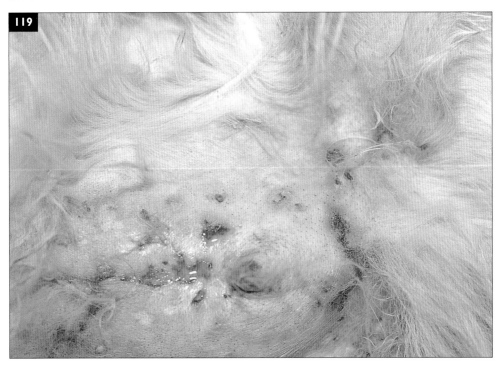

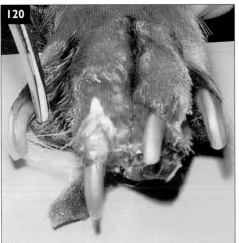

119, 120   Systemic lupus erythematosus. Ulcers and fistulas on the ventral abdomen (**119**) and paronychia (**120**) in a dog.

Systemic Lupus Erythematosus

Direct immunofluorescence testing
This will demonstrate the presence of immunoglobulin (IgA and/or IgM) or complement (C3) at the basement membrane zone in 50–90% of cases. However, these immunoreactants may be found in the basement membrane zone of animals having other skin diseases[1].

Hemogram
A hemogram may show anemia (non-regenerative or hemolytic), thrombocytopenia, leukopenia, or leukocytosis[3].

Cytologic analysis
Cytologic analysis of synovial fluid from animals with lameness may show increased numbers of non-degenerated neutrophils and occasional mononuclear cells[3].

Coombs test
This may or may not be positive.

Platelet factor-3 test
This may or may not be positive.

LE cell test
This test is not reliable. LE cells are polymorphonuclear neutrophils that have phagocytosed nuclei from dead and dying cells. The presence of LE cells is not a reliable feature of SLE in animals because there is a high incidence of both false-positive and false-negative results[2].

MAJOR AND MINOR SIGNS
In view of the difficulty in establishing a reliable diagnosis, a rating of the diagnostic signs has been suggested[5] (Table 2).

Definite SLE requires either two major signs or one major and two minor signs in addition to serologic evidence of SLE. Probable SLE requires one major or two minor signs together with serologic evidence

MANAGEMENT
Systemic corticosteroid, such as prednisone, prednisolone, or methylprednisolone (1.0–3.0 mg/kg PO q 12 h), is the initial therapy of choice. If significant improvement does not occur within 10 days, concurrent administration of azathioprine (2.0 mg/kg PO q 24 h, then q 48 h) can be instituted[1,3]. Do not use azathioprine in cats – use chlorambucil (0.2 mg/kg PO q 24 h, then q 48 h). Once clinical control has been achieved, the drug dosage schedules should be decreased to the lowest schedule that keeps the disease in remission. The prognosis for SLE is guarded as 40% of the cases die within 1 year either due to the disease or drug complications[3].

KEY POINT
- A disease that is very hard to diagnose definitively, particularly if the animal was previously exposed to steroid therapy.

Table 2 Rating of diagnostic signs for SLE[5]	
Major signs	*Minor signs*
Polyarthritis	Pyrexia of unknown
Dermatologic	origin
lesions	CNS signs, such
Coombs positive	as seizures
anemia	Pleuritis
Significant	(non-infective)
thrombocytopenia	
Glomerulonephritis	
Marked neutropenia	
Polymyositis	

Bullous Pemphigoid

DEFINITION
Bullous pemphigoid is a rare, vesicobullous and ulcerative condition affecting the skin and oral mucosa.

ETIOLOGY AND PATHOGENESIS
The condition is characterized by autoantibodies directed against antigen in the hemidesmosomes and, possibly, the basement membrane zone of the skin and the mucosa[1,2]. This results in disruption of dermoepidermal cohesion, separation and, subsequently, subepidermal vesicle formation. The vesicles quickly rupture and most animals present with ulcers and erosions[3]. The condition has been reported in both the dog and the cat.

CLINICAL FEATURES
Collie breeds appear to be predisposed[4], although case series are small, owing to the rarity of the condition. Most cases present with rapid or acute onset of ulcers and erosions (121), which may be confluent and, as a consequence, be very extensive. Predilection sites for lesions include the axillae and groins. Most cases have ulcerations within the oral cavity[4] (122). Pyrexia, septicemia, bacteremia, and dehydration, and even shock, may be anticipated as complications in acute cases, and animals are usually anorexic and depressed[4]. Occasional cases may have a more chronic course and in these cases, crusting lesions are more commonly seen than ulceration[3].

DIFFERENTIAL DIAGNOSES
- Pemphigus vulgaris
- Systemic lupus erythematosus
- Drug eruption
- Cutaneous neoplasia

DIAGNOSTIC TESTS
The history may suggest the potential for drug eruption and whether there is evidence of a polysystemic disease, which may suggest systemic lupus erythematosus. Clinical examination will confirm the absence of Nikolsky sign, and aspiration cytology will fail to demonstrate acantholysis. Definitive diagnosis usually rests on histopathologic examination of biopsy samples[2,4,5], although immunologic techniques may be necessary in some cases to confirm the diagnosis[6].

MANAGEMENT
The aim of treatment is to induce remission as quickly as possible. High doses of prednisolone (2.0–4.0 mg/kg PO q 12 h) are the cornerstone of most therapeutic protocols[3,5]. However, the high incidence of severe side-effects[5] means that if improvement in clinical condition cannot be quickly achieved, within 7–14 days, other adjunctive agents should be used in an attempt to reduce the dose of prednisolone. Typically, azathioprine (2.2 mg/kg PO q 48 h) or, possibly, chrysotherapy (aurothioglucose 1.0 mg/kg IM weekly or auranofin PO q 12 h) are used[5,7,8]. Once remission is attained, the drug doses are slowly tapered to the minimum required to maintain remission[5].

In some cases the dosage of medication necessary to maintain remission is still sufficient to produce unacceptable side-effects. Euthanasia may be necessary in these cases.

KEY POINTS
- A rare but potentially devastating disease.
- Needs aggressive management but a very guarded prognosis is necessary.

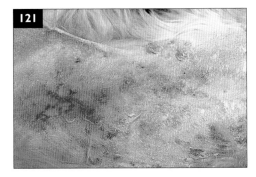

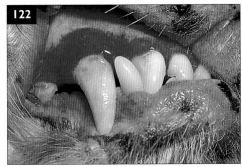

121, 122   Bullous pemphigoid. Ulcerations and erosions on the ventral abdomen (121) and within the oral cavity (122).

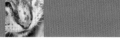

Sporotrichosis

DEFINITION
Sporotrichosis is a subacute or chronic pyo-granulomatous infectious disease of dogs and cats caused by the dimorphic fungus *Sporothrix schenckii*.

ETIOLOGY AND PATHOGENESIS
The organism is found worldwide and grows as a saprophytic mycelial fungus in moist organic debris[1]. Infection occurs via inoculation of the fungus into the skin by thorns or plant material, or by contamination of open wounds or broken skin with exudates from infected animals[1]. In a host the organism establishes infection in the yeast form. The number of organisms found in draining fluids of cats is much greater than other species, which increases the risk of transmission to other animals or humans[2]. Motile organisms have been found to penetrate intact human skin[3].

CLINICAL FEATURES
Typical lesions appear as papular or nodular swellings 3–5 weeks after inoculation[1]. Lesions become alopecic, crusted, and ulcerated, draining a reddish-brown serosanguineous fluid[2]. They are more common on the dorsal aspects of the head and trunk, but the extremities may also be involved (**123, 124**). Regional lymphadenopathy is common and affected lymph nodes may fistulate. Occasionally, lesions may extend along the lymphatics or become disseminated to bone, eyes, GI tract, CNS, and other visceral organs[1].

DIFFERENTIAL DIAGNOSES
- Cutaneous infections of systemic fungi
- Subcutaneous mycoses or algal infections
- Demodicosis
- Deep pyoderma
- Opportunistic mycobacterial infection
- Penetrating foreign bodies

DIAGNOSTIC TESTS
Impression smears or biopsies may reveal the round, oval or cigar-shaped yeast, which may be extracellular or within macrophages or inflammatory cells. Organisms are often present in small numbers and may be difficult to demonstrate with routine stains. Preferred stains for demonstration of the organism are PAS or GMS. Fluorescent antibody techniques are helpful for demonstration of the organisms. Diagnosis can also be made by culture or by inoculation of laboratory animals.

MANAGEMENT
Potassium or sodium iodide is the treatment of choice. In the dog, sodium iodide solution (44 mg/kg of a 20% PO q 8 h) is given for 7–8 weeks or 1 month beyond clinical cure[1]. The dose in cats is decreased (22 mg/kg q 8 h or q 12 h) due to the marked sensitivity of the feline species to iodine preparations[1]. Signs of iodide toxicity include fever, ptyalism, ocular and nasal discharges, anorexia, hyperexcitability, dry hair coat with excess scaling of the skin, vomiting or diarrhea, depression, twitching, hypothermia, and cardiovascular failure. Itraconazole (2.3 mg/kg PO q 12 h) is an alternative therapy if signs of iodide toxicity occur[1], and, in cats, may be preferable from the outset.

PUBLIC HEALTH SIGNIFICANCE
As there are documented cases of humans acquiring sporotrichosis by contact with ulcerated wounds or fluids from lesions, extreme care should be taken in handling infected animals, exudates, or contaminated materials. There is a greater risk associated with cats.

KEY POINT
- Zoonotic potential.

Sporotrichosis

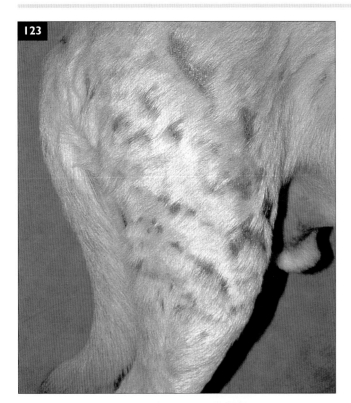

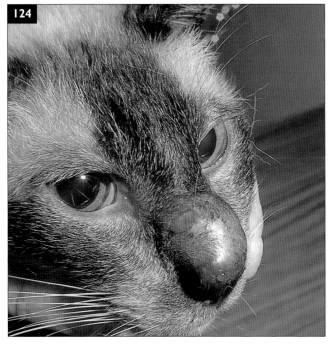

123, **124**   Sporotrichosis. Generalised cutaneous lesions in a dog (**123**); nodular form on the face of a cat (**124**).

Idiopathic Ear Margin Vasculitis

DEFINITION
Idiopathic ear margin vasculitis is a rare disease characterized by ulcerative lesions localized to the margins of the pinna.

ETIOLOGY AND PATHOGENESIS
The pathogenesis of this disease is unknown. However, it is probably an immune-mediated vasculitis caused by immune-complex disease (type III hypersensitivity)[1,2].

CLINICAL FEATURES
Dachshunds are predisposed to this condition, but other breeds may also be affected. Too few cases have been documented to determine if there is an age or sex predisposition. Affected animals first develop alopecia along the margins of the pinna. Then, skin in focal areas (0.2–2.0 cm/0.08–0.8 in) along the very edge of the pinna becomes darkened slightly and thickened and undergoes necrosis resulting in ulcers (**125**). Typically both ears are involved and each will have from one to eight lesions. Occasionally, 0.2–0.5 cm (0.08–0.2 in) ulcers will be noted on the inner aspects of the pinna. Lesions do not appear to be painful or pruritic and no other skin lesions or systemic signs are present. The ulcers will slowly enlarge if left untreated.

DIFFERENTIAL DIAGNOSES
- Frostbite
- Septic vasculitis
- Immune-mediated vasculitis secondary to other diseases
- Proliferative thrombovascular necrosis[2]
- Disseminated intravascular coagulation
- Cold agglutinin disease
- Cryoglobulinemia
- Ischemic necrosis associated with toxins

DIAGNOSTIC TESTS
Diagnosis is based on history, clinical findings, and histopathologic examination of biopsy samples. Several biopsies may be necessary to demonstrate the classic leukocytoclastic pattern of vasculitis.

MANAGEMENT
Dapsone (1.0 mg/kg PO q 8 h) stops the progression of lesions so that re-epithelialization occurs. Once the lesions have been controlled, the frequency of dosage can be reduced to the least amount necessary to maintain remission. Prednisone, prednisolone, or methylprednisolone (1.0–4.0 mg/kg PO q 12 h) may also result in resolution of lesions. However, some animals will only respond to the dapsone[3]. Tissues do not fill back in after undergoing necrosis, so that the ear margins will still have punched out areas present. Blood dyscrasias, thrombocytopenia, and hepatotoxicity may occur with dapsone therapy. Therefore, hemograms and chemistry profiles should be performed every 2 weeks during the first 6 weeks of therapy and monthly thereafter. Toxic changes are generally reversible if the dapsone administration is discontinued.

KEY POINT
- A rare dermatosis which may be difficult to manage effectively.

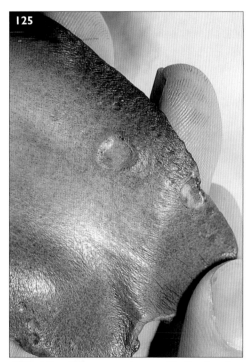

125 Idiopathic ear margin vasculitis. Focal, well-demarcated 'punched out' lesions on the pinna.

Papular and Pustular Dermatoses

GENERAL APPROACH
1 Superficial pyoderma is common and is frequently misdiagnosed.
2 Other causes of pustules include demodicosis, dermatophytosis, pemphigus foliaceus, calcinosis cutis, and drug eruption.
3 Pustules are uncommon in the dog and lots of pustules are, therefore, rare. Lots of well-formed pustules suggests pemphigus foliaceus rather than pyoderma, particularly if the pustules are in a peculiar place for pyoderma, such as the ventral aspect of the pinna or the lateral trunk.

GENERAL RULES
• Papules and a few pustules: swab for bacteriology
• Lots of pustules and only a few papules: biopsy

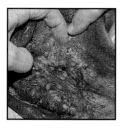
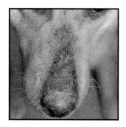
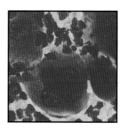
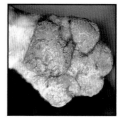

Superficial Pyoderma

DEFINITION

Superficial pyoderma is a cutaneous bacterial infection confined to the stratum corneum of the interfollicular skin and hair follicles.

ETIOLOGY AND PATHOGENESIS

Staphylococcus intermedius is the most frequent coagulase-positive *Staphylococcus* recovered from clinical samples taken from the affected skin of dogs with pyoderma[1,2]. Although *S. aureus* and, rarely, *S. hyicus* may be recovered from up to 10% of cases of canine pyoderma[3], *S. intermedius* is regarded as the principal canine cutaneous pathogen[3,4]. Coagulase-negative staphylococci, such as *S. epidermis* or *S. xylosus*, are occasionally recovered from clinical lesions in pure culture, but they are regarded, in general, as non-pathogenic[3,7].

Canine pyoderma is considered to be a secondary disease in which local changes in the cutaneous microclimate result in the development of conditions favorable for the growth and multiplication of pathogenic staphylococci[5,6]. Furthermore, some of the products of bacterial multiplication, such as protein A, may induce inflammatory changes within the epidermis, resulting in increased concentrations of exudates upon the skin surface, which may further favor bacterial multiplication[5,6]. The most common underlying causes of superficial pyoderma are ectoparasite infestations, hypersensitivities, and endocrinopathies.

CLINICAL FEATURES

Superficial pyoderma is usually pruritic and typically presents as an erythematous papulocrustous dermatitis. Pustules (126), either interfollicular or follicular in orientation, are usually heavily outnumbered by erythematous papules, crusted papules, epidermal collarettes, and patches of post-inflammatory hyperpigmentation (127). The most common site for superficial pyoderma to occur is on the glabrous skin of the groin and ventral abdomen. There may be patchy alopecia, particularly on the flanks of short-haired dogs, such as Doberman Pinschers, Boxers, and Great Danes (128, 129). Occasionally, unusual presentations may be encountered, such as dry, crusted lesions on the trunk, erythematous plaques in intertriginous regions, and erosions.

DIFFERENTIAL DIAGNOSES

- Demodicosis
- Dermatophytosis
- *Malassezia pachydermatis* infection
- Pemphigus foliaceus
- Zinc responsive dermatosis
- Dermatophilosis

DIAGNOSTIC TESTS

Identification of primary lesions, such as papules and pustules, greatly aids the diagnosis of superficial pyoderma, whereas the presence of secondary lesions, such as epidermal collarettes, post-inflammatory hyperpigmentation, and scale, are helpful but much less specific. Cytologic examination of the aspirated contents of pustules may allow identification of neutrophils, degenerate neutrophils, and intracellular cocci (130). Bacterial culture and sensitivity usually reveals a coagulase-positive *Staphylococcus*, typically *S. intermedius*. Histopathologic examination of appropriate biopsy samples will also allow diagnosis and elimination of the principal differential diagnoses.

MANAGEMENT

In some cases, where lesions are confined to the interfollicular skin, topical therapy with chlorhexidine or benzoyl peroxide may be sufficient to eliminate the infection. However, most cases of superficial pyoderma require systemic antibacterial therapy, although adjunctive topical therapy is usually indicated. Appropriate antibacterial agents for cases on first presentation include erythromycin (15 mg/kg PO q 8 h), lincomycin (22 mg/kg PO q 12 h), clindamycin (11 mg/kg PO q 24 h), oxacillin (20 mg/kg PO q 12 h), and trimethroprim- or ometoprim-potentiated sulfonamides (30 mg/kg PO q 12 or 24 h respectively).

Cases which are severe, or which have failed to respond to first-line therapy, should be subjected to bacteriologic culture and sensitivity testing and treated empirically, pending laboratory results, with trimethroprim- or ometoprim-potentiated sulfonamides (30 mg/kg PO q 12 or 24 h), cephalexin (25 mg/kg PO q 12 h), clavulanic acid-potentiated amoxycillin (25 mg/kg PO q 12 h), or enrofloxacin (5 mg/kg PO q 24 h).

Animals should be weighed to ensure the correct dosage is prescribed, closely monitored to ensure owner compliance, and treated for at least 7–10 days after clinical remission has been noted. In practical terms a 3-week course of appropriate antibacterial agents is a minimum.

Superficial Pyoderma

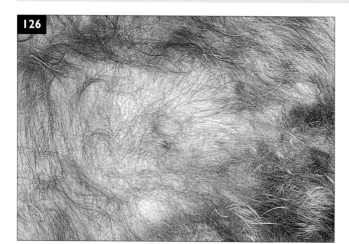

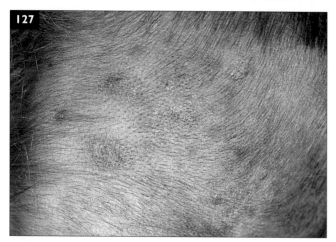

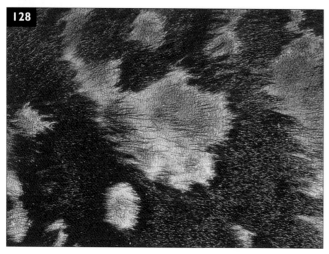

126–128 Superficial pyoderma. Discrete pustules on the ventral abdomen of a dog (**126**); papules, pustules, collarettes, and pigmentation (**127**); and patchy alopecia on the flank of a Great Dane (**128**).

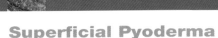

Superficial Pyoderma

Dogs which fail to respond should be subjected to bacteriologic culture and sensitivity, a re-evaluation of the diagnosis, and tests to identify likely underlying conditions. The most common underlying conditions are flea bite hypersensitivity, atopy, and hyperthyroidism.

KEY POINTS
- An underdiagnosed disease.
- Requires appropriate treatment for at least 3 weeks.
- Do not use steroids.
- Relapsing pyoderma requires a full work-up.

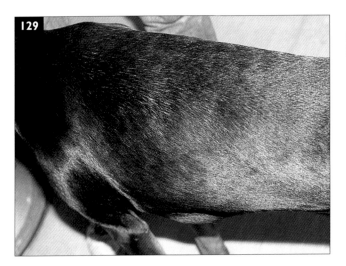

129 Superficial pyoderma. Patchy alopecia on the flank of a Doberman Pinscher.

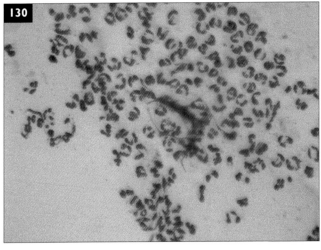

130 Photomicrograph of neutrophils and cocci, aspirated from a pustule. Compare this with the aspirate from pemphigus foliaceus (**137**).

Canine Acne (Chin and Muzzle Folliculitis and Furunculosis)

DEFINITION

Canine acne is a papular and/or pustular dermatosis associated with dilated hyperkeratotic follicles, furunculosis, and parafollicular inflammation.

ETIOLOGY AND PATHOGENESIS

The precipitating etiology and pathogenesis are unknown. The follicular plugging and parafollicular inflammation may predispose to follicular rupture, resulting in a foreign body reaction and, eventually, in some cases, secondary bacterial infection. The condition spontaneously resolves in many animals when they reach adulthood, although some individuals remain affected for life.

CLINICAL FEATURES

Canine acne occurs most commonly over the chin and lips of young, short-coated breeds of dogs such as Doberman Pinschers, English Bulldogs, Great Danes, Weimaraners, Rottweilers, and German Shorthaired Pointers. Lesions consist of follicular papules and/or pustules which may ulcerate and fistulate, draining a serosanguineous to seropurulent material (**131**). Follicles may rupture (furunculosis), and if the accompanying foreign body inflammation is extensive, small fibrous nodules may develop. Animals may suffer no discomfort if the lesions are minimal, although extensively affected areas may be sensitive and mildly pruritic.

DIFFERENTIAL DIAGNOSES

- Demodicosis
- Dermatophytosis
- Foreign body reaction

DIAGNOSTIC TESTS

The signalment and clinical signs are very suggestive. Skin scrapings should be taken to rule out demodicosis. Bacterial and dermatophyte culture and antibiotic sensitivity testing is indicated in cases which do not respond to empirical treatment.

MANAGEMENT

Affected areas may be cleaned daily with a benzoyl peroxide shampoo or gel to enhance removal of debris from the hair follicle and decrease the number of bacteria on the skin surface. The shampoo should be carefully rinsed from the affected area as benzoyl peroxide can be irritating in some cases. Mild cases may respond to just topical antibacterial and cleansing therapy, but more severely affected cases will benefit from topical glucocorticoids applied twice daily. If secondary infection occurs, systemic antibiotics for 3–6 weeks would be appropriate. A small number of cases require either continuous or episodic treatment for life.

KEY POINT

- Easy to overdiagnose. Do not forget the differential diagnoses.

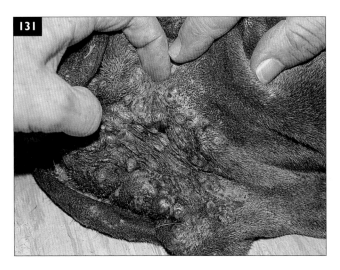

131 Canine acne. Fibrogranulomatous, cystic, and papular lesions due to canine acne.

Impetigo

DEFINITION
Impetigo is a superficial staphylococcal infection characterized by subcorneal pustules occurring on the glabrous or non-haired skin of young dogs.

ETIOLOGY AND PATHOGENESIS
Coagulase positive *Staphylococcus* spp. are usually isolated from pustules, but the underlying etiology is not understood. Poor management and poor hygiene have been implicated, but many affected animals come from clean environments.

CLINICAL FEATURES
Lesions appear as non-follicular pustules on the ventral abdomen (**132**) and occasionally the axilla in 2–9-month-old puppies. Pustules rupture resulting in small crusts or epidermal collarettes. Systemic signs of infection and pruritus are generally not a feature of the condition.

DIFFERENTIAL DIAGNOSES
• Demodicosis
• Dermatophytosis
• Contact irritant dermatitis

DIAGNOSTIC TESTS
Skin scrapings should be examined to rule out demodicosis. Examination of aspiration or impression smears of pustule contents will help to identify the etiology as staphylococcal. Dermatophyte culture should be performed in cases which fail to respond to antibacterial treatment.

MANAGEMENT
Mild cases may resolve spontaneously without treatment. If small numbers of lesions are present, topical antibacterial creams or ointments applied twice daily may be appropriate. If the affected area is large, then application of shampoos containing either chlorhexidine or ethyl lactate every other day for 7–14 days will generally result in resolution of lesions. If lesions are extensive, a 7–10 day course of systemic antibacterial treatment may be necessary.

KEY POINT
• An uncommon dermatosis.

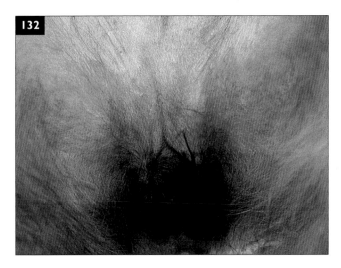

132 Impetigo. Small erythematous papules and pustules on the glabrous skin of a Collie pup.

Pemphigus Foliaceus

DEFINITION
Pemphigus foliaceus is an autoimmune disease in which autoantibodies are directed against components of the epidermis resulting in acantholysis and subcorneal vesicle formation[2].

ETIOLOGY AND PATHOGENESIS
Autoantibody (IgG) is formed against proteins bound to plakoglobin, a component of both desmosomes and adherans junctions[9]. These are the main intercellular bridges between the keratinocytes and are responsible for cell-to-cell cohesion. In addition, these sites are intimately linked to the intracellular cytoskeleton. If the assembly and function of these intercellular connections is defective, as a result of antibody binding to ligand, a loss of cohesion between the keratinocytes occurs. The associated changes in cytoskeleton result in acantholysis (rounding up) of individual keratinocytes and subsequent pustule formation. These primary lesions are transient owing to the thin canine and feline stratum corneum.

CLINICAL FEATURES
Pemphigus foliaceus is the most common form of pemphigus[1,4,10], and presents as a vesiculobullous or pustular dermatitis with secondary erythema, scale, alopecia, erosion, and crust formation. Epidermal collarettes are common[5]. Pemphigus foliaceus is usually a disease of gradual onset. It is variably pruritic and only rarely is it accompanied by systemic signs in the dog, even though generalized lesions may occur[7,8,10]. The disease is rare in the cat and, in this species, anorexia and pyrexia may be noted[7].

Usually, only the skin is affected and lesions on the mucocutaneous junctions and in the oral cavity are rare[5]. In most cases, lesions are symmetrical in distribution, usually commencing on the dorsal part of the muzzle[5] (**133**), face, and pinnae before slowly generalizing (**134**). In some instances, lesions may remain localized to small areas of the body, such as the pinnae (**135**). The footpads may become hyperkeratotic (**136**), and there may be erythema at the margins of the footpads[5]. Occasionally, the epithelium of the pads will slough and, rarely, lesions may be confined to the footpads[2,5,10].

DIFFERENTIAL DIAGNOSES
- Demodicosis
- Superficial pyoderma
- Zinc responsive dermatosis
- Dermatophytosis
- Actinic dermatosis
- Epitheliotropic lymphoma
- Drug eruption

DIAGNOSTIC TESTS
Consideration of history and clinical signs and the results of microscopic examination of skin scrapes will generally rule out demodicosis and dermatophytosis. The presence of primary lesions (pustules) is of great significance – a good place to look for them is the concave surface of the pinnae. Aspiration cytology may be practised on primary lesions, but not if there are only one or two: they should be biopsied to maximize the chances of a definitive diagnosis. Microscopic examination of cytologic samples may reveal rounded keratinocytes (acanthocytes) (**137**), and while these are highly suggestive of pemphigus foliaceus, they may be seen in cases of superficial pyoderma. In rare cases, there may be a positive Nikolsky sign: lateral digital pressure on the skin produces erosions. Histopathologic examination of biopsy material is diagnostic in some 80% of cases, and also rules out almost all of the differential diagnoses. Direct immunofluorescence or peroxidase/immunoperoxidase staining may be performed in cases where routine histopathologic examination is not diagnostic.

MANAGEMENT
The management of pemphigus foliaceus encompasses two aims: suppression of clinical signs and maintenance of clinical remission. Suppression of the clinical signs is achieved with immunosuppressive doses of prednisolone. Initial doses (1.1–2.2 mg/kg PO q 12 h) should be prescribed and if there is no improvement within 10–14 days, the dose should be increased (to 2.2 mg/kg, or even 3.3 mg/kg, PO q 12 h) and steroid-sparing regimes considered[3,10]. Animals should be closely monitored during induction for side-effects, and once remission is achieved the dose should be slowly tapered (to 0.25–2.2 mg/kg PO on alternate days). In one study, 42% of dogs could be maintained on alternate-day prednisolone[10]. The majority of feline cases respond well and are maintained comfortably in clinical remission with prednisolone therapy[7,10]. Some of the dogs which exhibited unacceptable side-effects to prednisolone or methylprednisolone may be controlled on alternate (or every third day) dexamethasone

Pemphigus Foliaceus

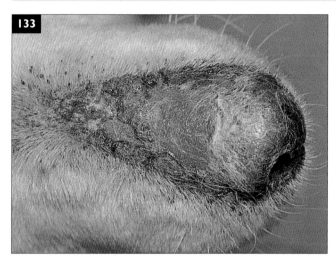

133–135 Pemphigus foliaceus. Localized lesions on the face of a German Shepherd Dog (**133**); generalized lesions on a cross-breed (**134**); lesions confined to the pinnae of a cat (**135**).

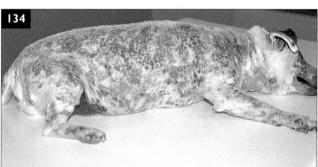

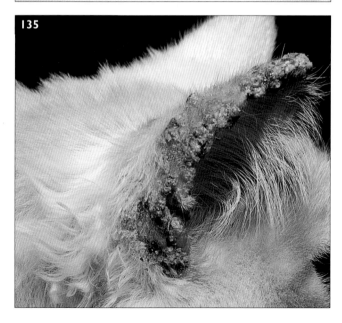

Pemphigus Foliaceus

(0.1 mg/kg). However, a significant proportion of dogs will fail to respond to glucocorticoid regimes or exhibit severe side-effects[10], and steroid-sparing regimes or alternative therapy must be considered[1,3,4].

Azathioprine is the most common agent employed for steroid-sparing or adjunctive treatment in autoimmune conditions[3]. The beneficial effects of azathioprine are not apparent for 3–5 weeks, and the aim is to use azathioprine alternated with prednisolone at the lowest doses necessary to maintain remission. Doses of 1–2 mg/kg PO q 24 h or on alternate days are usually well tolerated in dogs[10]. Azathioprine is contraindicated in cats. Bone marrow suppression or GI side-effects may occur, and animals should be closely monitored with biweekly blood counts for the first 8 weeks of therapy[3].

Aurothioglucose (gold salt therapy) has also been advocated as a steroid-sparing agent and as an adjunctive agent, and was useful in 23% of canine cases and 40% of feline cases in one study[10]. Sodium aurothiomalate is administered IM at an initial dose of 1 mg (dogs <10 kg and cats) or 5 mg (dogs >10 kg). If no side-effects are noted after 7 days, the dose is doubled. If no side-effects are observed, treatment is continued with weekly doses (1 mg/kg)[6]. The animals are closely monitored for side-effects, in particular, renal, hematologic, and dermatologic disease. Recently, an oral gold preparation (auranofin) has been described[10]. Dosage is between 0.05 and 0.2 mg/kg q 12 h, and side-effects appear to be much less frequent than with the parenteral forms of gold therapy.

KEY POINT
- Do not underestimate the difficulty in managing this disease. Some cases may be all but refractory.

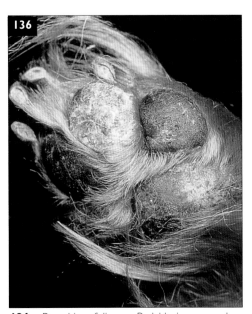

136   Pemphigus foliaceus. Pedal lesions on a dog.

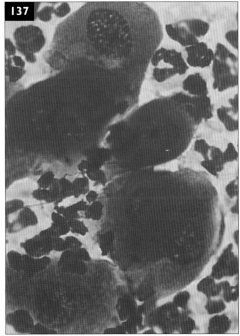

137   Acanthocytes (rounded up keratinocytes) with clustering neutrophils from a pustule in a case of pemphigus foliaceus.

Zinc Responsive Dermatosis

DEFINITION
Zinc responsive dermatosis in dogs occurs due to a relative or absolute deficiency of zinc in the diet or an impaired ability to absorb zinc from the gut. Naturally occurring zinc deficiency has not been reported in the cat.

ETIOLOGY AND PATHOGENESIS
Absolute dietary zinc deficiency is rare in animals fed high-quality, commercially-prepared diets[2]. More commonly, there is a relative deficiency due to interaction with other dietary components or an inability to utilize dietary zinc. Absorption of zinc from the gut is inhibited by iron, copper, and calcium, which compete with zinc for absorption. Intestinal phytate and inorganic phosphate bind zinc and thus hinder absorption[3]. Relative or absolute zinc deficiency is most likely to be seen in rapidly-growing animals, particularly giant breeds, fed inadequate diets or diets in which nutritional antagonism occurs, particularly due to high phytate content or oversupplementation with calcium.

Individuals of many breeds of dog, particularly Siberian Huskies and Alaskan Malamutes, are predisposed to zinc deficiency[4]. These animals appear unable to absorb adequate zinc, even when fed a nutritionally-balanced diet. A congenital inability to utilize zinc (lethal acrodermatitis) in English Bull Terriers has been reported[1].

CLINICAL FEATURES
In cases associated with relative dietary deficiency or dietary binding of zinc, the cutaneous signs predominate, although polylymphadenopathy may be detected. Well-demarcated areas of crusting, with an erythematous border, appear over the pressure points on the limbs and, in a more or less symmetrical manner, around the mouth and eyes[3] (**138**). The coat is dull and harsh and occasional areas of achromotrichia (loss of hair color) may be noted.

Lethal acrodermatitis (**139, 140**) of Bull Terriers may result in severe systemic signs, such as stunting, emaciation, and immunoincompetence[1].

DIFFERENTIAL DIAGNOSES
- Superficial pyoderma
- Demodicosis
- Dermatophytosis
- Pemphigus foliaceus

DIAGNOSTIC TESTS
The diagnosis of zinc responsive dermatosis must be based on the case history, clinical examination, dietary history (particularly the feeding of soya- or cereal-based diets), histopathologic examination of cutaneous biopsy specimens, and laboratory analysis of tissue zinc concentration[3]. The diagnostic value of leukocyte, serum, or hair zinc concentration alone is minimal.

MANAGEMENT
The prognosis for Bull Terriers with congenital acrodermatitis is very poor[1], whereas the prognosis for individuals exhibiting signs of zinc-responsive dermatosis is good. Zinc supplementation with oral zinc sulfate (10 mg/kg) or zinc methionate (1.7 mg/kg) once daily with food is the treatment of choice. If the supplement contains elemental zinc, it should be dosed at 2.5 mg/kg (of elemental zinc) PO q 24 h. Some animals require even higher doses than those detailed above before a response is seen.

Supplementation may be required for life in the Arctic breeds and other individuals, demonstrating an inability to absorb adequate zinc from normal diets. Animals exhibiting signs consequent upon a relative dietary deficiency require a nutritionally-balanced diet and oral supplementation only until the lesions have resolved.

KEY POINT
- May occur in dogs on a commercially-prepared diet.

Zinc Responsive Dermatosis

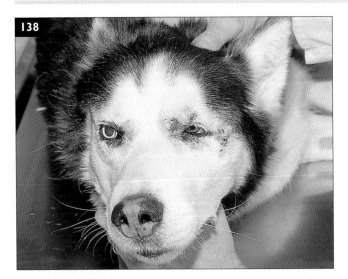

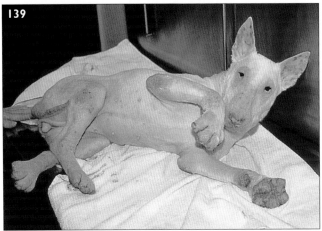

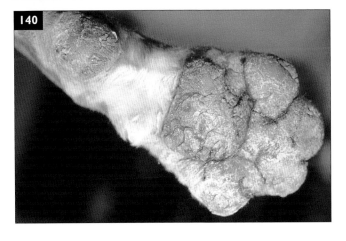

138–140   Zinc deficiency. Periorbital crusting (**138**); stunting (**139**) and chronic pododermatitis (**140**) in a Bull Terrier with lethal acrodermatitis. (Illustrations courtesy of H.W. Richardson.)

Canine Juvenile Cellulitis

(Juvenile Pyoderma, Puppy Strangles)

DEFINITION
Canine juvenile cellulitis is a granulomatous condition of puppies affecting the skin of the face, the pinnae, and the submandibular lymph nodes.

ETIOLOGY AND PATHOGENESIS
The etiology and pathogenesis of this condition are unknown. An immunologic abnormality may be involved as glucocorticoid therapy results in resolution of lesions. There is some evidence for an hereditary factor as some breeds, as well as particular lines within a breed, are predisposed[1,2].

CLINICAL FEATURES
The condition develops in puppies from 3–16 weeks or age. It occurs more frequently in Golden Retrievers, Dachshunds, Labrador Retrievers, Lhasa Apsos, and Gordon Setters[1-4]. Puppies are usually febrile, depressed, and anorexic. There is acute swelling of the muzzle, lips, and eyelids (**141**). Sterile pustules often develop in the skin of these areas as well as on the inner surface of the pinnae. After the pustules rupture, small ulcers, draining tracts, or crusts develop. Submandibular lymphadenopathy occurs and, occasionally, lymph nodes will abscessate and drain. Nodules over the trunk, preputial, and perineal areas, due to a pyogranulomatous panniculitis as well as sterile suppurative arthritis, have been reported in a small number of cases[2]. Permanent areas of alopecia and scarring may result if the lesions are extensive.

DIFFERENTIAL DIAGNOSES
- Angioedema due to an insect-bite reaction or vaccine
- Demodicosis
- Pyoderma
- Pemphigus foliaceus
- Adverse drug reaction

DIAGNOSTIC TESTS
Signalment and clinical signs are very suggestive. Skin scrapings and cytologic examination of the contents of an intact pustule will help to identify demodicosis or staphylococcal folliculitis, respectively. Bacterial culture of the contents of an intact pustule is important as gram-negative, in addition to gram-positive, bacteria may be secondary pathogens.

MANAGEMENT
Prednisolone (1–2 mg/kg PO q12 h) for 14–21 days, depending on the rate of resolution of the clinical signs. In most cases, significant improvement will be noted during the first 24–48 hours of treatment. Once lesions have resolved, the dosage may be reduced (q 48 h) to prevent relapse[3]. Warm soaks, twice daily, using aluminum acetate or chlorhexidine solutions can be helpful to keep the affected areas clean and to prevent the formation of crusts. If a secondary bacterial infection is suspected, systemic bactericidal antibacterial drugs can be used concurrently.

KEY POINT
- These cases require steroid therapy. Be sure to rule out demodicosis.

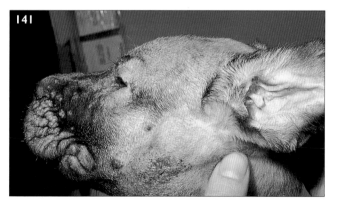

141   Juvenile pyoderma. Facial swelling in a pup.

Diseases Characterized by Sinus Formation

GENERAL APPROACH
1 Uncommon diseases, apart from bite wounds and foreign body penetration.
2 Biopsy and culture sensitivity are mandatory if there is no bite wound or no foreign body penetration.
3 Profuse or colored discharge from a sinus is not very common – bacterial culture and sensitivity (anaerobic culture also) are called for, and biopsy.
4 Foreign bodies may penetrate along tissue planes – contrast studies may be necessary.

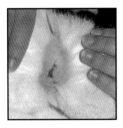
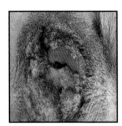
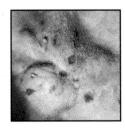
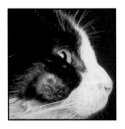

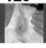

Bite Wounds

DEFINITION
Bite wounds occur following penetration of the skin by bites.

ETIOLOGY AND PATHOGENESIS
Penetration of the skin is usually followed by inoculation of oral flora or epidermal flora into the subcutis. The bruising accompanying the wound, and the failure of the discharge to drain through the small penetrations, facilitate abscess formation. The typical organisms in wounds resulting from dog bites are *Staphylococcus intermedius* and *Escherichia coli*[1], whereas in cat bites the usual isolates are *Pasteurella multocida*, *Bacteroides* spp., and β-hemolytic streptococci. One report found subcutaneous abscessation, and concomitant arthritis, in a colony of cats caused by bacterial L-forms[2].

CLINICAL FEATURES
Animals vary in their response to abscessation. In dogs the abscesses usually follow bites and these are usually on the limbs, head, and neck[3]. Cats are usually bitten on the head (**142, 143**), distal limb, or tail base. After the bite, the area surrounding the puncture is usually bruised and there may be some serous discharge or even bleeding. Dog bites are often sufficiently large that drainage is easy and abscessation is unusual. However, the small puncture wounds resulting from cat bites often seal and then present as an abscess after 2–4 days. Affected animals may be lethargic, inappetent, and in pain. Pyrexia may be noted. A soft, variably painful swelling develops which, if not lanced, bursts. The skin overlying the abscess may be necrotic and may slough. Cats may also develop a cellulitis from bite wounds. Typically, this occurs on a limb and is characterized by subcutaneous swelling resulting in pain and lameness. Careful examination of the affected area may reveal small crusts covering the puncture tracts.

DIFFERENTIAL DIAGNOSES
• Penetrating foreign body
• Demodicosis
• Panniculitis
• Feline leprosy and atypical mycobacterial infection
• Nocardiosis
• Subcutaneous and deep mycoses
• Cuterebriasis or dracunculiasis
• Neoplasia

DIAGNOSTIC TESTS
The clinical history is important. Abscessation following bite wounds is usually well documented in dogs. In cats, definitive histories are not common, but consideration of life style and the site of the abscess usually lead to diagnosis.

Recurrent abscess formation demands a thorough work up to establish the cause. Any underlying immunosuppression or endocrinopathy should be identified by appropriate tests. In cats, FeLV and FIV testing is important. Cytologic examination of discharge, bacterial (aerobic and anaerobic) and fungal culture of material from the cavity, and serology may all be employed in defining a diagnosis

MANAGEMENT
Abscesses should be drained surgically and lavaged. Once the abscess is drained, animals usually recover promptly. Postoperative antibacterial agents, such as amoxycillin, are usually administered for 4–5 days. The same principles are applied to the management of dog bite wounds, although a broad-spectrum, penicillinase-resistant antibacterial agent should be used, rather than amoxycillin.

KEY POINTS
• Bite wounds may be contaminated.
• Failure to respond promptly should be treated seriously.

Bite Wounds

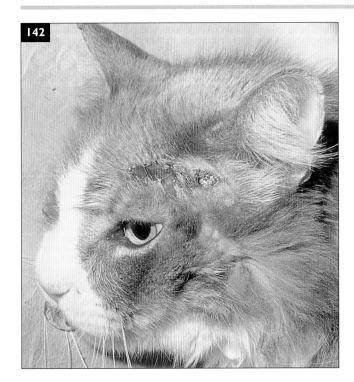

142 Bite wound on the head of a cat.

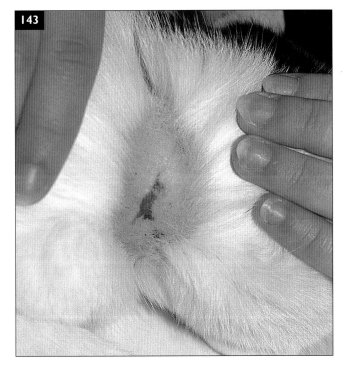

143 Cat bite abscess on the neck.

Deep Pyoderma

DEFINITION
Deep pyoderma occurs when infection is present beneath the basement membrane, i.e. in the dermis.

ETIOLOGY AND PATHOGENESIS
Deep pyoderma may occur as a consequence of superficial (or pyotraumatic) pyoderma, following extension of infection through ruptured follicle walls (furunculosis). However, direct inoculation from contaminated bite wounds or penetrating foreign bodies is the most common etiology, particularly in the cat. Many cases are idiopathic, but with the exception of deep pyoderma following foreign body penetration or bite wounds, cases of deep pyoderma, particularly in the dog, should be considered secondary to demodicosis or immunosuppression until proved otherwise. Endocrinopathies, in particular, should be considered.

As with the other classifications of pyoderma, the principal organism recovered from lesions is *Staphylococcus intermedius,* but other microorganisms, particularly gram-negative bacteria, may be found. Culture and sensitivity is mandatory when investigating deep pyoderma.

CLINICAL FEATURES
In contrast to superficial pyoderma, the deep infections are easily recognized. Ulcers, sinus formation, and cellulitis are commonly seen. Treatment is often difficult and prolonged, and management is helped by classification into a number of subgroups, many of which are described in their own right elsewhere:

- Localized deep folliculitis and furunculosis
- Deep pyoderma
- Nasal pyoderma
- Foreign body sinus (page 126)
- Canine acne (page 111)
- Callus pyoderma (page 134)
- Interdigital pyoderma
- Anal furunculosis (page 125)
- Bite wounds and subsequent abcessation (page 120)
- German Shepherd Dog pyoderma (page 84)

Localized deep folliculitis and furunculosis
These are thought to be a complication of pyotraumatic dermatitis or superficial pyoderma. Animals, typically Labrador and Golden Retrievers, present with a pruritic, exudative, erythematous thickened patch (**144**). The major differential diagnosis is pyotraumatic dermatitis (page 29). Localized deep folliculitis and furunculosis may be differentiated clinically by having a thickened feel and the presence of satellite lesions – both uncommon in pyotraumatic dermatitis.

Deep pyoderma
This usually occurs as a result of underlying disease or foreign body penetration. However, idiopathic cases will be seen which fit no well-recognized syndrome, but fulfil the criteria for deep pyoderma such as ulceration and sinus formation (**145, 146**).

Nasal pyoderma
This is a dermatosis affecting the dorsal muzzle but not the nasal planum. The peracute form presents as inflammatory papules which rapidly coalesce and progress to an erythematous, eroded, granuloproliferative plaque which is extremely painful. These lesions have been traditionally associated with rooting behavior. More recently the possibility that they represent peracute inflammatory reactions to arthropod and insect bites and stings has been proposed (see pages 164 and 166). The more chronic form of the dermatosis is characterized by crusted papules (**147**) and occasionally by sinus formation.

DIFFERENTIAL DIAGNOSES
- Demodicosis
- Deep or superficial fungal infection
- Panniculitis
- Nocardiosis
- Immune-mediated disease (such as discoid lupus erythematosus and pemphigus foliaceus in the case of nasal pyoderma)

DIAGNOSTIC TESTS
In addition to treating the infection, a determined search for underlying disease should be made. Demodicosis should always be considered until ruled out by skin scrapings. Other causes such as hypothyroidism and hyperadrenocorticism should also be considered. Misuse of glucocorticoids for the symptomatic control of pruritic dermatoses, such as atopy, or internal disease, such as musculoskeletal problems, may also be contributory. Bacterial culture and sensitivity testing is mandatory.

MANAGEMENT
Failure to identify an underlying cause mandates symptomatic treatment. The affected

Deep Pyoderma

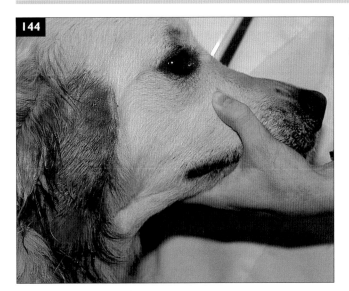

144   Localized folliculitis and furunculosis on the head of a Golden Retriever.

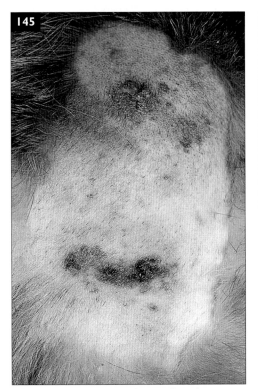

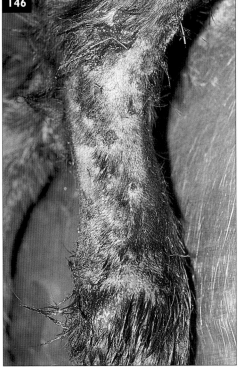

145   Localized deep pyoderma, clipped out. Note the focal erythema and sinus formation in the main lesion, but also the two smaller lesions seen easily only after clipping.

146   Multiple sinus formation and deep pyoderma on the distal limb of a cross-bred dog.

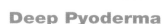

Deep Pyoderma

areas should be clipped out, and a body clip given if lesions are extensive. Whirlpool baths are helpful, if available. Antibacterial shampoos (chlorhexidine particularly) are useful. Systemic treatment according to sensitivity testing is required until lesions have resolved. In practice this usually means 8–12 weeks of therapy. Owners should be warned that in idiopathic cases relapse is possible. In cases of repeated relapse, long-term antibacterial strategies may be necessary.

KEY POINTS
- Culture and sensitivity testing are mandatory.
- Search for underlying disease.
- Do not forget demodicosis.

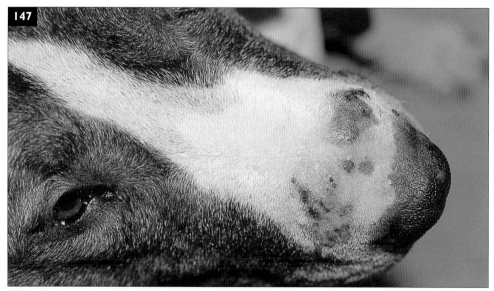

147 Nasal pyoderma. Note the crusting on the nose but the failure of the lesions to affect the nasal planum. This is a key point in trying to differentiate pyoderma from immune-mediated disease.

Anal Furunculosis (Perianal Fistulas)

DEFINITION
Anal furunculosis is characterized by chronic draining sinus tracts involving the perianal and perirectal tissues.

ETIOLOGY AND PATHOGENESIS
The cause of anal furunculosis is unknown. Most affected animals have a broad-based tail and low tail carriage. It has been hypothesized that this reduces anal ventilation and results in a fecal film over the perianal area. This predisposes to infection and abscessation of the circumanal glands and hair follicles in the perianal skin, resulting in fistula formation[1]. Day (1993)[2] has identified infiltration by eosinophils into ductal tissue and aggregates of T lymphocytes within the depths of the tissue, suggesting that complex immunologic processes are at play in these dogs.

CLINICAL FEATURES
The condition is most common in German Shepherd Dogs, but has also been diagnosed in Irish Setters and Labrador Retrievers as well as in an English Setter and a Dandie Dinmont Terrier[3]. Historically, the most common complaint is tenesmus or straining to defecate. Dyschezia (painful defecation), weight loss, matting of hair surrounding the anus, foul odor, diarrhea, and frequent licking of the anal area may also be noted. The perineum is often very painful and many animals will have to be sedated in order to adequately evaluate the extent of the lesions. On physical examination the perianal area is often covered with a foul-smelling exudate and fecal material. Erythema as well as varying numbers of shallow ulcers and fistulous tracts may be present (**148**). In severe cases there may be 360 degree ulceration of the perianal area[4].

DIFFERENTIAL DIAGNOSES
- Anal sac disease
- Anal or rectal neoplasia
- Rectal foreign bodies
- Anal pruritus secondary to *Malassezia pachydermatis* or atopy

DIAGNOSTIC TESTS
The diagnosis is based on history and clinical findings.

MANAGEMENT
Surgical procedures are the treatment of choice. Several techniques are described with or without tail amputation[5,6].

KEY POINTS
- Pathognomonic presentation.
- Very difficult to manage.

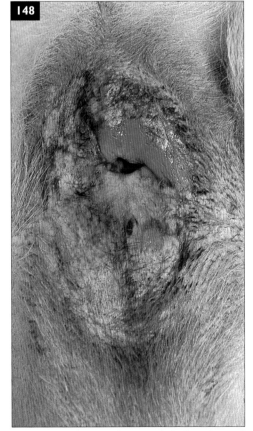

148   Perianal fistulas. Discrete foci of erosion and ulceration are apparent around the anal ring in this German Shepherd Dog.

Foreign Body Sinus

DEFINITION
Foreign bodies inoculated into the dermis provoke a vigorous inflammatory response that may result in sinus formation

ETIOLOGY AND PATHOGENESIS
Foreign body granulomas and sinus formation result when the inciting stimulus is not removed by phagocytosis[1]. The list of causal agents is long but plant awns, such as foxtails (*Hordeum jubatum*) in North America and *Hordeum murinum* in Europe, are responsible for the majority of lesions (**149**). Other exogenous foreign bodies include suture material, vaccine adjuvant, pieces of vegetation, insect mouthparts or stings, and airgun pellets. Endogenous foreign bodies include keratin, free lipid, calcium salts, and urate deposition. The foreign body sinus may get progressively longer as the inoculated agent migrates along tissue planes.

CLINICAL FEATURES
Nodules and a draining sinus are typical (**150**). The most common sites for exogenous foreign body penetrations are the dorsal interdigital regions (**151**) and the anterior aspects of the distal limbs. Local lymphadenopathy is common, but systemic signs are rare unless distant or deep migration (possibly into body cavities) has occurred, resulting in draining tracts. Secondary bacterial infection associated with awn penetration is common. Other forms of foreign bodies may result in papules, nodules, abscesses, and draining tracts.

DIFFERENTIAL DIAGNOSES
- Demodicosis
- Panniculitis
- Feline leprosy and atypical mycobacterial infection
- Nocardiosis
- Subcutaneous and deep mycoses
- Cuterebriasis or dracunculiasis
- Acral granuloma
- Neoplasia

DIAGNOSIS
Consideration of the history and clinical signs will narrow the diagnosis down and appropriate laboratory tests will rule out infectious agents. Surgical exploration and contrast radiography may be indicated in cases of deep penetration or migration. Biochemical investigation of renal and hepatic and endocrine function may be indicated if an endogenous foreign body suggests metastatic calcification or urate deposition.

MANAGEMENT
Drainage, plus débridement if indicated, for exogenous foreign bodies[1]. It must be appreciated that pieces of vegetation (particularly grass awns) may migrate from one body cavity to the next, which makes exploration of the tracts a potentially major piece of surgery. Systemic antibacterial treatment is indicated in most cases. Endogenous foreign bodies usually mandate medical management rather than simple surgical removal, although this may play a part.

KEY POINT
- Most cases are straightforward, but be prepared for the complicated one.

Foreign Body Sinus

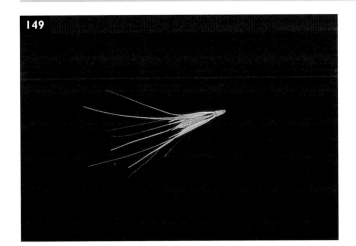

149   Foxtail.

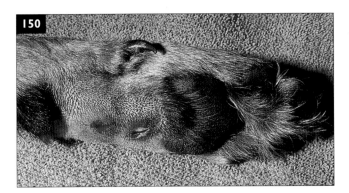

150   Foreign body sinus. Note the swollen, erythematous margins around the tracts.

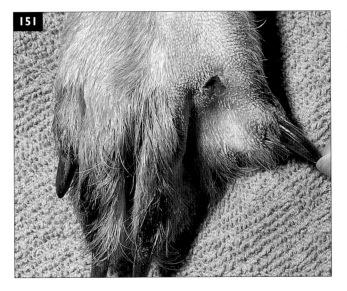

151   Foreign body penetration in the interdigital region due to a foxtail.

Atypical Mycobacterial Infections

DEFINITION
Cutaneous infection with mycobacteria of the atypical (Runyon's Group IV) class, such as *Mycobacterium fortuitum, M. chelonei, M. phlei, M. smegmatis*, and *M. vaccae*.

ETIOLOGY AND PATHOGENESIS
Atypical mycobacteria are ubiquitous[1]. Cats are affected much more commonly than dogs[4], and most cases result from traumatic inoculation of the organism by bites and penetrating wounds[2,5]. However, the inguinal region is the most commonly affected site and this is not an area which is frequently traumatized during cat fights. Traumatic penetration by contaminated inanimate objects is most probably the cause in these cases[5].

CLINICAL FEATURES
Animals typically present with chronic nodules, draining tracts, and subcutaneous granulomas[2] (**152**). Most lesions in cats are on the ventral abdomen and around the base of the tail[5], and there are often multiple fistulas. The affected areas may be markedly firm on palpation[5]. Systemic signs are minimal; pain and lymphadenopathy are variable[2].

DIFFERENTIAL DIAGNOSES
- Penetrating foreign body
- Demodicosis
- Panniculitis
- Feline leprosy
- Nocardiosis
- Subcutaneous and deep mycoses
- Cuterebriasis or dracunculiasis
- Neoplasia

DIAGNOSTIC TESTS
Clinical suspicion may be raised by the chronic history, resistance to systemic antibacterial agents, and failure to demonstrate a foreign body. Culture and sensitivity testing is feasible, but laboratories must be advised to test for atypical mycobacteria. Histopathologic examination of excised tissue may be diagnostic if special stains are utilized, although organisms may not always be seen[2]. Cats should be screened for immunosuppressive viral infections such as FeLV or FIV.

MANAGEMENT
Surgical excision or debulking, in combination with systemic antibacterial treatment, offers the best chance of success. Antibacterial treatment should be based on sensitivity testing, but agents such as potentiated sulfonamides, amikacin, gentamycin, kanamycin, and enrofloxacin may be indicated[2,4,5]. The susceptibility of the organisms to antibacterial agents varies from species to species, with *M. smegmatis* being most sensitive, even to doxycycline, *M. fortuitum* being sensitive only to amikacin and fluoroquinolones, while *M. chelonae* is often sensitive only to amikacin[3]. Cases may go into remission with treatment, only to relapse when it is withdrawn, and a very guarded prognosis is warranted.

KEY POINT
- Much more common in some countries than others. Local knowledge is important.

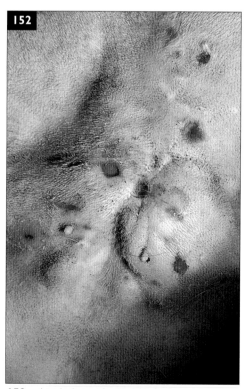

152 Atypical mycobacterial infection. Pyogranulomatous panniculitis in the groins and ventral abdomen due to *Mycobacterium smegmatis*.

Feline Leprosy

DEFINITION
Feline leprosy is a cutaneous infection caused by infection with *Mycobacterium lepraemurium*.

ETIOLOGY AND PATHOGENESIS
The causal agent, *M. lepraemurium*, is inoculated by bites. The seasonal nature of cases – most occur during the autumn and winter – and the knowledge that arthropods can transmit mycobacteria has been interpreted as suggesting an insect vector[1]. The natural host is unknown. The immune status of the cat, and the type of host response to the bacilli, dictates the clinical course and the signs of the disease[1,2].

CLINICAL FEATURES
There are regional differences in the seasonal frequency of feline leprosy, although the occurrence of the disease is worldwide[1,2]. Young adult cats are predisposed[2]. The most frequent sites for lesions to occur are the head and limbs. Clinical signs vary, with single or multiple cutaneous nodules being apparent (**153**), which may or may not ulcerate[2]. Occasionally, local lymphadenopathy is noted.

DIFFERENTIAL DIAGNOSES
- Penetrating foreign body
- Demodicosis
- Panniculitis
- Nocardiosis
- Subcutaneous and deep mycoses
- Cuterebriasis or dracunculiasis
- Neoplasia

DIAGNOSTIC TESTS
Diagnosis is made on the basis of histopathologic observation of a granulomatous response in association with the presence of acid-fast bacilli[2], and on culture.

MANAGEMENT
Clofazimine has been reported as useful in the management of feline leprosy[3]. A course of this antibacterial drug (8 mg/kg/day for 6 weeks and then twice weekly for 6 weeks, or 2–3 mg/kg/day for 5–8 months) was reported to induce remission in three cats[3].

KEY POINT
- An ubiquitous but rare infection.

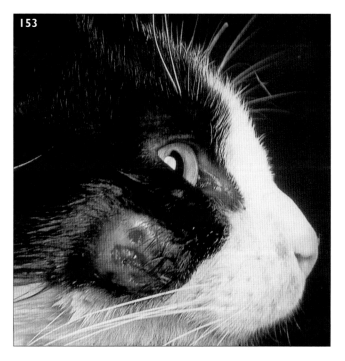

153   Feline leprosy. A discrete, erythematous nodule on the lateral aspect of the face of a cat.

Dermoid Sinus

DEFINITION
Dermoid sinus results from a persistent congenital connection between the dura and the skin of the dorsal midline.

ETIOLOGY AND PATHOGENESIS
Dermoid sinus results from incomplete separation of the ectoderm and the neural tube during embryogenesis[1]. The defect is congenital. The sinus usually passes from the dura to the skin of the dorsal midline by way of the interarcuate ligaments[1], but may sometimes pass through a defect in the dorsal arch[2]. Accumulation of keratinaceous debris and sebum may result in an inflammatory process. Bacterial infection may occur within the tract. Neurologic signs may accompany inflammation or infection.

CLINICAL FEATURES
There is no sex predisposition, but Rhodesian Ridgebacks are predisposed[1,3]. Rarely, other breeds may be affected, such as Boxers, Shih Tzus, and Yorkshire Terriers[2,4]. The clinical signs may be minimal – a whorl of hair in the dorsal midline, for example. Sometimes, hairs or even discharge may be apparent emerging from the sinus (**154**). Neurologic signs may be dramatic[2].

DIFFERENTIAL DIAGNOSES
- Foreign body penetration
- Injection reaction

DIAGNOSIS
The clinical signs are very suggestive. Radiography and contrast radiography may be necessary to delineate the sinus tract and define the diagnosis.

MANAGEMENT
Surgical excision of the tract and associated debris is the treatment of choice.

KEY POINT
- Pathognomonic presentation in Rhodesian Ridgeback.

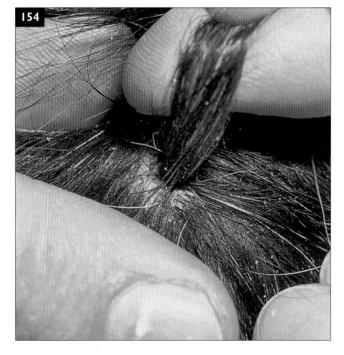

154 Dermoid sinus. A discrete tuft of hair is plainly visible emerging from the sinus in the dorsal midline.

Blastomycosis

DEFINITION
Blastomycosis is a systemic fungal disease caused by the dimorphic fungus *Blastomyces dermatitidis*.

ETIOLOGY AND PATHOGENESIS
Blastomycosis primarily occurs in North America with an endemic region that includes areas of the eastern seaboard, southern Canada, the Great Lakes region, and the Mississippi, Missouri, Ohio, and St. Lawrence river valleys[1,2]. Soil, especially sandy, acid soil near river valleys and impoundments, serves as the reservoir for the mycelial phase of the organism[3]. The major mode of transmission of *B. dermatitidis* is believed to be inhalation of spores from mycelial growth in the soil[4]. High humidity and/or fog is thought to facilitate transmission by aerosolizing and carrying spores to the host[4]. Spores are deposited in the alveoli, where they are phagocytized by macrophages and then transform from the mycelial phase to the yeast phase and further replicate[2]. The infection may be contained within the lung and its associated lymph nodes if the host immune system mounts an appropriate response. If not, dissemination will occur via hematogenous or lymphatic routes to other organ systems, such as cutaneous, ocular, skeletal, urogenital, and CNS[2].

CLINICAL FEATURES
Large breed, male dogs that are 2–4 years of age, living near river valleys or lakes in endemic areas, are predisposed[4]. Late summer and early autumn have been found to be periods of higher risk for infection[4]. Clinical signs vary depending on the length of infection and which organ systems are involved. Clinical features in decreasing order of occurrence are anorexia 72%, lethargy 70%, shortness of breath 60%, chronic cough 58%, weight loss 58%, skin lesions 40%, ocular lesions 40%, lameness 20%, and seizures 2%[1,2,3]. Skin lesions are generally multiple but, occasionally, will be single. They may appear as small abscesses which drain with the formation of ulcers and fistulous tracts (**155**), or they may appear granulomatous and proliferative. Exudates from within abscesses or from draining tracts may be either serosanguineous or purulent.

Blastomycosis is very rare in the cat and most reported cases have had disseminated lesions. Respiratory, cutaneous, ocular, and CNS signs have been reported[2].

DIFFERENTIAL DIAGNOSES
- Cryptococcosis
- Cutaneous infections of other opportunistic fungi and algae
- Sporotrichosis
- Demodectic mange with secondary pyoderma
- Opportunistic mycobacterial infection
- Cutaneous histiocytosis
- Neoplasia

DIAGNOSTIC TESTS
Impression smears and aspirates will result in demonstration of the organism (5–20 μm, broad-based, budding yeast with a thick, refractile, double-contoured cell wall) in 84% of cases[2]. Histopathologic examination of biopsy samples is diagnostic. Serologic techniques may also be used to aid the diagnosis. Agar gel immunodiffusion has a sensitivity and specificity in the dog of over 90% and is the serologic test most frequently used[2]. Recently an ELISA has been developed which has a sensitivity of 100% and a specificity of 97%[1].

MANAGEMENT
Itraconazole (5 mg/kg PO q 12 h) for 4 days then q 24 h for 30 days beyond clinical resolution of lesions[5]. Most cases will require 90–120 days of therapy. Cats are treated q 12 h as they do not seem to absorb the drug as well as dogs[5]. Itraconazole is as effective as amphotericin B alone, amphotericin B plus ketoconazole, or ketoconazole alone, and is less toxic[5].

KEY POINT
- Rare dermatosis which mandates aggressive treatment.

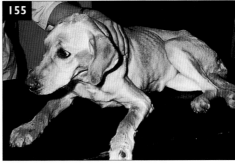

155 Blastomycosis. Note the emaciated condition of this dog. A discharging sinus is visible on the left foot.

Subcutaneous Mycoses

DEFINITION
Subcutaneous mycoses occur as a consequence of the local inoculation of saprophytic fungi.

ETIOLOGY AND PATHOGENESIS
Contamination of penetrating wounds is thought to account for the majority of these cases[2]. Infections are usually localized by the host response which results in a granuloma. Causative agents include *Sporothrix schenckii*, *Prototheca* spp., members of the Class Phaeohyphomycoses such as *Drechslera spicifera*, and members of the Class Mucoraceae such as *Mucor* spp. and *Rhizopus* spp.[1].

CLINICAL FEATURES
Chronic, non-responsive localized (**156**) or generalized nodules and thickening associated with shallow ulcers or fistulas are characteristic of the subcutaneous mycoses[1-5]. They may spread locally, along lymphatics[3]. Systemic dissemination is unusual but if it occurs, respiratory or GI signs may occur, accompanied by signs of pain and weight loss.

DIFFERENTIAL DIAGNOSES
• Penetrating foreign body
• Demodicosis
• Panniculitis
• Feline leprosy and atypical mycobacterial infection
• Nocardiosis
• Deep mycoses
• Cuterebriasis or dracunculiasis
• Neoplasia

DIAGNOSTIC TESTS
Clinical history of a refractory draining tract will raise suspicion. Cytologic examination of exudate may, in some circumstances, reveal organisms (for example, *Prototheca* spp., *D. spicfera*, and the Phycomycetes), but histopathologic examination of excised tissue and appropriate culture will give a definitive diagnosis.

MANAGEMENT
Sodium iodide (1 ml of 20% solution/4.5 kg PO q 12 h) is the treatment of choice for sporotrichosis[1,3]. Complete surgical excision is advocated for the other subcutaneous mycoses, followed by amphotericin B for the actinomycetes[1]. A guarded prognosis should be given. Itraconazole (10 mg/kg PO q 24 h) has been effective in the management of *D. spicifera*.

KEY POINT
• Rare dermatosis which mandates aggressive treatment.

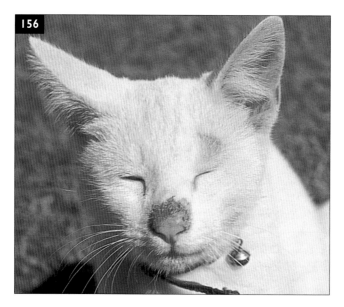

156

156 Sporotrichosis. Discrete erythematous nodule on the face of a cat with *Sprorothrix schenckii* infection following foreign body inoculation.

Diseases Characterized by Crust and Scale

GENERAL APPROACH

1 This group of diseases is characterized by secondary lesions – crust and scale.
2 The list of differential diagnoses could be huge – try and limit the investigation to the diseases most commonly seen.
3 When faced with a large list of differential diagnoses, at least in the early stages of the work up, it is helpful to consider broad groups of diseases, rather than specific differentials, i.e. could this disease be due to:
   - ectoparasites
   - infections
   - nutritional or congenital disorders
   - allergic diseases
   - immune-mediated diseases
   - other disorders.

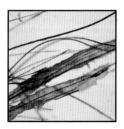
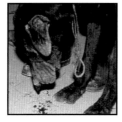
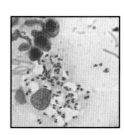
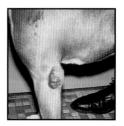

Callus Formation

DEFINITION
A callus is a defined area of hyperkeratosis, which is sometimes lichenified and typically occurs over bony pressure points.

ETIOLOGY AND PATHOGENESIS
The hyperkeratosis and thickening of the skin are due to irritation, and result from frictional contact with a hard surface on the exterior of the skin and pressure from an underlying bony prominence.

CLINICAL FEATURES
Callus development occurs more frequently in large, short-haired breeds that sleep on hard surfaces, such as concrete, wood, brick, or rock. Lesions usually develop on the lateral aspect of the elbows or hocks (**157**). They may also develop on the sternum of deep-chested dogs or dogs with short legs in which the sternum may continually contact objects such as stairs. Callosities appear as focal areas of alopecia and hyperkeratosis with a light gray surface. Entrapment of hair and/or sebum in a callus may result in a foreign body reaction with draining tracts and secondary infection (**158**).

DIFFERENTIAL DIAGNOSES
- Demodicosis
- Neoplasia
- Dermatophytosis
- Deep pyoderma
- Zinc responsive dermatosis

DIAGNOSTIC TESTS
Diagnosis is generally based on the history and clinical features.

MANAGEMENT
The animal's sleeping habits should be modified so that it rests on soft bedding material, such as foam rubber padding. Callus size may be reduced by daily application of a preparation containing 6.6% salicylic acid, 5% sodium lactate, and 5% urea, which promotes desquamation of the stratum corneum. Twice daily treatment with flucinolone acetonide in dimethyl sulfoxide hastens the process by reducing inflammation and decreasing basal cell turnover rates.

If callus formation is present, then systemic treatment with bactericidal antibacterial agents is indicated, based on culture and sensitivity testing. Treatment should be continued until the lesions have resolved and this may take many weeks.

KEY POINT
- Management is a key issue in the control of this problem.

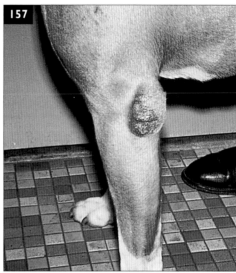

157 Elbow callus. Large, pigmented, deeply convoluted lesions on the lateral aspect of elbows are typical of callus.

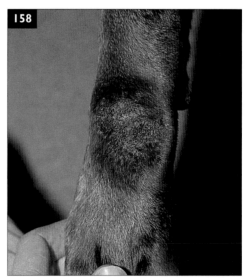

158 Callus pyoderma overlying the hock of a Bull Terrier.

Sebaceous Adenitis

DEFINITION

Sebaceous adenitis is an uncommon disease of dogs characterized by a thinning of the hair coat and increased adherent scale formation.

ETIOLOGY AND PATHOGENESIS

The etiology and pathogenesis are unknown. In Standard Poodles the disease is hereditary and appears to be autosomal recessive in transmission[1]. Theories concerning pathogenesis include either an autoimmune response to sebaceous gland antigens, or a primary structural defect of the sebaceous gland or its duct, which allows the leakage of sebum into the dermis where it provokes a foreign body reaction[1]. During the early stages of the disease, a mild perifolliculitis is present. Later, a nodular granulomatous inflammatory reaction occurs around the sebaceous gland, which results in its destruction. End-stage follicles evidence a parafollicular fibrosis, which is often accompanied by keratin plugging of the follicular infundibula. It is not known if there is a causal relationship between the sebaceous gland changes and the abnormal follicular keratinization, or if these are simply coexisting features of a common inheritable process[2]. Alopecia associated with sebaceous gland adenitis is thought to be a consequence of the parafollicular fibrosis interfering with stem cells of the follicle[1].

CLINICAL FEATURES

Sebaceous gland adenitis occurs in young-adult to middle-aged dogs, with no sex predilection. There is a breed predilection for Standard Poodles, Akitas, Hungarian Vizslas, and Samoyeds[1–3]. However, the disease has also been reported in the Airedale, American Eskimo Dog, Cocker Spaniel, Rough Collie, Miniature Dachshund, Dalmation, Doberman Pinscher, German Shepherd Dog, Golden Retriever, Hovawart, Irish Setter, Labrador Retriever, Lhasa Apso, Maltese Terrier, Miniature Pinscher, Miniature Poodle, Old English Sheepdog, Pomeranian, Scottish Terrier, Shih Tzu, Springer Spaniel, St Bernard, Toy Poodle, and Weimaraner[1]. Appearance, distribution, and severity of lesions varies from breed to breed, and from animal to animal within a breed.

In Standard Poodles the first signs of clinical disease generally appear in young-adult to middle-aged animals, and 90% of affected animals are between 1.5 and 5 years of age[1]. Lesions first start on the top of the neck, head, back, or ears. Initially, they appear as scaling and thinning of the hair or focal areas of alopecia. There are usually prominent follicular casts – tightly adherent follicular debris around the base of the hair shaft (**159**). As the condition progresses, more areas of skin become involved, and severe scaling with characteristic tightly adherent silver-white scales

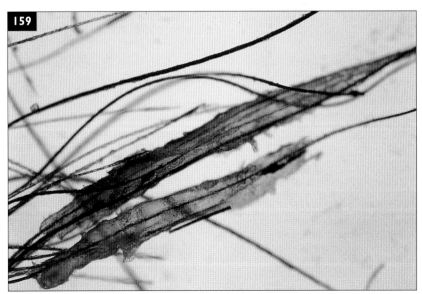

159 Follicular casts on hair shafts. These are evidence of abnormal function in the hair canal.

Sebaceous Adenitis

incorporating small tufts of matted hair appear (**160, 161**). This is accompanied by a further thinning of the coat in involved areas. In severe cases a secondary bacterial folliculitis may develop. Samoyeds have lesions similar to Standard Poodles, except that the scale tends to build up into plaque-like lesions[2].

Akitas exhibit scaling similar to Standard Poodles, but often have a more extensive alopecia, seborrhea, and superficial bacterial folliculitis or deep bacterial folliculitis and furunculosis. They may also manifest systemic signs of malaise, fever, and weight loss[2].

Hungarian Vizslas and other short-coated breeds have clinical signs that are initially characterized by multifocal annular and serpiginous areas of alopecia and fine white scaling that occur progressively over the head, ears, and trunk[2,3].

DIFFERENTIAL DIAGNOSES
- Vitamin A responsive dermatitis
- Dermatophytosis
- Demodicosis
- Superficial pyoderma
- Zinc responsive dermatosis
- Endocrinopathies
- Color dilute alopecia
- Epitheliotropic lymphoma

DIAGNOSTIC TESTS
Histopathologic examination of skin biopsies reveals a multifocal inflammatory infiltrate of histiocytes, lymphocytes, neutrophils, and plasma cells around the sebaceous glands and other adnexal structures in early disease[1–3]. Advanced cases will have moderate acanthosis, hyperkeratosis, follicular keratosis, and absence of sebaceous glands[2,3].

MANAGEMENT
Therapy is palliative and response to various medications is variable. Early or mild cases may be helped by keratolytic shampoos, emollient rinses, and omega-3 and omega-6 fatty acid dietary supplements[4]. More severe or advanced cases may be helped by spraying or rinsing daily or every 2–3 days with a mixture of 50–75% propylene glycol in water. The synthetic retinoids isotretinoin or etretinate (1–2 mg/kg PO q 24 h) may result in improvement in some cases[3,4]. Hungarian Vizslas have a better response to isotretinoin than other breeds. Cyclosporine (5 mg/kg PO q 12 h) has been reported to help some animals that have not been responsive to the retinoids[5].

The use of systemic glucocorticoid agents, such as prednisolone, at anti-inflammatory doses (0.5–0.7 mg/kg PO q 12 h) may be of value if cases are diagnosed early. Once the follicular damage has occurred and the inflammatory reaction has ameliorated, they are of less value.

As sebaceous adenitis in Standard Poodles is a genetic disease, its prevalence can be decreased by identifying and not breeding animals who are carriers or who are affected with the disease. To assist owners and breeders in identification of both normal and affected animals, the Sebaceous Adenitis Registry for Standard Poodles has been established. Current information about this can be obtained by contacting the Institute for Genetic Disease Control, P.O. Box 222, Davis, CA 95617, USA.

KEY POINTS
- Diagnosis is only made by histopathologic examination of multiple (more than 5) biopsy samples.
- Management involves considerable effort, and good client communication is imperative.

Sebaceous Adenitis

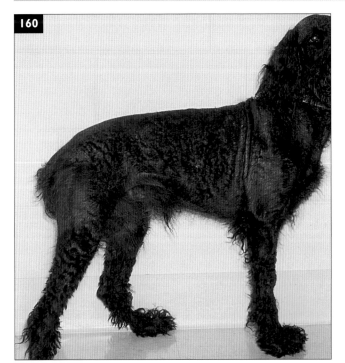

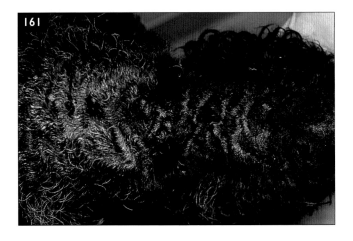

160, 161   Sebaceous adenitis. Note the patchy alopecia and scale.

Feline Acne

DEFINITION
Feline acne is a multifactorial skin disease characterized by comedo formation on the chin and lips.

ETIOLOGY AND PATHOGENESIS
Feline acne may be idiopathic or the condition may develop due to multiple factors that result in a localized keratinization defect of hair follicles and hyperplasia of the sebaceous glands. Diseases and conditions which may predispose to the development of acne include demodicosis, dermatophytosis, virus infections (FeLV or FIV and upper respiratory viruses), irritant contact dermatitis, atopic dermatitis, and stress of moving to a new location[1]. The hair follicles become distended with lipid and keratinous debris, resulting in the classic comedones (blackheads) of acne. If these follicles rupture and release keratin and sebaceous material into the dermis, a foreign body reaction with inflammation will develop. Many bacteria are often found in the follicular plugs and their presence can lead to infection and further inflammation.

CLINICAL FEATURES
Feline acne can occur in cats of any age and there is no breed or sex predisposition[2]. Lesions generally occur on the lower lips, chin, and occasionally the upper lips. Comedones, especially around the lateral commissures of the mouth and the lower lip, are the predominant findings (**162**). Initially, these lesions are not pruritic, but they may be noticed by the owner. If the condition progresses, erythematous crusted papules, folliculitis, and furunculosis may develop which can result in pruritus and scarring. Alopecia, erythema, and swelling of the chin is seen in severe cases[1,2]. In Persian cats the lesion may affect the face as well as the chin (**163**). Excoriations from scratching may occur in cases with severe inflammation. When secondary bacterial infections are present, *Pasteurella multocida*, β-hemolytic streptococci, and coagulase-positive *Staphylococcus* spp. have been isolated[1].

DIFFERENTIAL DIAGNOSES
• Contact dermatitis
• Eosinophilic granuloma
• Pyoderma
• *Malassezia* dermatitis
• Dermatophytosis
• Demodicosis
• Trauma
• Dietary intolerance
• Atopic dermatitis

DIAGNOSTIC TESTS
Microscopic examination of skin scrapings and impression smears of follicular plugs, dermatophyte culture, and bacterial culture and sensitivity will rule out infectious causes. Histopathologic examination of biopsy samples will confirm the diagnosis

MANAGEMENT
Clients should be forewarned that feline acne is a condition that generally is not cured, but just controlled with periodic or continuous treatment.

If there is an underlying predisposing condition, such as demodicosis or dermatophytosis, it should be addressed with specific treatment.

Treatment for idiopathic feline acne will vary with the type and severity of lesions. Small numbers of asymptomatic comedones may not require any treatment. Larger numbers of comedones with seborrhea and some swelling of the chin will benefit from the antibacterial and follicular flushing actions of alternate day or twice weekly benzoyl peroxide gel or shampoo. Benzoyl peroxide may be irritating to some cats and should be discontinued if erythema develops. This is less likely to happen if the concentration of the benzoyl peroxide is kept to 3% or less[1]. Alternative shampoos would be those containing ethyl lactate, sulfur-salicylic acid, and chlorhexidine.

If bacteria are found on impression smears, topical antibacterial preparations containing mupirocin may be helpful. If bacterial folliculitis or furunculosis is present, systemic antibiotics, such as clavulanated amoxicillin or cephalosporins, for 2–6 weeks would be appropriate.

The comedolytic activity of topical vitamin A products (0.05% retinoic acid cream) applied daily at first and then on alternate days or twice weekly has been beneficial in some cases[1]. This product may also cause irritation and its use should be monitored closely.

If there is severe inflammation resulting from a foreign body reaction to keratin and sebum of ruptured hair follicles, a course of systemic corticosteroids (prednisone, prednisolone, or methylprednisolone (1–2 mg/kg PO q 24 h)) for 10–14 days is indicated.

Isotretinoin (2 mg/kg PO q 24 h) has been advocated for the treatment and control of refractory cases[1]. It acts by decreasing the activity of sebaceous glands and normalising

Feline Acne

keratinization within hair follicles, and therapeutic benefits have been observed in 30% of treated cases. Clinical response should occur within 1 month[1]. Once improvement is seen, the isotretinoin dose may be reduced to twice weekly for control. Side-effects of its use in cats include conjunctivitis, periocular crusting, vomiting, and diarrhea[1]. Monthly laboratory screenings are suggested when it is used over prolonged periods[1]. It is *extremely teratogenic* and appropriate caution should be observed for both animals and humans.

KEY POINT
- Although apparently pathognomonic, the clinical signs may also reflect demodicosis or dermatophytosis. All cases should be subjected to skin scrapings and fungal culture.

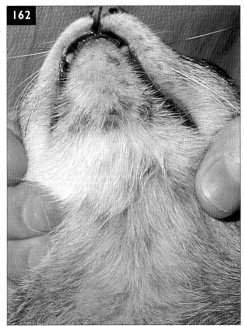

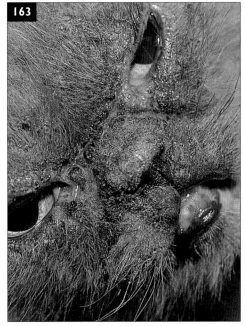

162 Feline acne. Characteristic appearance of multiple comedones on the rostral aspect of the mandible.

163 Persian cat with severe lesions of feline acne affecting the rostral chin and face.

Idiopathic Seborrhea of Cocker Spaniels

DEFINITION
Idiopathic seborrhea in Cocker Spaniels is a common, possibly familial, dermatosis associated with abnormal basal epidermal cell kinetics.

ETIOLOGY AND PATHOGENESIS
Compared with normal dogs, basal epidermal cells of the epithelium and hair follicle of affected dogs undergo accelerated cellular kinetics[1–3]. Specifically, there is an increase in the proliferative pool of actively dividing basal cells, a shortened cell cycle, and an increased transit time between basal layer and granulosa. The hair follicle and sebaceous gland are similarly affected. The result is an increase in cell turnover which is characterized by shedding of variable-sized rafts of adherent squames in conjunction with a variable degree of oiliness and alopecia. Secondary pyoderma and *Malassezia pachydermatis* dermatitis are common complications.

CLINICAL FEATURES
Most animals display some clinical signs of abnormal keratinization from an early age. There may be a spectrum of signs which vary from individual to individual. Mildly affected dogs exhibit an increase in retention of greasy scale around the nipples, in the lip folds, and in the external ear canals. More severely affected animals exhibit lesions in the skin folds of the neck and may develop lesions on the trunk. Severely affected dogs are malodorous, greasy, alopecic, and pruritic with a papular scaling and occasionally crusting dermatosis (**164, 165**). Overt otitis externa is common.

DIFFERENTIAL DIAGNOSES
- Dietary deficiency
- Ectoparasite infestation
- Atopy
- Pyoderma
- *Malassezia pachydermatis* infection
- Dietary intolerance
- Hypersensitivities
- Endocrinopathies

DIAGNOSTIC TESTS
Diagnosis of the disease is based on history and ruling out all other causes of the dermatosis[4,5]. The history of some degree of skin disease or recurrent otitis externa from an early age is suggestive. Details of management should identify idiosyncratic and potentially deficient diets. Skin scrapes and tape strips will reveal ectoparasites, secondary bacteria, and *M. pachydermatis*. Trial therapy with systemic antibacterial agents will help to assess the degree of pyoderma. Restricted diets and intradermal skin testing will rule out hypersensitivities. Dynamic endocrine testing to assess thyroid and adrenal status may be indicated.

MANAGEMENT
Failure to identify a definitive cause condemns the animal to a lifetime of symptomatic therapy. Every effort must be made to identify an underlying disease. Management of the idiopathic disease in Cocker Spaniels has traditionally been based around the use of tar and salicylic acid shampoo 2–3 times per week to remove crust and scale, degrease the skin, and suppress keratinization[4,5]. Aggressive control of fleas, suppressing secondary pyoderma, and treating the otitis externa are also important[4,5].

Just as in other complex diseases, the management of this condition must be tailored to the individual and topical therapeutics are useful. Clinicians should institute treatment with mild jupicol and wood tar-based shampoos. Gradually, if needed, more potent shampoo regimes may be utilized, typically in ascending order of decreasing keratolytic activity:

- Jupicol and wood tar shampoos
- Coal tar shampoos
- Sulfur, salicylic acid, and tar shampoos
- Benzoyl peroxide
- Selenium sulfide

Only if topical regimes fail should systemic treatment with glucocorticoids or retinoids be contemplated. Above all, remember to control pyoderma as staphylococcal infections may result in serious deterioration in these cases.

Recently, the role of *M. pachydermatis* in the symptomatology has been appreciated, and antimalassezial treatment is now an important part of the clinician's armamentarium. Oral sunflower oil (1.5 ml/kg PO q 24 h) may prove useful[6]. The use of synthetic derivatives of retinoic acid, particularly etretinate (1 mg/kg PO q 24 h), has been reported[7], and this form of treatment may be very useful in the future as a means of suppressing the accelerated cellular kinetics and associated defects in keratinization which underlie the condition.

KEY POINT
- A common condition – do not overdiagnose it.
- Try and avoid the use of systemic steroids in these cases.

Idiopathic Seborrhea of Cocker Spaniels

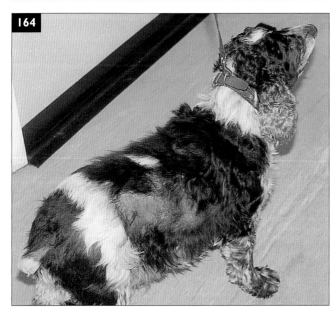

164, 165 Idiopathic defects in keratinization (primary seborrhea) are often accompanied by patches of alopecia and scale (**164**). These patches may be erythematous and pruritic, a sign often associated with *Malassezia pachydermatis* infection (**165**).

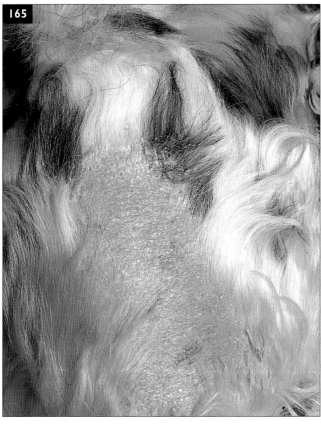

Actinic Dermatoses

DEFINITION
Actinic dermatosis is skin damage resulting from prolonged exposure to light in the wavelength 200–400 nm.

ETIOLOGY AND PATHOGENESIS
Ultraviolet light is divided into UV-A (320–400 nm) and UV-B (290–320 nm). UV-A penetrates into the deep dermis while UV-B penetrates only to the upper dermis[1]. Exposure to UV light results, progressively, in erythema, heat, edema, pain, and pruritus[1]. Chronic actinic cutaneous inflammation may result in inflammatory, locally proliferative lesions. Chronic exposure also may result in the induction of cutaneous tumor[1,2]. Chronic exposure to UV-B results in a progressive decrease in epidermal Langerhans cell numbers[2]. Reduced immune surveillance may result in local oncogenic changes escaping detection and resulting in neoplasia.

CLINICAL FEATURES
Both dogs and cats may be affected. Actinic lesions develop in lightly pigmented, lightly haired, or alopecic areas of the body, such as the face, lower flanks, and ventrum. The tips of the pinnae, above the hairline, are particularly susceptible (**166**) and in white-haired cats, actinic changes may be detected even in animals resident in Western Europe. There is local thickening and a fine scale develops. Scarring and curling of the distal pinnae may be noted and eventually an ulcerative, invasive squamous cell carcinoma develops. In areas of the world with very high levels of actinic radiation, cats may also develop lesions on the rhinarium.

In light-colored dogs the most common site of actinic radiation damage is the rostral face, immediately caudal to the planum nasale (**167**). There is erythema, fine scale, and progressive alopecia. There may be loss of pigmentation and scarring. In dogs which habitually sleep in the sun, lesions may develop on the lower flank, ventrum, scrotum, and limbs[3]. Many cases become secondarily infected with *Staphylococcus intermedius*.

DIFFERENTIAL DIAGNOSES
- Demodicosis
- Dermatophytosis
- Discoid lupus erythematosus
- Superficial pyoderma
- Pemphigus foliaceus or erythematosus
- Dermatomyositis
- Uveodermatologic syndrome
- Drug eruption
- Cutaneous neoplasia

DIAGNOSTIC TESTS
Local knowledge of climate and breeds at risk will greatly aid diagnosis. Observation that lightly pigmented skin is affected whereas adjacent pigmented skin is unaffected is very suggestive of an actinic dermatosis. Microscopic examination of skin scrapings will allow demodicosis to be ruled out. Fungal culture will allow dermatophytosis to be ruled out. Biopsy samples will reveal changes consistent with actinic dermatitis, such as superficial dermal fibrosis and follicular keratosis[3,4].

MANAGEMENT
Elimination of secondary pyoderma is important. Sun avoidance measures may be helpful, although they are difficult to institute for free-roaming cats. Local sun protection may be achieved with heavy T-shirts (fitted over the trunk) or PABA sun-blocking cream. Tattooing may be considered in some cases. In cats with pinnal lesions, the distal pinnae may be amputated to below the hair line as a preventive measure.

KEY POINT
- Treat these dermatoses seriously. Neoplastic transformation may occur.

Actinic Dermatoses

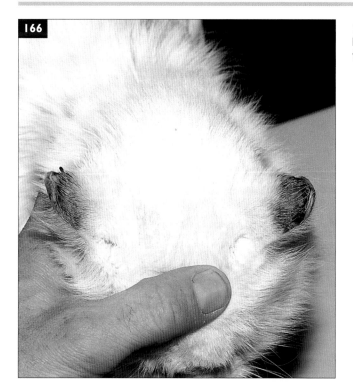

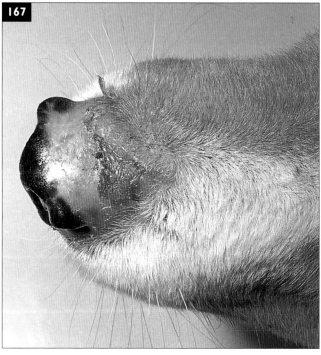

166, 167 Actinic dermatitis. Pinnal lesions in a cat (**166**) and facial lesions in a dog (**167**).

Leishmaniasis

DEFINITION
Canine leishmaniasis is a serious systemic disease with a diversity of clinical presentations resulting from an infection by a diphasic protozoan.

ETIOLOGY AND PATHOGENESIS
Leishmaniasis is epizootic in certain parts of the Mediterranean basin (Spain, Portugal, France, Italy, Greece, and northern Africa) as well as in southern Russia, India, China, and eastern Africa[1,2]. Although there are many species of *Leishmania* affecting both dogs and humans, the species primarily responsible for disease in these areas is *L. donovani*[2,3]. The disease is also epizootic in central and South America with *L. donovani* responsible for visceral lesions and *L. braziliensis* and *L. tropicana* resulting in infections characterized by small cutaneous nodules, ulcers, or mucocutaneous lesions[1,2]. Isolated outbreaks of the disease have also been reported in Oklahoma, Ohio, and Texas[1].

Leishmania spp. complete their life cycles in two hosts: a vertebrate (Carnivora, Rodentia, Edentsata) which acts as the reservoir, and an insect, the phlebotomine sand fly, which acts as the vector. The life cycle begins when a female fly feeds on an infected vertebrate host and ingests a small number of amastigotes. The amistigotes multiply and become flagellated promastigotes in the gut of the sand fly. The promastigotes migrate to the esophagus and pharynx of the insect attracted by chemotaxic substances in the fly's crop[4]. When a fly feeds on another vertebrate host, promastigotes that have become lodged in the proboscis are transferred. Once in the new host, the promastigotes lose their flagellae and again change into amastigotes, which are phagocytized by and multiply in cutaneous macrophages. Eventually, they reach high enough numbers that the cell bursts. Free organisms are again phagocytized by other macrophages, and the amastigotes, whether in the interior of the macrophages or free swimming, disseminate to bone marrow, skin, liver, pancreas, kidneys, adrenal glands, digestive tract, eyes, testes, bone, and joints[4]. Onset of clinical signs can vary from 1 month to 7 years[2]. The parasite causes tissue damage via means of two pathogenic mechanisms:
- The production of non-suppurative inflammatory granulomas, which are responsible for skin, hepatic, enteric, and osseous lesions.
- The production of circulating immune complexes that lodge in the blood vessels, renal glomeruli, and joints, resulting in vasculitis, glomerulonephritis, ocular lesions, and lameness.

CLINICAL FEATURES
Historically, affected dogs are noted to have one or more of the following, in decreasing order of incidence:
- Decreased endurance
- Weight loss
- Somnolence
- Polydipsia
- Anorexia
- Diarrhea
- Vomiting
- Polyphagia
- Epistaxis
- Melena
- Sneezing and coughing[2,4,5]

Skin lesions are one of the most frequently noted abnormalities on physical examination. Lesions that have been described include:
- Exfoliative dermatitis (**168, 169**)
- Ulcerations
- Onychogryposis
- Focal alopecia predominately on the head and pinnae
- Dry and dull hair coat
- Sterile pustular dermatitis
- Paronychia
- Diffuse erythema
- Nasal depigmentation
- Nasal and digital hyperkeratosis
- Nodules
- Erythematous plaques[3,4]

Other physical examination findings listed in decreasing order of incidence include:
- Lymphadenomegaly
- Cachexia
- Lameness
- Fever
- Conjunctivitis
- Enlarged spleen
- Rhinitis
- Keratitis
- Icterus
- Blepharitis
- Uveitis
- Panophthalmitis[2,4,5]

Leishmaniasis

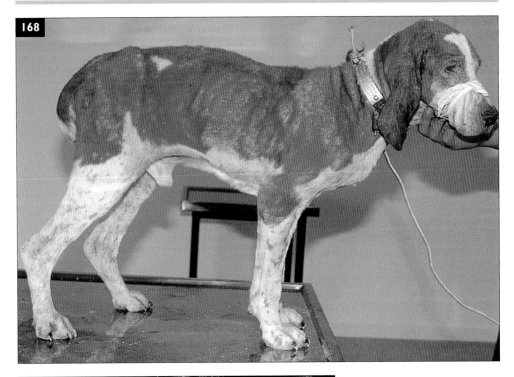

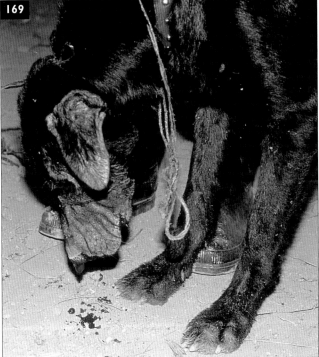

168, 169   Canine leishmaniasis. Emaciation is common (**168**). Hyperkeratosis and systemic disease are also features of leishmaniasis. Note the epistaxis in this dog (**169**).

Leishmaniasis

DIFFERENTIAL DIAGNOSES
- Pemphigus foliaceus
- Systemic lupus erythematosus
- Sebaceous adenitis
- Zinc responsive dermatitis
- Bacterial folliculitis
- Dermatophytosis
- Demodicosis
- Superficial necrolytic dermatitis
- Epitheliotropic lymphoma

DIAGNOSTIC TESTS
Clinical examination and the knowledge that the affected animal lives in, or has come from, an area where leishmaniasis is prevalent will raise clinical suspicion. Detection of organisms in the macrophages obtained via bone marrow or lymph node aspirates (**170**) will confirm the diagnosis, as will detection of organisms in liver or skin biopsies. Diagnosis can also be based on serologic techniques, such as complement fixation, IFA, direct hemagglutination, and ELISA methodology[2].

MANAGEMENT
Prior to initiation of treatment it must be determined if the health legislation of the country concerned permits treatment, as euthanasia of infected dogs is necessary in some countries. It is also important to determine if the patient's condition is such that it will allow for a reasonable chance of successful treatment.

At present, pentavalent antimonials, especially meglumine antimonate (100 mg/kg SC or IV) and sodium stibogluconate (10–50 mg/kg SC or IV), are considered the most effective drugs for the treatment of canine leishmaniasis[3,5]. (IM injections are not recommended as they may result in abscess formation and muscle fibrosis[2].) Dogs, are treated daily for 10–30 days or are given 2 or 3 courses of 10–15 days of therapy separated by 10–15 day intervals. Cases which do not have organ failure generally respond well with clearing of lesions within a few weeks. However, many cases relapse within a few months to 1 year and need to be retreated[5].

KEY POINTS
- A disease that is difficult to diagnose and to treat.
- Potentially zoonotic.

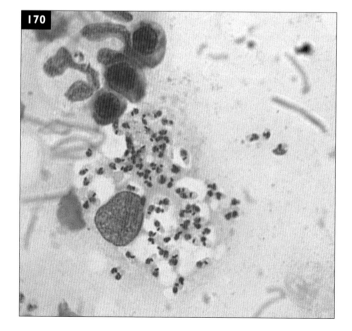

170   *Leishmania* organisms in a lymph node aspirate.

Cutaneous Horn

DEFINITION
Cutaneous horns are localized, benign outgrowths of horny tissue with the appearance of small horns.

ETIOLOGY AND PATHOGENESIS
The etiology of many cutaneous horns is unknown. In some cases they may be associated with underlying cutaneous neoplasia, follicular cysts, or papillomavirus infection. Multiple cutaneous horns have been reported in the cat, associated with FeLV infection[1].

CLINICAL FEATURES
Cutaneous horns are localized and non-pruritic (**171**). Multiple lesions may be seen in some individuals. In animals with long coats the horns may not be immediately apparent and it is not until they are groomed that the lesions are noticed. In cats, cutaneous horns may affect the footpads[1]. There is no breed, age, or sex incidence. The horn may be 3–5 cm (1.2–2.0 in) in length, firm to the touch, and not easily removed from the underlying skin. If pulled off, they tend to regrow.

DIFFERENTIAL DIAGNOSES
- Papilloma
- Crusted, ulcerative neoplasms
- Infundibular keratinizing acanthoma

DIAGNOSTIC TESTS
The clinical appearance of the lesion is pathognomonic. Affected cats should be screened for FeLV infection.

MANAGEMENT
Surgical excision is curative, although the horn and underlying tissue should be submitted for histopathologic examination in an attempt to identify any underlying cause.

KEY POINT
- Benign lesions which require removal.

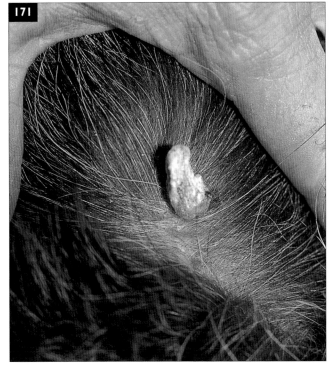

171 Cutaneous horn.

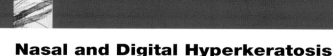

Nasal and Digital Hyperkeratosis

DEFINITION
Nasal hyperkeratosis is associated with excessive amounts of horny tissue confined to the planum nasale. Digital hyperkeratosis presents similarly and affects the footpads.

ETIOLOGY AND PATHOGENESIS
Hyperkeratosis occurs as a consequence of increased production of, or retention of, keratinized tissue. This abnormal keratinization may be the result of an inborn error of metabolism, as occurs in ichthyosis. Familial footpad hyperkeratosis has been reported in Dogues de Bordeaux[1].

Nasal and digital hyperkeratosis may occur in the same individual. Canine distemper virus infection may result in nasodigital hyperkeratosis and was very common, although it is seen less frequently now. Systemic disease, such as pemphigus foliaceus and dietary deficiency, in particular, zinc, may also result in pedal, nasal, or nasodigital hyperkeratosis. Spontaneous idiopathic disease, particularly of the older dog, is the most common clinical presentation.

CLINICAL FEATURES
Nasal hyperkeratosis is confined to the planum nasale and presents as a variably thickened, fissured accumulation of dry, horny tissue (**172**). Pedal hyperkeratosis is more variable in presentation (**173**, **174**). In old dogs with idiopathic disease, the periphery of the footpads is more severely affected and this pattern of hyperkeratosis is also seen in metabolic epidermal necrosis, although in the latter condition there are usually lesions elsewhere in addition to signs of systemic disease. Pemphigus foliaceus may result in footpad hyperkeratosis, and in some cases the pedal lesion may be the only signs of disease[2].

DIFFERENTIAL DIAGNOSES
- Canine distemper virus infection
- Pemphigus foliaceus
- Zinc responsive dermatosis
- Metabolic epidermal necrosis

DIAGNOSTIC TESTS
Consideration of the vaccinal history, and the risks of exposure to the virus, is particularly important *vis-à-vis* a diagnosis of canine distemper virus infection. Dietary history will raise suspicions of absolute or relative zinc deficiency, and consideration of the clinical signs and history will suggest the presence, or otherwise, of systemic disease. Ichthyosis is congenital. Histopathologic examination of biopsy samples is the most useful diagnostic tool.

MANAGEMENT
If a specific disease can be identified, then it should be managed accordingly. The management of idiopathic disease can be difficult because of the nature of the lesions and the tendency of the animal to lick topically applied agents. Local application of keratolytic and keratoplastic agents, such as preparations containing 60% salicyclic acid, 5% urea, and 5% sodium lactate, may be of value, as may application of petroleum jelly[3]. Topical application of 50% propylene glycol may also be useful in more severe cases[1]. Topical tretinoin gel may also be of value in severe cases[4]. The fissures in the hyperkeratotic tissue may become infected and in these cases, systemic glucocorticoid and antibacterial treatment will be necessary.

KEY POINT
- A frustrating disease to manage.

Nasal and Digital Hyperkeratosis

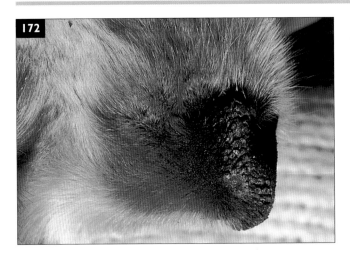

172   Nasal hyperkeratosis in a Cocker Spaniel.

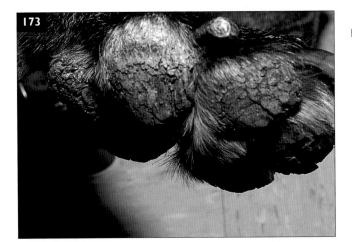

173, 174   Digital hyperkeratosis.

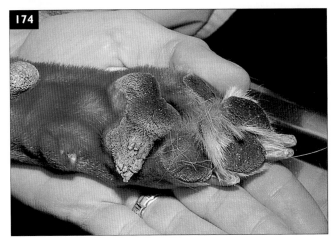

Vitamin A Responsive Dermatosis

DEFINITION
Vitamin A responsive dermatosis is a rare dermatosis characterized by epidermal hyperkeratosis and markedly disproportionate follicular hyperkeratosis.

ETIOLOGY AND PATHOGENESIS
The etiology of the dermatosis is not known. Retinoic acid is essential for a wide range of cell and tissue functions, but its cutaneous role is particularly directed towards the proliferation and differentiation of keratinocytes where it regulates the expression of keratins[1]. However, even though the clinical signs resolve with vitamin A supplementation, there is no evidence that affected animals are fed diets deficient in vitamin A.

CLINICAL FEATURES
The dermatosis is almost entirely confined to Cocker Spaniels[2]. The clinical signs usually begin between 2 and 5 years of age. Animals exhibit a generalized scaling of gradually deteriorating severity. Pruritus and a malodorous skin are common complaints[2]. Animals also exhibit focal, frond-like, often erythematous, crusted plaques, particularly on the lateral thorax and ventrum (**175**).

DIFFERENTIAL DIAGNOSES
- Scabies
- Flea bite hypersensitivity
- Atopy
- Dietary intolerance
- Idiopathic defects in keratinization

DIAGNOSTIC TESTS
Although the clinical and historical features of the dermatosis might suggest vitamin A responsive dermatosis, the diagnosis can be confirmed on the basis of histopathologic examination of biopsy samples.

MANAGEMENT
The dermatosis responds to oral medication with vitamin A (10,000 units) daily[2]. Clinical signs resolve within 4–6 weeks, and affected dogs may be maintained in remission provided daily supplementation is continued.

KEY POINT
- A rare dermatosis ultimately diagnosed by response to supplementary vitamin A.

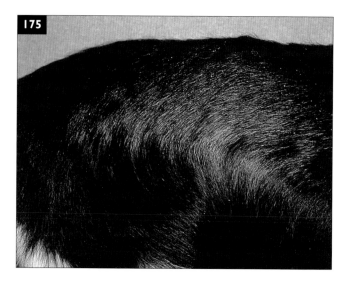

175 Vitamin A responsive dermatosis. Alopecia and focal accumulations of scale are typical of this condition.

Canine Distemper

DEFINITION
Canine distemper is a systemic viral condition that may cause skin lesions in addition to those in internal organs.

ETIOLOGY AND PATHOGENESIS
The causal agent is a paramyxovirus which is transmitted in infected droplets and aerosol from infected animals. Viral multiplication occurs in lymphoid tissue before dissemination to other tissues.

CLINICAL FEATURES
The prominent clinical signs of this condition are systemic illness associated with the respiratory, GI, and central nervous systems. Some dogs may develop an erythematous papulopustular dermatitis on the ventral abdomen during this acute stage. Nasal and footpad hyperkeratosis may develop in some animals. Due to this hyperkeratosis, the footpads become progressively harder, flattened, and smooth (**176**). If the animal recovers from the disease, the footpad lesions will generally resolve while the nasal hyperkeratosis remains.

DIFFERENTIAL DIAGNOSES
- Idiopathic nasal digital hyperkeratosis
- Pemphigus foliaceus
- Vitamin A responsive dermatosis
- Zinc responsive dermatosis
- Lethal acrodermatitis of Bull Terriers
- Superficial necrolytic dermatitis

DIAGNOSTIC TESTS
The diagnosis of canine distemper is based on history and clinical findings. As the clinical signs of canine distemper can be quite vague and varied, the changes in the pads may serve as a diagnostic aid.

MANAGEMENT
No specific treatment, other than supportive care, is available.

KEY POINT
- Controlled with vaccination.

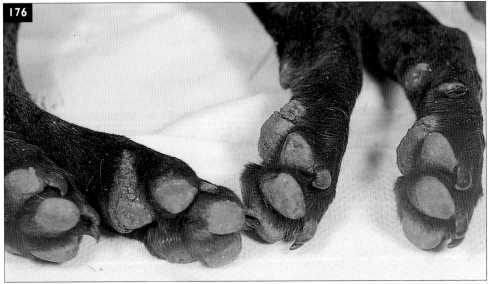

176 Canine distemper virus infection. Digital hyperkeratosis of all the footpads.

Erythema Multiforme

DEFINITION
Erythema multiforme is a rare, immune-mediated dermatosis with an unpredictable clinical manifestation[1].

ETIOLOGY AND PATHOGENESIS
The immune-mediated hypersensitivity may occur in association with infections or neoplasia, although most reports describe drug eruption, particularly to sulfonamides[1-4]. Lesions are associated with the deposition of immunoglobulin and complement with cellular destruction by cytotoxic lymphocytes[1]. The disease presents in two forms, erythema multiforme major and minor[1]. The more serious form is associated with signs of systemic disease and, often, extensive ulceration, whereas the minor variant is rarely associated with either systemic signs or ulceration[1].

CLINICAL FEATURES
Unless there are extensive ulcerations, the clinical signs of erythema multiforme often are present for days or weeks before a definitive diagnosis is made. Lesions of erythema multiforme minor have included erythematous macules, papules, plaques, wheals, and ulcers, often arranged in annular, arcuate, or polycyclic shapes[2] (**177**). Erythema multiforme major typically presents as a vesiculobullous disorder with extensive erosions, crusting, and even depigmentation[3,4].

DIFFERENTIAL DIAGNOSES
• Superficial and deep pyoderma
• Superficial and deep mycoses
• Demodicosis
• Pemphigus foliaceus and vulgaris
• Bullous pemphigoid
• Drug eruption
• Systemic lupus erythematosus
• Epitheliotropic lymphoma

DIAGNOSTIC TESTS
Clinical history and physical examination may suggest the diagnosis, but histopathologic examination of biopsy samples provides the definitive diagnosis[2].

MANAGEMENT
If the source of the offending antigen can be identified and removed, then erythema multiforme minor has a fair prognosis and most cases improve[2]. In severe cases, intravenous fluid therapy may be necessary in order to combat dehydration and shock. Every effort must be made to identify an underlying disease and the importance of drug eruption cannot be overemphasized.

KEY POINT
• Drug eruption is the most common cause of this condition.

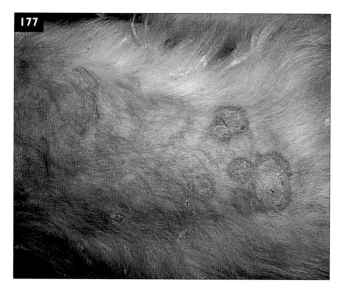

177 Erythema multiforme. Multiple papules, crusts, and erosions.

Pigmentary Abnormalities

GENERAL APPROACH
1 Many of the conditions are associated with permanent pigmentary disturbances.
2 Diagnosis can be difficult and treatment unrewarding.

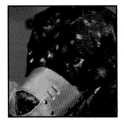
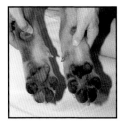
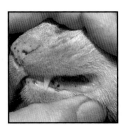
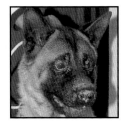

Color-dilution Alopecia

(Color-mutant Alopecia, Blue Doberman Syndrome)

DEFINITION
Color-dilution alopecia is an inherited disorder of color-diluted dogs characterized by alopecia developing in the areas of the dilute-colored hair.

ETIOLOGY AND PATHOGENESIS
Color-dilution alopecia is thought to occur because of changes in genes in the D locus[1,2]. As some animals with color dilution do not develop the condition, there appear to be other alleles or factors responsible[1-3]. Affected animals have many large, irregularly shaped melanin granules in the basal keratinocytes, hair matrix cells, and the hair shafts[1,3]. It has been suggested that hair matrix cells are affected by the cytotoxic effects of melanin precursors, which results in cessation of hair growth and, eventually, follicular dysplasia[1]. The extensive melanin clumping in hair and associated distortion of the cuticular-cortical structure of the hair are thought to lead to fragility and breaking of hair shafts at these sites[3].

CLINICAL FEATURES
Color-dilution alopecia has been diagnosed mainly in Blue Doberman Pinschers leading to the early name of Blue Doberman syndrome. However, the syndrome has also been diagnosed in other breeds with blue color dilution, including the Dachshund, Great Dane, Whippet, Italian Greyhound, Chow Chow, Standard Poodle, Yorkshire Terrier, Miniature Pinscher, Chihuahua, Bernese Mountain Dog, Shetland Sheepdog, Schipperke, Silky Terrier, Boston Terrier, Saluki, Newfoundland, and mixed-breed dogs[1,2,4]. The syndrome has also been diagnosed in the Fawn Doberman Pinscher, Fawn Irish Setter, and Red Doberman Pinscher[1,2,4]. The syndrome appears in approximately 93% of Blue and 83% of Fawn Doberman Pinschers[1].

Onset generally occurs in animals 4 months to 3 years of age. However, it has developed in some animals as late as 6 years of age[4]. Affected animals initially manifest a gradual onset of a dull, dry, brittle, poor-quality coat with fractured hair (**178, 179**). As the condition progresses, a moth-eaten partial alopecia develops, which may continue to worsen until there is total alopecia of dilute-colored hair. Follicular papules often develop and may advance to comedo formation or secondary bacterial folliculitis. As the condition becomes chronic, the affected skin can become hyperpigmented and seborrheic. The severity of the syndrome varies with lighter-colored animals developing the most extensive lesions.

DIFFERENTIAL DIAGNOSES
- Hyperadrenocorticism
- Hypothyroidism
- Follicular dysplasia
- Demodicosis

DIAGNOSTIC TESTS
Clinical examination will raise suspicion of the disorder. Microscopic examination of affected hair may demonstrate uneven distribution and clumping of melanin (**180**) that may cause distortion of the hair shaft. Histopathologic examination of biopsy samples will confirm the diagnosis.

MANAGEMENT
There is no specific treatment that will alter the course of the syndrome. In some animals, weekly bathing with benzoyl peroxide shampoo to reduce comedo formation and seborrhea may be beneficial. Systemic antibiotics would be appropriate if a secondary bacterial folliculitis is present.

KEY POINTS
- Diagnosis depends on histopathologic examination and this may be difficult.
- The chronic nature of the disease demands careful and exhaustive work up.

Color-dilution Alopecia

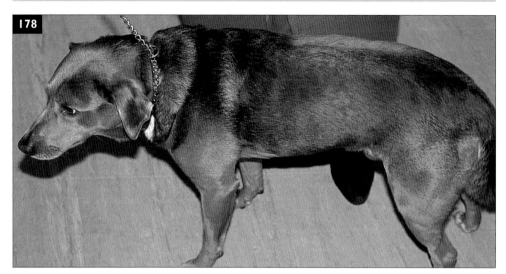

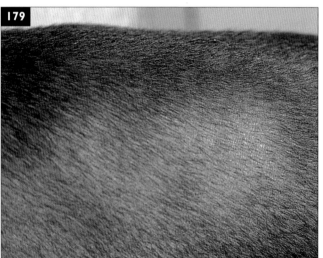

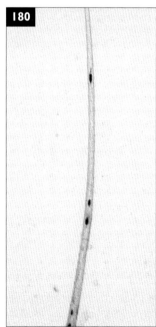

178, 179   Color-dilution alopecia in a dilute-blue cross-bred (**178**) and a Red Doberman Pinscher (**179**).

180   Photomicrograph of a hair from a color-dilute Doberman Pinscher. Note the clumping of the pigment granules.

Vitiligo

DEFINITION
Vitiligo is an acquired disorder characterized by selective destruction of melanocytes in skin and hair matrix cells, which results in leucoderma (depigmentation of skin) and leucotrichia (depigmentation of hair).

ETIOLOGY AND PATHOGENESIS
Vitiligo is thought to result from an aberration of immune surveillance which allows the development of antimelanocytic antibodies. These antibodies have been demonstrated in dogs and cats with vitiligo, but not in normal animals[1]. Additional theories in humans revolve around the possibility that there is either a neurochemical mediator that destroys melanocytes or inhibits melanin production, or that there is an intermediate metabolite in melanin syntheses that causes melanocyte destruction[2].

CLINICAL FEATURES
There is a marked breed predisposition for vitiligo in the Belgian Tervuren. Other dogs that appear to be at increased risk include the German Shepherd Dog, Rottweiler, and Doberman Pinscher. It has also been diagnosed in various other breeds and has been reported in Siamese cats[1,3]. Vitiligo generally appears in young adulthood as asymptomatic macules on the planum nasale, lips, muzzle, buccal mucosa (**181**), and footpads. Leucoderma and, in some cases leucotrichia (**182**) occur in affected areas[4]. Progression of lesions is variable, with lesions of some animals repigmenting, while others have permanent depigmentation[4]. Idiopathic depigmentation of the nose can develop and may be a form of vitiligo. Lay terms for this are 'Dudley nose' and 'snow nose'. There appears to be a predisposition for this in the Golden Retriever, Yellow Labrador Retriever, and Arctic breeds such as the Siberian Husky and Alaskan Malamute[3].

DIFFERENTIAL DIAGNOSES
- Canine uveodermatologic syndrome
- Discoid lupus erythematosus
- Dermatomyositis
- Systemic lupus erythematosus

DIAGNOSTIC TESTS
Diagnosis is based on history, physical examination, and microscopic examination of skin biopsy samples.

MANAGEMENT
There is no treatment that has been shown to be of benefit.

KEY POINT
- Vitiligo is quite common – client education is important.

Vitiligo

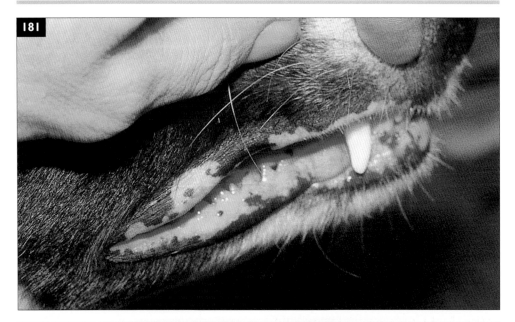

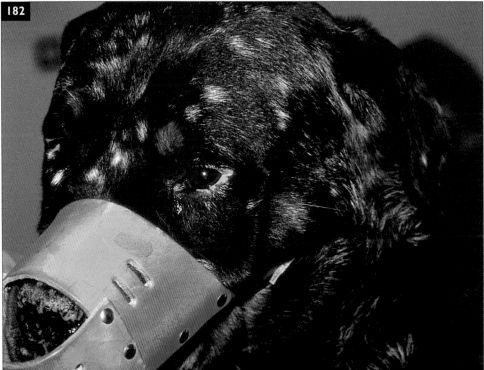

181, 182   Vitiligo. Loss of pigment on the lips of a Border Collie (**181**); patchy leucotrichia on the head of a Rottweiler (**182**).

Canine Uveodermatologic Syndrome

(Vogt–Koyanagi–Harada-like (VKH) Syndrome)

DEFINITION

Canine uveodermatologic syndrome is a rare canine condition that is believed to be an immune-mediated antimelanocyte disease resulting in ocular, dermal, and hair abnormalities[1-4].

ETIOLOGY AND PATHOGENESIS

Although the underlying mechanism of immunoregulatory dysfunction has not been elucidated, it is known in humans that a type IV or cell-mediated hypersensitivity exists against melanin and melanocytes[1,3]. Distinct subpopulations of cytotoxic T lymphocytes with activity against melanocytes have been identified[3]. Similar mechanisms have been proposed for the dog[1-3].

CLINICAL FEATURES

Although the condition has been reported in many different breeds of dogs, Akitas, Samoyeds, Siberian Huskies, Alaskan Malamutes, Chow Chows, and their related crossbreeds appear to be at increased risk[1,3]. Ocular signs generally precede skin changes and consist initially of bilateral uveitis to severe panuveitis. Later, retinal detachment, posterior synechia with secondary glaucoma, and cataracts may develop. Skin and hair abnormalities consist of depigmentation that often involves the eyelids, nasal planum, lips, scrotum, vulva, and pads of the feet (**183, 184**), as well as variable erythema, ulceration, and crusting of skin in the depigmented areas[1,3]. Pruritus may be a feature and lymphadenopathy is common[1]. Initial onset of lesions has been noted in animals ranging from 13 months to 6 years of age[3].

DIFFERENTIAL DIAGNOSES

* Discoid lupus erythematosus
* Systemic lupus erythematosus
* Pemphigus foliaceus
* Pemphigus erythematosus
* Vitiligo
* Dermatomyositis

DIAGNOSTIC TESTS

Diagnosis is based on history, ophthalmic examination, physical examination, and histopathologic examination of skin biopsy samples.

MANAGEMENT

Topical or subconjunctival corticosteroids and topical cycloplegics are beneficial in patients with anterior uveitis[3]. Prednisolone, methylprednisolone, or prednisone (0.5–2.0 mg/kg PO q 12 h) is usually required to resolve the uveitis and dermatologic lesions. After resolution of lesions, the dose can be tapered, although long-term therapy is often required to maintain remission. Azathioprine (2 mg/kg PO q 24 h) with tapering after clinical resolution (to 0.5 mg/kg PO q 24 h) may allow for a reduction of the corticosteroid dose. In some patients it may be possible to discontinue the corticosteroids and rely on azathioprine alone[3].

KEY POINT

* This condition requires aggressive treatment and demands definitive diagnosis.

Canine Uveodermatologic Syndrome

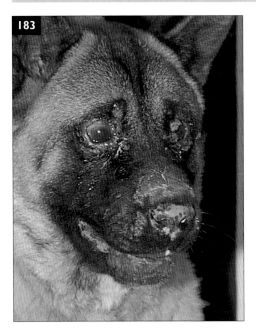

183, 184   Canine uveodermatologic syndrome. Loss of pigment on the nasal planum and nose (**183**) and on the footpads (**184**).

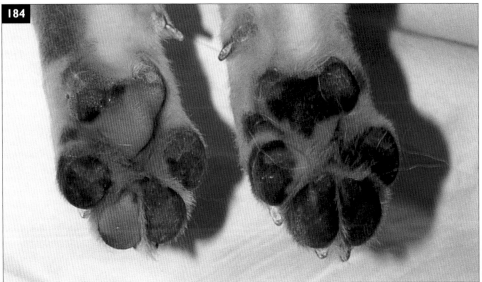

Lentigo and Lentiginosis Profusa

DEFINITION
A lentigo is a brown, circular macule due to an increased number of melanocytes at the dermoepidermal junction, without evidence of focal proliferation[1].

ETIOLOGY AND PATHOGENESIS
The etiology of lentigines is not known, although the role of a papillomavirus has been postulated in the canine disease[2]. While there is a biochemical relationship established between inflammatory reactions and post-inflammatory hyperpigmentation[3], there is no suggestion that lentiginous disorders have a similar etiology. A hereditary pattern of lentiginosis profusa was reported in Pugs and an autosomal dominant mode of transmission demonstrated[4]. Lentigo in orange cats has been reported[5], but no theories as to pathogenesis were offered.

CLINICAL FEATURES
In the heritable disorder in Pugs, the macules were first noted between 1 and 4 years of age. The lesions were discrete, well-demarcated, slightly raised, and non-pruritic, and were found on the distal limbs, although lesser numbers were present on the proximal limbs and trunk[4]. The macules gradually enlarged to reach a size of approximately 10 mm (0.4 in) in diameter and then remained static. With time, the density of coloration faded[4,6]. In orange cats the lesions were first noted on the lips (**185**), and most animals were affected before 12 months of age[5]. In most cases the lentigines spread locally to affect the eyelids and nasal regions. Pruritus was not noted. There is one case recorded of an adult silver short-hair cat which developed non-pruritic generalized lesions[7].

DIFFERENTIAL DIAGNOSES
• Superficial pyoderma
• Demodicosis
• Pigmented neoplasms

DIAGNOSTIC TESTS
The clinical appearance of these lesions is usually sufficient to make a diagnosis. Histopathologic examination of biopsy samples will allow a definitive diagnosis.

MANAGEMENT
Dermabrasion has been used in humans[8], but is not indicated in animals where no associated clinical signs are noted.

KEY POINT
• Benign lesion requiring client education rather than treatment.

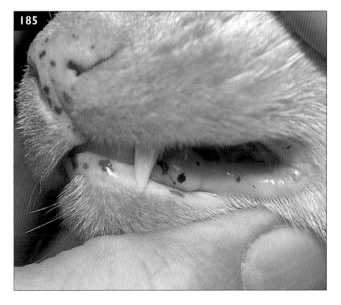

185 Lentigines on the lower lip of a cat.

Environmental Dermatoses

GENERAL APPROACH

1. Often the presentation is acute and the available history is poor – careful examination is important.
2. Many cases are short-lived but some signs may be chronic.

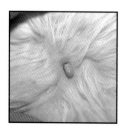
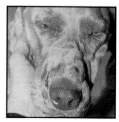
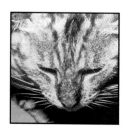
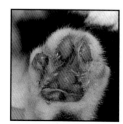

Tick Infestation

DEFINITION
Tick infestation is the presence of, or attachment of, either ixodic or argasid ticks on an animal.

ETIOLOGY AND PATHOGENESIS
Based on taxonomic classifications, ticks are generally divided into two Classes: hard (ixodic) and soft (argasid). Most clinical problems are due to infestations with ixodic ticks. Several species are capable of infestation, including *Rhipicephalus sanguineus* (brown dog tick or kennel tick), *Dermacentor variabilis* (American dog tick, wood tick), *D. andersoni* (Rocky Mountain wood tick), *D. occidentalis* (Pacific or West Coast tick), *Amblyomma maculatum* (Gulf Coast tick), *A. americanum* (Lone Star tick), *Ixodes dammini* (deer tick), *I. scapularis* (black legged tick), *I. pacificus* (found in California and Oregon, USA), and *I. ricinus* (castor bean tick, found in Europe)[1,2].

Ticks from both Classes pass through four stages: egg, larva (seed tick), nymph, and adult. The larva, nymph, and adult of both sexes feed on blood and lymph, with the female stages becoming distended after engorgement. In general, the ixodic ticks are three-host ticks with the larva and nymph stages primarily feeding on small rodents[1]. A three-host tick, *R. sanguineus* can complete its life cycle on the dog. It is a common tick that may be found worldwide[1].

The various ticks can transmit certain diseases or organisms:

- *R. sanguineus*: *Babesia gibsoni*, *Coxiella burnetii*, *Ehrlichia canis*, *Hepatozoan canis*, *Pasteurella tularensis*.
- *D. andersoni*: *B. canis*, *C. burnetti*, Rocky Mountain spotted fever.
- *D. variabilis*: *P. tularensis*, Rocky Mountain spotted fever.
- *A. americanum*: Rocky Mountain spotted fever.
- *A. maculatum*: *Leptospira pomona*.
- *I. dammini*, *pacificus*, and *ricinus*: *Borrelia burgdorferi* (Lyme disease)[1,3].

The argasid tick of clinical importance in dogs and cats is the spinous ear tick, *Otobius megnini*, which is found worldwide in warm, moist climates. This is a one-host tick, but only the larva and nymph stages are parasitic[2].

CLINICAL FEATURES
Ticks of various stages of the life cycle may be seen attached to the skin (**186**). Erythema may be present in the skin adjacent to the attached tick (**187**). This may result in the area being mildly pruritic. Crusting and a small nodule may develop at the site where a tick was removed. This is due to an immunologically mediated inflammatory reaction to the tick saliva rather than the commonly held belief that the head of the tick or mouthparts have been left in the skin[4]. Otitis externa may result from the irritation of large numbers of spinous ear ticks in the canal. Tick paralysis may occur due to a neurotoxin in the saliva of engorging females of several species of ixodic ticks, particularly those of the genus *Dermacenor*[1]. This appears clinically as an ascending flaccid lower motor neuron paralysis.

DIAGNOSTIC TESTS
The observation of ticks during physical or otic examination confirms the diagnosis.

MANAGEMENT
Ticks can be removed by grasping them with either a forceps or gloved fingers and applying slow traction until they are pulled free. In many cases a small amount of skin will be pulled off and still be attached to the tick mouthparts. Permethrin dips, sprays, or concentrated drops may be applied to dogs if there is a heavy infestation. Permethrin products also have the advantage of having repellent activities. The application of fipronil spray will result in rapid killing of ticks and is useful in periods of anticipated challenge, particularly considering the 4-week efficacy period. Collars containing amitraz are also available for use in the control of tick infestations in dogs. These collars do not repel or prevent ticks from becoming attached; however, the ticks die and drop off the animal soon after they start feeding.

Because of cat grooming patterns, tick infestations are less common in cats. Pyrethrin products labeled for use in cats would be appropriate if infestations do occur, and fipronil would also be indicated.

The premises need to be treated with a product such as chlorpyrifos if *R. sanguineus* is responsible for the infestation. This is because the entire life cycle of this tick can be completed on the dog, which results in large numbers of all life stages in the animal's immediate surroundings.

KEY POINT
- The prolonged, intimate, contact between the tick and its host provides plenty of opportunity for exchange of infection.

Tick Infestation

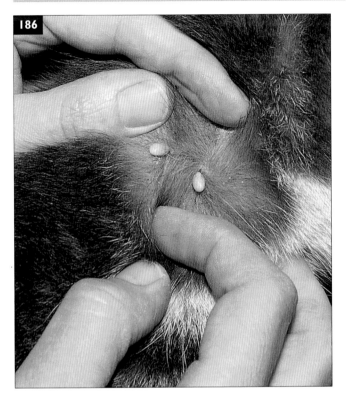

186 Tick infestation. Two ticks, not yet engorged, on the neck of a cat.

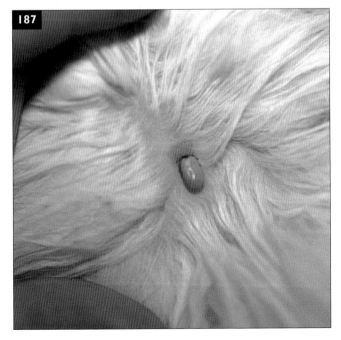

187 A tick, and an erythematous reaction to it, on the neck of a cat.

Bee Stings and Spider Bites

DEFINITION

Local or systemic reactions to toxins or foreign bodies introduced by bites or stings.

ETIOLOGY AND PATHOGENESIS

The stings of bees and other Hymenoptera contain phospholipases, hyaluronidases, and bradykinin-like mediators[1]. These agents are responsible for the local vasodilation and sensation of pain which follow stings. Spiders (and some caterpillars) may cause localized reactions, either through implantation of spicules or through bites which introduce a variety of necro- and neurotoxins[2,3].

CLINICAL FEATURES

Most reactions to insect and arthropod toxins are localized and are characterized by erythema, edema, and transient pain. In cats, sudden, soft, regional edema of the distal forelimb is a common site for stings, presumably a consequence of the cat 'playing' with the insect. In dogs it is usually the soft tissue of the face which exhibit signs, with edema and angioedema of the eyelids and muzzle being seen (**188**). Occasionally, generalized urticaria may be seen and systemic reactions (anaphylactic in nature) have been reported[4]. Peracute nasal dermatitis in dogs, which is associated with eosinophilic furunculosis[5], may be a reaction to insect stings[6] (**189**). Occasionally, the bite of an arthropod is followed by the development of a granulomatous response at the site[7]. The bites of spiders are inherently more dangerous than those of the Hymenoptera, with the potential for severe localized vasculitis, tissue necrosis, and systemic reactions[3,6].

DIFFERENTIAL DIAGNOSES (OF LOCALIZED REACTIONS)

- Nasal pyoderma
- Urticaria
- Dermatophytosis
- Immune-mediated dermatoses and drug eruption

DIAGNOSTIC TESTS

Clinical history of a peracute onset following the bite or sting will eliminate most of the differential diagnoses. Often the insect or spider is not seen and a bite or sting is inferred rather than documented. Histopathologic examination of biopsy samples is often necessary to eliminate acute nasal pyoderma from the eosinophilic furunculosis.

MANAGEMENT

Systemic glucocorticoids, at anti-inflammatory doses, are indicated once the diagnosis is established. Systemic antihistamines may be of value in cases characterized by edema and urticaria. Local bathing with wet dressings may be of value in cases of peracute nasal eosinophilic furunculosis. Sedation may be indicated to prevent the dog causing severe self-trauma. The owner should be warned that some loss of hair and scarring are inevitable.

KEY POINT

- Treat peracute eosinophilic folliculitis aggressively.

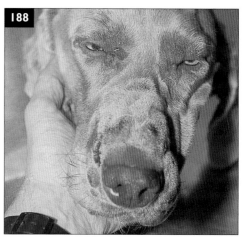

188 Urticaria. Symmetrical swelling of the face following a sting from a bee.

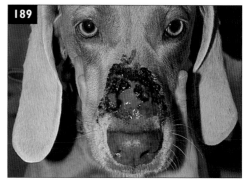

189 Peracute eosinophilic furunculosis following stings from a bee.

Dermatoses Caused by Body Fluids

DEFINITION
Dermatoses caused by chronic exposure to urine, feces, saliva, or tears.

ETIOLOGY AND PATHOGENESIS
Chronic exposure to any bodily fluid results in surface maceration, erythema, secondary infection, and alopecia. Common examples are facial fold inflammation in Persian cats and fold dermatitis in Spaniels.

CLINICAL FEATURES
These dermatoses are usually focal, with little tendency to spread. The lesions usually extend from the source of the discharge and follow local skin folds (**190, 191**). The affected areas are erythematous, alopecic, and often malodorous. Secondary infection is common. Pruritus is variable.

DIFFERENTIAL DIAGNOSES
- Fold dermatitis
- Demodicosis
- *Malassezia pachydermatis* dermatitis
- Mucocutaneous candidiasis

DIAGNOSTIC TESTS
Breed association and clinical site will allow recognition of fold dermatitis. Microscopic examination of skin scrapes and tape strips will demonstrate ectoparasites and yeast, respectively. Care should be taken to rule out systemic disease, as not all cases are entirely anatomical.

MANAGEMENT
The management of these diseases is directed towards attending to the underlying cause of the discharge and symptomatic treatment of the dermatosis. Once the cause of the discharge is effectively treated, the dermatologic lesions resolve and further treatment is not necessary. In debilitated animals the onset of urine scald may be delayed if petrolatum is applied to the areas of skin adjacent to the urogenital orifices. Placing the animals on mesh floors may help. Unfortunately, some of the underlying conditions are difficult to treat definitively and long-term symptomatic treatment may be indicated.

KEY POINT
- Identification of the underlying cause is mandatory.

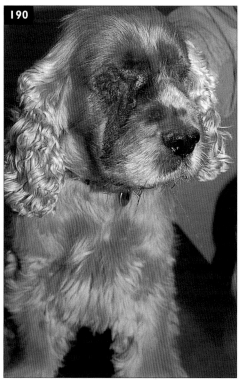

190   Epiphora secondary to hypothyroidism has resulted in periocular alopecia and hyperpigmentation.

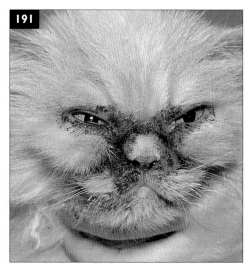

191   Facial fold dermatitis in a Persian cat following chronic epiphora.

Fly and Mosquito Bite Dermatoses

DEFINITION
A papular or papulocrustous reaction to the bites of flies and mosquitoes.

ETIOLOGY AND PATHOGENESIS
Fly bite dermatitis is usually caused by the stable fly *Stomoxys calcitrans,* and is considered to be a non-specific reaction to the pain and injury caused by the bite. Similarly, the clinical signs of insect bite dermatosis in dogs is thought to be caused by bites of the mosquito, bush fly, sand fly, or buffalo fly. In contrast to the canine dermatosis, feline mosquito bite hypersensitivity is caused by a Type 1 reaction to substances within saliva which are injected into the skin when the mosquito bites.

CLINICAL FEATURES
Fly bite dermatitis is a crusting, pruritic dermatosis which affects the tips of the pinnae of dogs during the summer months. In Rough Collies, Shetland Sheepdogs, and other breeds in which the tips of the pinnae bend over, the bites occur on the fold, whereas in those breeds with erect ears the lesions occur at the tips of the pinnae. Lesions consist of erythema, hair loss, and hemorrhagic crusting resulting from oozing of blood and serum.

Insect bite dermatitis is most commonly seen in short-coated dogs, such as Weimaraners, Doberman Pinschers, German Shorthaired Pointers, and Bull Terriers, which are kept outdoors, especially in warm climates. Papules and crusted papules are followed by focal alopecia (**192**). The lesions are usually confined to the dorsal and lateral surfaces of the trunk and upper limbs. Buffalo gnat bites will result in circular 1 cm (0.4 in) areas of erythema on the non-haired areas of the ventral abdomen.

Feline mosquito bite hypersensitivity (**193**) affects cats of any breed during the summer months in warm climates[1,2]. Typically, there is papular eruption on the outer and inner aspects of the pinnae and on the nose. Erosions, crusting, scaling and, sometimes, depigmentation may follow. Cats often exhibit a mild pyrexia. Hyperkeratosis of all the pads of all four feet, preceded by swelling, tenderness, erythema and, sometimes, fissuring of the pads, is seen in most cases. There is peripheral lymphadenopathy. Rarely, the condition will be accompanied by a corneal eosinophilic granuloma.

DIFFERENTIAL DIAGNOSES
- Squamous cell carcinoma
- Scabies
- Superficial pyoderma
- Demodicosis
- Urticaria
- Pemphigus foliaceus
- Feline eosinophilic granuloma complex
- Notoedric mange
- Pemphigus erythematosus
- Systemic lupus erythematosus
- Atopic dermatitis

DIAGNOSIS
The seasonal and environmental nature of the dermatosis means that many individuals are affected year after year. A history of exposure is often known, particularly for fly bite dermatosis of the pinnae. Microscopic examination of skin scrapes will eliminate *Demodex canis* from the differential of insect bite dermatitis. Superficial pyoderma is characterized by papules, pustules, and epidermal collarettes. The combination of the clinical signs described for the cat is pathognomonic.

MANAGEMENT
Ideally, these dermatoses are managed by preventing animals being exposed to the insects, although in reality it is often impossible to enforce. The bites of *S. calcitrans* may be deterred by the use of insect repellents such as DEET. Flies and mosquitoes may be excluded from closed areas by fine mesh. Most cases resolve spontaneously when the attentions of the insects are prevented, although in some instances it may be necessary to use systemic glucocorticoids to induce remission.

KEY POINT
- Control of the condition is difficult unless management changes are invoked.

Fly and Mosquito Bite Dermatoses

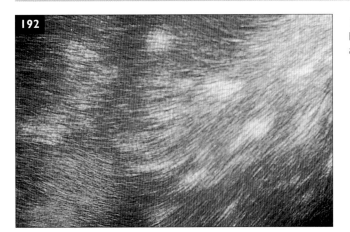

192 Insect bite dermatitis. Patchy alopecia on the flanks of a Wire-haired Pointer.

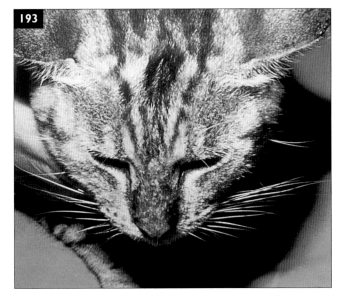

193 Feline mosquito bite hypersensitivity. (Illustration courtesy of Dr K. Mason.)

Burns

DEFINITION
Burns are tissue damage resulting from thermal or chemical insult.

ETIOLOGY AND PATHOGENESIS
Direct heat burns result from contact with a hot object or substance. The most common direct heat burn is the 'clipper burn', which results from a hot clipper blade contacting the skin. Less frequently, direct heat burns develop from situations such as cats walking over hot stove burners, contact with hot exhaust parts of cars and wood or coal heaters, poor supervision of paralytic animals on heating pads, hot liquids spilled on animals, and malfunction of hair-drying equipment. Flame burns may result from fires in homes or automobile accidents. Electrical burns may be seen in and around the oral cavity when a young dog chews an electrical cord.

The severity of a burn is related to the maximum temperature the tissue attains and the duration of the overheating. These in turn are dependent on such variables as the temperature and mass of the burning agent; the mass, specific heat, and thermal conductivity of the burned body; the temperature of the environment in which post-burn cooling takes place; and the amount of heat convection in the surrounding medium. Body tissues, of which water is the main component, are characterized by high specific heat, which means that a large amount of heat is required to raise the temperature of tissue, and low thermal conductivity, which means the heat will be slow to dissipate. The clinical relevance of this is that the duration of tissue overheating extends beyond the contact time with the burning agent. Therefore, *immediate cooling of the burned area can shorten the duration of tissue overheating, thereby decreasing tissue damage.*

Minimal overheating of tissue causes inapparent, reversible cell damage. Further overheating will produce foci of irreversibly damaged cells scattered among reversibly damaged and non-injured cells. Finally, when a critical threshold is exceeded, necrosis of the entire tissue occurs. Because transition from healthy skin to necrotic skin is gradual, regeneration of skin defects proceeds from partly damaged rather than healthy tissue, and this results in a longer healing time when compared with mechanical injuries of the same depth.

Severe burns may also result in shock as well as hemostatic, liver, kidney, erythron, respiratory, and immunologic disorders[1,2].

CLINICAL FEATURES
The clinical appearance of a burn will vary depending on the etiology and severity of the burn. The human classification of burns is not appropriate for dogs and cats as the skin of dogs and cats is thinner and does not blister as easily. Burns in these species are best classified as either partial thickness or full thickness. Partial-thickness burns are characterized by incomplete destruction of the skin and clinically are distinguished by erythema, local edema, occasional small vesicles, evidence of persistent capillary circulation, and partial sensation to touch (**194**). Full-thickness burns are characterized by complete destruction of all elements of the skin, including adenexa and nerves. Clinically, they are distinguished by lack of superficial blood flow, insensitivity to touch, and easy epilation of hair. It may take 10–14 days before the skin shows a color change and separation of necrotic skin begins (**195**).

DIAGNOSTIC TESTS
Diagnosis is based on history and clinical features.

MANAGEMENT
Minor burns
Standard principles for the treatment of small traumatic lesions of the skin may be applied to minor burns, as experimental studies in animals and clinical studies in humans have not demonstrated a particular treatment for minor burns that has distinct advantages[3].

Severe burns
Clients should be encouraged to apply ice-water packs (ice and water in a plastic sack) to the burn site if it has occurred within 2 hours and the animal will permit this action. Exposed tissue may be gently overlaid or loosely wrapped with old towels, pillow cases, or strips of sheets. Owners should be instructed to spend minimal time on these endeavors, as they are not as critical as veterinary management of possible shock.

On initial examination, airways should be examined to assure they are patent and significant hemorrhage should be controlled. Then evaluation and, if necessary, treatment for shock should be instituted according to standard principles[4].

Cooling the affected areas is appropriate if the burn occurred within the past 2 hours. Cooling reduces pain, depth of the burn wound,

Burns

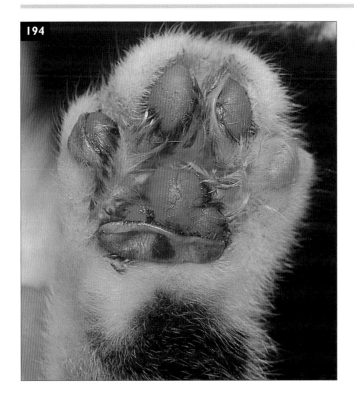

194   Slough of the skin over the pad secondary to scald.

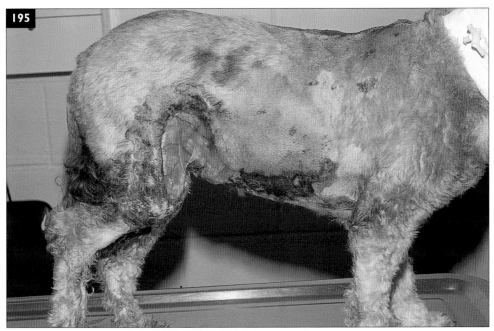

195   Extensive burns in a dog 13 days after the injury occurred.

Burns

edema and mortality. If appropriate, the skin should be cooled by compresses or immersion in water (3–17°C/37.4–62.6°F) for approximately 30 minutes[5].

Cleaning and débridement is important. Hair should be clipped from all of the affected areas and other contamination and debris should be rinsed off by flushing with saline or washing with povidone–iodine soap. All tissue that is devitalized (determined by a change in the color of tissue, lack of sensation to touch, lack of capillary circulation, and easy epilation of hair) should be excised as it serves as a good growth medium for bacteria. Final confirmation of the extent of burn wounds may not be completely possible until about 10 days post burn, when separation of normal and necrotic tissue becomes obvious. Immersion of the affected areas in a whirlpool bath for 15–20 minutes twice daily is effective for the removal of exudate and helpful for the loosening and removal of necrotic tissue.

Topical antibacterial treatment is useful. Silver sulfadiazine cream is an effective and practical antibacterial drug for topical therapy. Besides having antibacterial properties, it is non-irritating to exposed tissues, has no systemic side-effects, and is easily applied to the wound, which is then bandaged with loose mesh gauze. Dressings are changed twice daily. During changes, necessary débridement is performed, and old medications along with any exudate is removed by irrigation with saline or immersion in a whirlpool bath.

Use of biologic and synthetic dressings and skin grafts should be considered. Biologic dressings, such as specially prepared pig skin and synthetic dressings made of either silicon polymers, polyurethane, or polyvinyl chloride polymers, provide benefit by maintaining a water layer on the surface of the wound that aids re-epithelialization, clears surface bacteria, and minimizes fibrosis, inflammation, heat loss, and pain[2]. They are most effective when infection and eschar are minimal. Because the skin of dogs and cats is very elastic and has loose subcutaneous tissue, skin defects can often be closed by direct apposition of one of several reconstructive techniques making use of skin flaps. If the defect is too large for direct apposition or a skin flap, a free autogenous graft of either full or partial thickness may be used.

Systemic antibacterial treatment in the management of burn wounds is questionable. Studies in animals and human burn patients show that systemic antibiotic therapy does not favorably influence mortality, fever, or rate of healing[3]. Their use should be limited to confirmed cases of bacterial septicemia and selection should be determined by sensitivity tests.

KEY POINT

• Animals with extensive burns will require intensive therapy over a long period of time. Clients must be warned of this fact.

Myiasis

DEFINITION

Myiasis is the infestation of organs or tissue by fly larvae that feed on necrotic or living tissue of the host.

ETIOLOGY AND PATHOGENESIS

Lesions are generally associated with larvae of flies that produce facultative myiasis in contaminated skin wounds. Typically, they are from the genera *Musca, Calliphora, Phaenicia, Lucilia, Phormia,* and *Sarcophaga*[1]. They go through four developmental stages: egg, larva, pupa, and adult. For facultative myiasis to develop in a warm-blooded animal, there must be a factor such as traumatized skin, ocular discharge, neglected wound, or fecal soiling to attract the female fly and the deposition of eggs. Larval stages can move independently over the surface of a wound ingesting secretions, exudate, dead cells, and debris, but not live tissue. However, they can induce irritation, injure cells, and provoke exudation.

Obligatory myiasis is due to the screw-worm fly *Cochliomyia hominivorax*[1]. This fly is dependent on fresh wounds as a site for larval development. These larvae can liquefy and devour viable tissues thereby enlarging the wound. They occur infrequently in North America, but are of major importance in Central and South America[1].

CLINICAL FEATURES

Affected animals will be noted to have predisposing factors, such as matting of the hair coat or a thick coat, which hinders drying of the skin resulting in maceration, necrotic tissue from wounds or neoplasia, urine or fecal soiling of the hair coat, fold dermatitis, or ocular discharge. Larvae can be found under the matted hair or in the wounds. They produce punched-out lesions in the tissues and may tunnel in diseased tissues producing cavities (**196**). Often a foul odor is associated with the condition.

DIAGNOSTIC TESTS

Diagnosis is based on clinical findings of maggot-infested wounds.

MANAGEMENT

Hair and mats should be clipped from infested areas. The area can be flushed with either Burrow's solution or a dilute chlorhexidine solution to clean debris and larvae from the wound. Flushing around deeply imbedded larvae may cause them to float free. If not, they will have to be removed with a forceps. Necrotic tissue, if present, should be removed and the wound dressed with silver sulfadiazine to control infection. Appropriate treatment should be administered for any systemic signs.

The client should be informed that the animal's wounds should be kept clean and, if possible, the animal housed in a fly-free environment until healing occurs. They should also be made aware of predisposing conditions so that steps can be taken to prevent reoccurrence.

KEY POINT

• Look for the underlying cause in these cases.

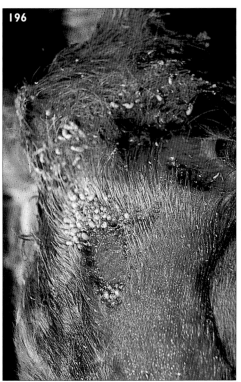

196   Myiasis. Focal, punched-out ulcers are often found in these cases when the overlying matted hair and crust is removed.

Frostbite

DEFINITION
Frostbite is tissue damage that results from freezing.

ETIOLOGY AND PATHOGENESIS
Frostbite occurs with prolonged exposure to freezing temperatures and is more likely to occur if the animal is also exposed to windy conditions or if there is wetting of a body area. The pathogenesis involves direct cold injury to the cell, indirect cold injury by formation of ice crystals, and impaired circulation with hypoxia.

CLINICAL FEATURES
Lesions typically occur in areas where hair coat is sparse. In cats the tips of the ears, tail, and footpads are most commonly affected, while in dogs it is more often the scrotum and footpads (197). Cats with mild frostbite may be asymptomatic with the only noticeable feature being a delayed lightening of hair color on the tips of the ears and curling of the pinnae. The acute phase of more severely damaged tissue is characterized by being cool to the touch, pale, and hypoesthetic. With thawing, the affected areas become erythematous, painful, edematous and, eventually, may either develop scaling or necrosis.

DIFFERENTIAL DIAGNOSES
• Vasculitis
• Squamous cell carcinoma
• Disseminated intravascular coagulation
• Cold agglutinin disease
• Cryoglobulinemia
• Ischemic necrosis associated with toxins

DIAGNOSTIC TESTS
Diagnosis is based on history and clinical findings.

MANAGEMENT
Mild cases of frostbite may not require any treatment or only the application of a bland ointment. If there is deep freezing of tissues, the case should be handled in such a way as to avoid thawing and refreezing as this greatly increases tissue damage. Initial treatment should consist of rapid thawing in warm water (38–44°C/100.4–111.2°F)[1]. After warming, the patient should be carefully monitored to ensure that self-mutilation does not occur. Irreversibly damaged tissue demarcates in 7–14 days. Further therapeutic management of necrotic tissue and resulting defect parallels that of thermal injury.

KEY POINT
• Careful management of severe cases is necessary if further tissue damage is to be avoided.

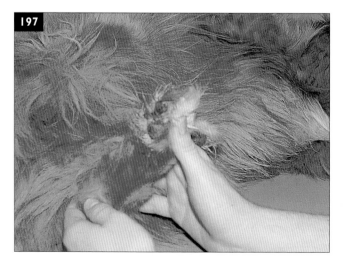

197 Frost bite. Note the pallor of the feet.

Endocrine Dermatoses

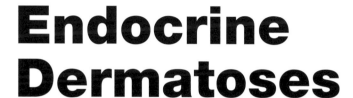

GENERAL APPROACH

1 Not all diseases with symmetrical lesions are endocrine in origin.
2 Many of these diseases are difficult to diagnose and treat.

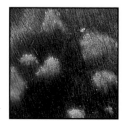
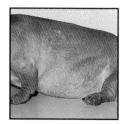
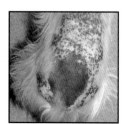
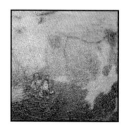

Hypothyroidism

DEFINITION

Hypothyroidism is the clinical syndrome, generally featuring alopecia, that occurs when the thyroid gland fails to produce and release thyroid hormones. It is classified as primary, secondary, or tertiary depending on whether the abnormality is at the level of the thyroid gland, pituitary gland, or hypothalamus.

THYROID PHYSIOLOGY

Thyrotropin-releasing hormone (TRH) is produced and released from the hypothalamus. It stimulates the synthesis and release of thyrotropin (TSH) from the adenohypophysis of the pituitary. TSH in turn stimulates the production and release of thyroid hormones from the thyroid gland. Variations in circulating concentrations of thyroid hormones regulate release of TSH by negative feedback mechanisms. When thyroid hormone concentrations are high, TRH is ineffective in stimulating TSH secretion. Conversely, when thyroid hormone concentrations decrease, this feedback inhibition is removed and secretion increases in response to the unopposed actions of TRH[1].

In a healthy euthyroid animal, all of the 3,5,3',5'tetraiodothyronine (thyroxine, T_4) is produced by the thyroid gland, while only 20% of the 3,5,3'triiodothyronine (T_3) and 5% of 3,3',5 triiodothyronine ('reverse' T_3, rT_3) are of thyroidal origin[2]. The majority of T_3 and rT_3 is derived from extrathyroidal deiodination of T_4 in peripheral tissues. It has been determined that T_4 is a prohormone, T_3 is the major metabolically active thyroid hormone, and rT_3 is metabolically inactive. Thyroid hormone is necessary for the initiation of the anagen (growth) phase of the hair cycle and normal cell metabolism of the skin[3].

Circulating levels of T_4 and T_3 may be lowered due to non-thyroidal factors, such as a variety of illnesses (renal failure, liver disease, diabetes mellitus, hyperadrenocorticism, systemic infection, pyoderma, and demodicosis), 'euthyroid sick syndrome', and drugs (glucocorticoids, anticonvulsants, phenylbutazone, and sulfonamides)[4,5]. The lowering of thyroid hormone levels is thought to be a normal adaptation to either the medication or the disease and does not reflect thyroid dysfunction.

ETIOLOGY AND PATHOGENESIS

In dogs, more than 90% of clinical cases of hypothyroidism are caused by primary destruction of the thyroid gland[6]. Lymphocytic thyroiditis and idiopathic thyroid necrosis and atrophy are cited as the two main causes of acquired primary hypothyroidism[7]. Lymphocytic thyroiditis is thought to be an autoimmune disorder reflecting abnormalities in humoral and cell-mediated autoimmunity[7].

CLINICAL FEATURES

The clinical signs of canine hypothyroidism are extremely variable and may include both systemic signs and dermatologic signs. Systemic signs associated with hypothyroidism include lethargy, mental dullness, weight gain (**198**), heat seeking, reproductive failure, bradycardia and, rarely, myopathies and neuropathies. Dermatologic features include bilaterally symmetrical alopecia (**199–201**), a dry, brittle, lusterless hair coat, seborrhea, poor hair growth after clipping, hyperpigmentation, and recurrent pyoderma (**202, 203**).

DIFFERENTIAL DIAGNOSES

- Hyperadrenocorticism
- Growth hormone responsive dermatosis
- Sebaceous adenitis
- Color-dilution alopecia
- Sertoli cell tumor
- Seasonal flank alopecia
- Telogen effluvium/anagen defluxion
- Dermatophytosis
- Demodicosis
- Pattern baldness
- Sex hormone disorders
- Superficial pyoderma

DIAGNOSTIC TESTS

Because various drugs and non-thyroidal illness can lower basal levels of serum T_4, T_3 and free T_4, they are not reliable tests for the conformation of hypothyroidism in the canine[4]. The administration of exogenous bovine TSH (0.1 U/kg (maximum dose 5 U) IV or, alternatively, 1 U for animals weighing 15 kg (33 lb) or less and 2 U for animals over 15 kg (33lb)) will cause a significant rise in T_4 levels, with levels within normal range, in animals who have non-thyroidal illness, whereas truly hypothyroid dogs will have a minimal increase in the T_4 post stimulation[4]. As the availability of TSH to use for the stimulation of animals is extremely limited, this procedure is not practical for most veterinarians. Validated TSH assays are now becoming available and offer the most promise. Values for this test would be expected to be elevated in animals with primary hypothyroidism. Response to a therapeutic trial of L-thyroxine has been advocated to confirm a clinical diagnosis of hypothyroidism in situations where diagnostic testing is inconclusive or un-

Hypothyroidism

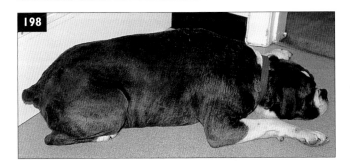

198–201   Hypothyroidism. Lethargy, dullness, and alopecia in a Boxer (**198**); symmetrical alopecia in an Airedale (**199**); alopecic tail (**200**); alopecia on the flank (201).

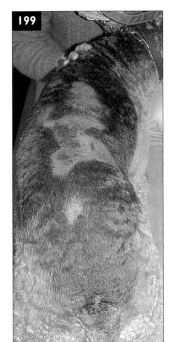

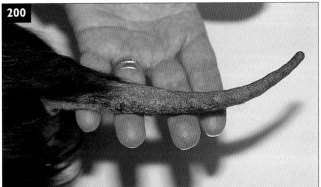

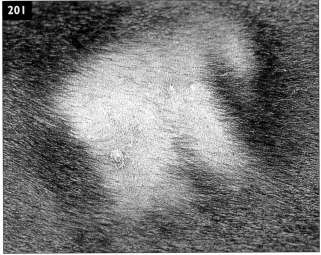

Hypothyroidism

available, or where expense is a concern for the client[4]. Trial therapy is to be avoided if possible as it may be misleading. This is because the metabolic effects of thyroxine may result in some hair regrowth and improvement in clinical signs regardless of their cause[3,8].

MANAGEMENT
Life-long treatment with levothyroxine (0.02 mg/kg PO q12 h)[3]. An alternative dosing regime

is 0.5 mg/m^2. Dosing on the basis of m^2 minimizes the underdosing of small dogs and overdosing of large dogs[8].

KEY POINTS
- An underdiagnosed clinical syndrome – its frequency in general practice exceeds that of diabetes mellitus.
- Diagnosis is difficult, but prospects are improving.

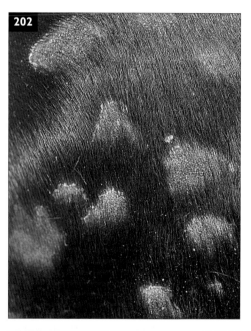

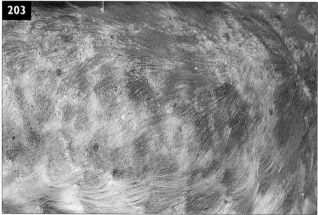

202, 203   Hypothyroidism. Secondary infection with minimal inflammation (**202**); secondary folliculitis and associated patchy alopecia (**203**).

Hyperadrenocorticism

DEFINITION

Hyperadrenocorticism (HAC) results from prolonged exposure to elevated serum cortisol concentrations.

ETIOLOGY AND PATHOGENESIS

HAC may be spontaneous or iatrogenic. Most cases (80–85%) of spontaneous HAC in the dog result from adrenocortical hyperplasia consequent upon excessive secretion of adrenocorticotrophic hormone from the pituitary (pituitary-dependent hyperadrenocorticism – PDH). Approximately 15–20% are due to adrenal neoplasia[1]. HAC is extremely rare in the cat[2].

There are no breed, age, or sex predispositions to iatrogenic disease. Most cases result from long-term, high-dose administration of glucocorticoid, either PO or by depot injection. The risk of inducing iatrogenic HAC may be minimized by administering oral prednisone (or prednisolone or methylprednisolone) on an alternate day basis[3]. Rarely, cases have been reported due to topical administration, such as ophthalmic or otic medication[4,5].

CLINICAL FEATURES

Animals of any age may be affected and there is a steadily increasing risk with age, leveling off between 7–9 years of age[1]. There appears to be no sex predisposition to HAC, but females are predisposed to adrenal neoplasia[6]. Terriers in particular are predisposed to HAC, Dachshunds to adrenal tumors, Boxers to pituitary neoplasia, and both Toy and Miniature Poodles to idiopathic adrenal hyperplasia[1].

Dogs with HAC may exhibit a number of clinical signs. Commonly noted clinical signs are pu/pd, a pendulous abdomen (**204**) with hepatomegaly (**205**), polyphagia, lethargy, and muscular weakness[6,7]. Dermatologic signs include secondary pyoderma and demodicosis, truncal or facial alopecia (**206, 207**), thinning of the skin (**208–210**), particularly on the abdomen, comedone formation, and calcinosis cutis[7,8]. Some dogs may exhibit only one clinical sign, making diagnosis difficult.

DIFFERENTIAL DIAGNOSES

- Hypothyroidism
- Sertoli cell neoplasia
- Adrenal sex hormone dermatoses (growth hormone responsive dermatosis)
- Follicular dysplasia
- Diabetes mellitus

DIAGNOSTIC TESTS

The most common hematologic abnormality in dogs is eosinopenia, and while other changes include a stress neutrophilia and lymphopenia and often an erythrocytosis, they are not diagnostic[6,7]. Common biochemical changes are elevations in alkaline phosphatase, cholesterol, and sometimes glucose but, again, these are non-diagnostic[6,7]. Basal cortisol concentrations are of no value in the diagnosis of HAC. Histopathologic examination of biopsy samples may be helpful in some cases, perhaps as many as 67%[9], but in many instances the cutaneous changes are non-diagnostic.

ACTH test

This tests the capacity of the adrenal glands to secrete cortisol. A basal blood is taken and 0.25 mg synthetic ACTH injected, either IV or IM[10], and a second blood taken after 90 minutes. Both samples are submitted for cortisol assay. Irrespective of the first cortisol concentration, the second should be between 270 and 690 nmol/l (9.7–25 μg/dl). Cortisol concentrations in excess of 690 nmol/l (>25 μg/dl) suggest HAC but cannot discriminate between adrenal or pituitary etiologies. Furthermore, some dogs with adrenal tumors respond normally. Dogs with iatrogenic HAC show very reduced response to the ACTH test.

Low-dose dexamethasone (LDD) suppression test

This tests the pituitary–adrenal axis which is abnormally resistant to dexamethasone suppression in spontaneous HAC[6]. A basal blood is taken, dexamethasone injected (0.01 mg/kg IV) and subsequent samples are taken after 4 and 8 hours. All three samples are submitted for cortisol assay. In normal dogs the administration of dexamethasone suppresses the serum cortisol concentration for the duration of the 8-hour test period such that after 4 hours it is less than 50% of the first sample and after 8 hours it is less than 40 nmol/l (1.4 μg/dl). In about 30% dogs there is adequate suppression at 4 hours but 'escape' at 8 hours with cortisol concentrations rising again, and this pattern is diagnostic for PDH. In most cases of adrenal neoplasia, and some 25% of spontaneous HAC cases, there is no suppression whatsoever, and in other cases there may be suppression but it does not fall below 50% of baseline. These and other abnormal responses are confirmatory for

Hyperadrenocorticism

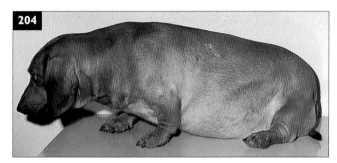

204–206 Hyperadrenocorticism in dogs. Abdominal enlargement and muscle weakness in a Dachshund (**204**); hepatomegaly and dropped abdomen (**205**); facial alopecia (**206**).

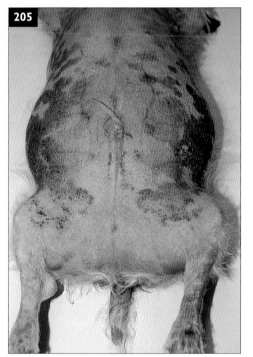

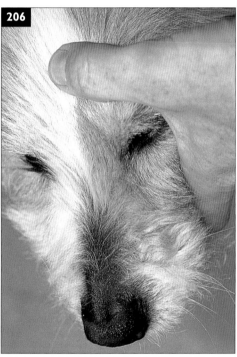

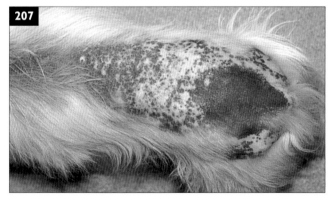

207 Hyperadrenocorticism in dogs. Dorsal alopecia.

Hyperadrenocorticism

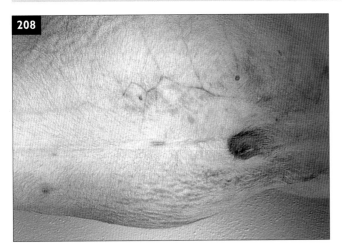

208   Hyperadrenocorticism in dogs. Abdominal enlargement due to hepatomegaly. Note the thin skin.

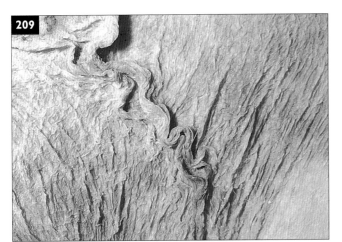

209   Hyperadrenocorticism in dogs. Prominent abdominal veins and tenting due to loss of dermal tissue and thinning of the epidermis.

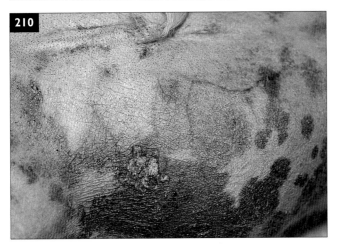

210   Hyperadrenocorticism in dogs. Prominent abdominal vasculature and patch of calcinosis cutis.

Hyperadrenocorticism

HAC, but do not indicate etiology and high-dose dexamethasone testing is indicated.

High-dose dexamethasone (HDD) suppression test

This tests the resistance of the pituitary–adrenal axis to high doses of dexamethasone, since in dogs with PDH the resistance documented with the LDD can be overridden. A basal blood sample is taken and dexamethasone injected (1 mg/kg IV). Subsequent blood samples are taken after 4 and 8 hours and submitted for cortisol assay. Any significant suppression (>50%) is diagnostic for PDH. Resistance to HDD is seen in about 15% cases of PDH and the majority of dogs with adrenal neoplasia[6].

Discrimination of the 15% cases of PDH from adrenal neoplasia can be difficult, although plasma ACTH assay, radiography, diagnostic imaging of the adrenal glands, or performing an ACTH test after loading doses of o'p'DDD (and noting suppression of cortisol) should be helpful[6,10–13].

MANAGEMENT

The treatment of choice for PDH is o'p'DDD (Lysodren). An induction dose (30–50 mg/kg q 24 h) is given for 10 days, at which point an ACTH test is run to assess the adrenal reserve. Both basal and post-ACTH cortisol concentrations should be in the normal resting range[9]. Rarely, induction with o'p'DDD may cause such precipitate falls in serum cortisol that an Addisonian crisis develops, with signs such as lethargy, weakness, vomiting, and diarrhea. The incidence and severity of these side-effects may be reduced by administering prednisone (or prednisolone) (0.2 mg/kg/day). Severe side-effects to o'p'DDD induction may dictate withdrawal of o'p'DDD and a temporary increase in glucocorticoid supplementation[9].

After the first 10 days of therapy, about 15% of dogs with PDH will still have elevated post-ACTH cortisol concentrations, and induction doses of o'p'DDD must be continued until the ACTH test is suppressed adequately. About 30% of dogs will have subnormal pre- and post-ACTH cortisol concentrations, and in these cases o'p'DDD is withheld until normal cortisol concentrations are recovered. At this point, maintenance doses of o'p'DDD are given (30–50 mg/kg/week) in 2 or 3 divided doses. Some dogs prove very hard to stabilize, some relapse, and some develop signs of mineralocorticoid deficiency. Readers are referred to specialist references for these cases[6].

Adrenal neoplasia may be managed by surgical resection[14,15]. Alternatively, medical therapy with o'p'DDD may be utilized. Very high dose o'p'DDD therapy (50–90 mg/kg/day) for up to 11 weeks (with regular ACTH tests to assess response) may be necessary to reduce serum cortisol concentrations to normal levels in these cases. Furthermore, higher maintenance doses of o'p'DDD are necessary to maintain remission. Nonetheless, in those animals without metastatic disease, the medical option provides an effective alternative to surgery[16].

Recently the use of L-deprenyl has been described for the treatment of PDH[17]. Although there are as yet very few clinical trials of this agent, early indications are that it may be useful, particularly in very small dogs and in early or mild cases of HAC.

KEY POINT

- An underdiagnosed clinical condition. In practice, its frequency should approximate that of diabetes mellitus.

Pituitary Dwarfism

DEFINITION
Pituitary dwarfism is a hereditary hypopituitarism resulting in a failure of growth plus variable coat, thyroidal, adrenocortical, and gonadal abnormalities.

ETIOLOGY AND PATHOGENESIS
The presence of a cyst (Rathke's cleft cyst) in the pituitary gland, resulting in varying degrees of anterior pituitary insufficiency, is responsible for the majority of cases. However, the condition has been described in dogs with either hypoplastic or normal anterior pituitary glands[1,2]. The condition is thought to be inherited as a simple autosomal recessive condition[3,4].

CLINICAL FEATURES
Pituitary dwarfism is seen primarily in German Shepherd Dogs and Carnelian Bear Dogs[3,5]. Affected dogs often appear normal during the first 2–3 months of life. After this time a failure to properly grow in stature and a retention of puppy coat become apparent (**211**). Partial loss of the puppy coat then occurs, resulting in a bilateral symmetrical alopecia over the neck, caudolateral aspects of the thighs and, occasionally, the trunk. Growth of primary hair is generally limited to the face and distal extremities. The skin becomes hyperpigmented, hypotonic, and scaly, and comedones may develop. Gonadal status may be altered with testicular atrophy occurring in males and anestrus in females. Affected animals may also show evidence of personality changes, such as aggressiveness and fear biting[1]. Clinical signs of hypothyroidism and adrenocortical insufficiency will be noted if there is a lack of TSH or ACTH. The condition is generally compatible with life, but most animals only live to 3–8 years of age[6].

DIFFERENTIAL DIAGNOSES
- Congenital hypothyroidism
- Malnutrition
- Skeletal dysplasias
- Gonadal dysgenesis
- Severe metabolic diseases

DIAGNOSTIC TESTS
History and clinical findings are usually diagnostic of an endocrinopathy. Failure to see an increase in plasma growth hormone levels (normal levels 1–2 ng/ml) after the injection of xylazine (0.1–0.3 mg/kg IV) or clonidine (0.01–0.03 mg/kg IV)[3]. Severe prolonged hypoglycaemia occurs after injection of regular insulin (0.025 U/kg IV)[3,4].

Histopathologic examination of biopsy material which reveals evidence of a decreased amount and size of elastin fibres is highly suggestive. Appropriate evaluations of thyroidal, adrenal, and gonadal status will allow a definitive diagnosis.

MANAGEMENT
Bovine somatotropin (10 IU SC) every other day for 30 days with retreatment necessary every 3 months to 3 years[3-7]. Repeated injections of bovine somatotropin has the potential to result in hypersensitivity reactions or diabetes mellitus[7]. Improvement in the skin and hair will generally be noted within 6–8 weeks. An increase in stature is generally not achieved as the growth plates close rapidly[1]. Appropriate therapy for adrenocortical insufficiency and/or hypothyroidism should be instituted if they are present.

KEY POINT
- A well-recognised disease, but very uncommon.

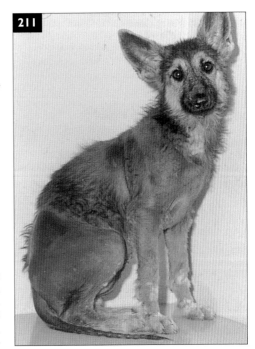

211 Pituitary dwarf.

Canine Familial Dermatomyositis

DEFINITION

Dermatomyositis is a hereditary inflammatory disease of skin and muscle which is characterized by symmetrical scarring alopecia about the face and limbs and atrophy of the muscles of mastication[1].

ETIOLOGY AND PATHOGENESIS

The etiopathogenesis of dermatomyositis in dogs is unknown. It is familial in Collies and Shetland Sheepdogs and breeding studies in Collies supports an autosomal dominant mode of inheritance with variable expressivity[2,3].

CLINICAL FEATURES

The disease occurs more commonly in Collies and Shetland Sheepdogs, but has also been reported to occur in the Welsh Corgi, Chow Chow, German Shepherd Dog, and Kuvasz[4]. Lesions generally develop before animals are 6 months of age, but can occasionally develop in adults. The typical distribution pattern for lesions is the face (especially the bridge of the nose, around the eyes, and the tips of the ears (**212**)), carpal and tarsal areas (**213**), digits, and tip of the tail. A scarring alopecia, erythema, scaling, and mild crusting are the most common findings. Occasionally, vesicles, papules, pustules, and ulcers may be found[2]. The rate of development and progression of lesions is quite variable as they often wax and wane and may undergo spontaneous regression. Muscle involvement occurs after the development of skin lesions and correlates with the severity of skin lesions[2]. It is often minimal and limited to temporal and masseter atrophy. Severely affected dogs have difficulty in eating, drinking, and swallowing, and may evidence growth retardation, megaesophagus, lameness, widespread muscle atrophy, and infertility[2]. Pruritus and pain are generally not features of the disease.

DIFFERENTIAL DIAGNOSES

- Discoid lupus erythematosus
- Dermatophytosis
- Epidermolysis bullosa
- Demodicosis
- Facial pyoderma

DIAGNOSTIC TESTS

Diagnosis is based on history, physical examination, compatible histologic changes in skin biopsies, and electromyography abnormalities consisting of positive sharp waves, fibrillation potentials, and bizarre high-frequency discharges of affected muscles[3].

MANAGEMENT

As the lesions of dermatomyosits can wax and wane on their own it is difficult to determine the effectiveness of any particular treatment. No treatment may be needed for cases with minimal lesions as they may spontaneously resolve in many cases. Oral vitamin E (200–800 IU/day) or marine lipid supplements may provide some improvement for skin lesions, but not the muscle lesions[2]. Prednisolone (1 mg/kg PO q 24 h) can be used for the treatment of lesions when they flare. Prolonged use of prednisolone is discouraged as it may cause aggravation of the muscle atrophy. Pentoxifylline (400 mg q 24–48 h) has been suggested as a possible treatment[2]. As this drug is a gastric irritant, it must be given with food. There is a lag period of 2–3 months before clinical benefits are noted. One author (PJM) has seen improvement in some dogs when they were treated with a combination of tetracycline (250 mg q 8 h in animals less than 10 kg, and 500 mg q 8 h in animals over 10 kg) and niacinamide (250 mg q 8 h in animals less than 10 kg, and 500 mg q 8 h in animals over 10 kg).

The various treatments suggested should not be expected to result in complete resolution of lesions as they only minimise the development of new lesions and lessen the severity of those present. This is a heritable disease and affected dogs and their offspring should not be used for breeding.

KEY POINT

- A well-recognized disease that is not easy to diagnose or manage.

Canine Familial Dermatomyositis

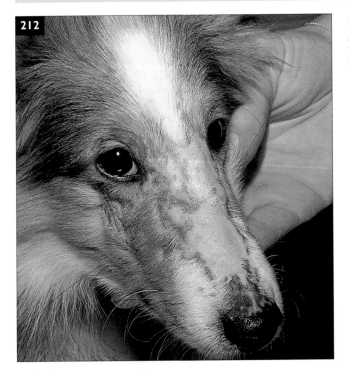

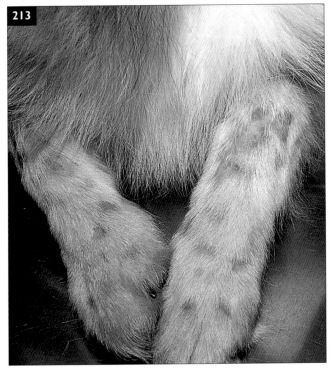

212, 213   Dermatomyositis in a Rough Collie demonstrating the alopecia and scale formation.

Sertoli Cell and other Testicular Neoplasia

DEFINITION
Sertoli cell neoplasms, seminomas, and interstitial cell tumors are potentially malignant neoplasms of the testicle arising, respectively, from the sustenticular cells, germinal cells, and cells of Leydig.

ETIOLOGY AND PATHOGENESIS
The etiology of testicular neoplasia is unknown. Cryptorchidism predisposes to Sertoli cell neoplasia and Sertoli cell tumors appear in retained abdominal or inguinal testes earlier than in scrotal testes[2,6]. Functional (estrogen secreting) Sertoli cell tumors occur in about 30% of cases and are more common in retained testes than in scrotal testes[6]. Alopecia may also be noted, in addition to the signs of feminization[2,6]. Symmetrical alopecia is commonly seen in association with Sertoli cell neoplasia, but rarely with other testicular neoplasia[2,6]. Malignant transformation with metastasis occurs in about 10% of cases of Sertoli cell tumor and about 5% of seminoma cases[2,6].

CLINICAL FEATURES
Boxers and, perhaps, Cairn Terriers, Border Collies, Shetland Sheepdogs, and Pekingese, are predisposed to testicular neoplasia[2,6], and they are affected at an earlier age (mean 7.2 years) than other breeds (mean 9–10 years)[2,6]. Interstitial cell tumors are the most common testicular tumors in dogs[2]. They are usually very small, often not palpable, and are confined to scrotal testes. Interstitial cell tumors are often associated with testosterone production, and prostatomegaly, perianal gland hyperplasia, perineal hernia, and tail gland hyperplasia (hyperandrogenism) may be noted[2,3,7]. Rarely, feminization is reported[5]. Most seminomas are scrotal in location, are usually palpable, and are very rarely associated with clinical signs other than testicular enlargement. Seminomas may, occasionally, metastasize[2]. Sertoli cell tumors are usually palpable if scrotal. However, systemic signs are usually associated with tumors in a non-scrotal location[2]. Symmetrical alopecia and hyperpigmentation may be seen, along with gynaecomastia and a pendulous penile sheath (**214**). A linear erythematous band may be noted along the ventral midline of the sheath (**215**). The hyperestrogenemia may be associated with signs such as squatting to urinate or attraction to male dogs. In addition, profound bone marrow depression may be noted in dogs with Sertoli cell neoplasia, and rarely other testicular tumors, and this may be severe enough to cause death[4,5].

DIFFERENTIAL DIAGNOSES
- Hypothyroidism.
- Hyperadrenocorticism.
- Adrenal sex hormone production.

DIAGNOSTIC TESTS
Physical examination will often reveal a scrotal or inguinal enlargement, or suggest cryptorchidism.

MANAGEMENT
Castration is indicated if testicular neoplasia is suspected. Signs of feminization can be expected to resolve 2–6 weeks after castration unless functional metastases are present[1,6]. Perianal gland hypertrophy and prostatomegaly, and tail gland hypertrophy, will also resolve after castration.

KEY POINT
- Always examine/palpate the scrotum in male dogs.

Sertoli Cell and other Testicular Neoplasia

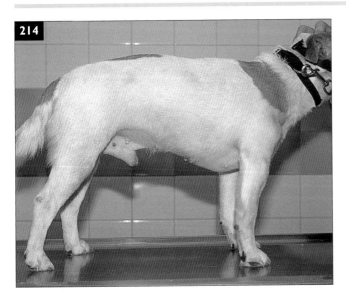

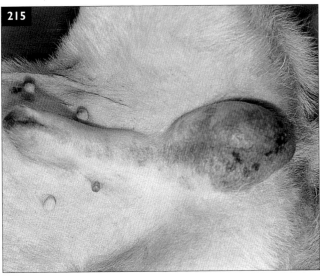

214, 215 Sertoli cell tumor. Note the downward pointing of the sheath (**214**) and the enlarged scrotum (due to a neoplastic testis) and the linear erythematous line along the sheath (**215**).

Dermatoses Responsive to Neutering

DEFINITION
These are rare dermatoses characterized by varying degrees of symmetrical alopecia and abnormalities in keratinization

ETIOLOGY AND PATHOGENESIS
The etiology of these conditions is not known. In one series of six cases of castration-responsive dermatosis[1], all had elevated serum concentrations of estradiol 17β. The source of this elevation was not reported. Defining these conditions has proved difficult because, for example, the inability to demonstrate abnormalities in circulating gonadal hormones in many cases may reflect simply the failure to assay the hormone involved. Alternatively, these conditions may reflect changes in follicular receptor expression or imbalance in sex hormones due to adrenal sex hormone production or the suspension of anagen initiation for a nonendocrinological reason. Hyperestrogenism may be associated with ovarian cysts or developmental abnormalities of the reproductive tract and, occasionally, by iatrogenic administration of estrogens. Hypoestrogenism has been proposed to reflect early neutering of bitches but there is some doubt as to the validity of this observation.

CLINICAL FEATURES
Keeshonds, Alaskan Malamutes, Pomeranians, and Miniature Poodles are most commonly affected by castration-responsive dermatosis. The disease often presents as bilaterally symmetrical alopecia (**216**), frequently affecting the neck, flanks, ventrum, and perineum[1,2]. The hair coat is usually completely absent in affected areas, although sometimes a rather woolly secondary haircoat remains. Animals may exhibit quite profuse scale and the remaining hair may exhibit a change in color, generally appearing paler than previously.

Hyperestrogenism is rare and there is no breed predisposition. Affected bitches usually exhibit ventral alopecia with the neck and perineum also affected[3]. The alopecic skin may be hyperpigmented and lichenified with comedones and an accumulation of greasy exudate[3,4], and there may be vulval enlargement[3]. Chronic cases may exhibit ceruminous otitis externa in addition to a generalized defect in keratinization characterized by greasy scale. The condition may be caused by ovarian cysts or pseudohermaphroditism[4,5] or, rarely, by iatrogenic administration of estrogens, typically for stress incontinence,

Hypoestrogenism is seen particularly in Dachshunds and Boxers[4]. There is diffuse thinning of the coat along the ventral abdomen and perineum, extending onto the caudal aspects of the thighs.

DIFFERENTIAL DIAGNOSES
- Hypothyroidism
- Hyperadrenocorticism
- Adrenal sex hormone production (growth hormone responsive dermatosis)
- Demodicosis
- Dermatophytosis
- Follicular dysplasia
- *Malassezia* dermatitis
- Defects in keratinization

DIAGNOSTIC TESTS
Clinical examination, historical features, skin scrapes, tape strips, and histopathologic examination of biopsy samples will allow the differential diagnosis to be narrowed to the endocrinopathies. In entire bitches a history of anestrus, polyestrus, or continuous estrus may suggest hyperestrogenism. Thyroid and adrenal disease is ruled out by dynamic assay. Elevated serum concentrations of estradiol 17β may suggest castration responsive dermatosis.

MANAGEMENT
Where appropriate, animals should be neutered. Owners should be cautioned that the surgery is irreversible and may not have any beneficial effects on the dermatosis.

KEY POINT
- Theories on etiology, classification, and management of disease in this area are far from satisfactory.

Dermatoses Responsive to Neutering

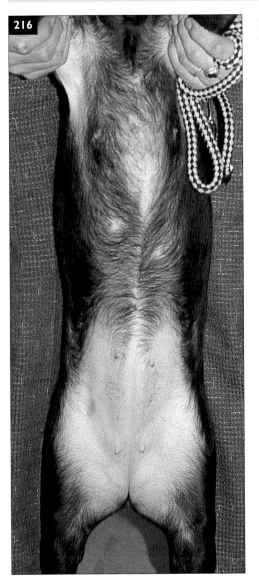

216   Symmetrical alopecia associated with a dermatosis responsive to neutering.

Dermatoses Related to Adrenal Sex Hormones

(Growth Hormone Responsive Dermatoses)

DEFINITION
Dermatoses due to sex hormone production by the zona reticularis in the adrenal glands.

ETIOLOGY AND PATHOGENESIS
Acquired or congenital deficiency in 11β-hydroxylase, 21-hydroxylase, or 3β-hydroxysteroid dehydrogenase has been proposed to result in accumulation of progesterone, 17-hydroxypregnenalone, or dehydroepiandrosterone, respectively[1,3]. There may also be a reduction in the synthesis of cortisone and aldosterone, stimulating ACTH secretion and resulting in adrenal hyperplasia and further increasing the concentration of circulating sex hormones. Binding of these hormones to certain, susceptible hair follicles results in alopecia[1,3].

CLINICAL FEATURES
Pomeranians, Chow Chows, Keeshonds, Samoyeds, and Poodles are predisposed[1]. Most animals are affected between 1 and 2 years of age, although older animals may also be presented. Either sex may be affected and the dermatosis may occur before or after neutering. The clinical signs are confined to symmetrical alopecia of the trunk, caudal thighs, and cervical regions (**217, 218**). Animals are not systemically affected. Alopecia may eventually affect the entire trunk, sparing the head and limbs[1]. Primary hairs are lost at first, but with time the secondary hairs also disappear. Hair may fail to regrow after clipping and, paradoxically, some affected cases exhibit local regrowth of hair after biopsy or local trauma[1].

DIFFERENTIAL DIAGNOSES
- Hypothyroidism
- Hyperadrenocorticism
- Castration responsive dermatosis
- Follicular dysplasia
- Cyclic flank alopecia
- Telogen or anagen defluxion

DIAGNOSTIC TESTS
After a full blood and biochemical screen, a dynamic thyroid and adrenal test should be performed, i.e. TSH and low-dose dexamethasone tests. Histopathologic examination of biopsy material will allow rule out of follicular dysplasia and defluxion, but is unlikely to differentiate between the endocrinopathies. ACTH testing should be performed using a dose of cosyntropin (synthetic ACTH) (0.5 IU/kg IV) and taking samples after 60 minutes[1,2]. Post-ACTH elevations in serum concentration of sex hormones is diagnostic.

MANAGEMENT
Entire animals should be neutered. Failure to regrow hair after neutering, or making the diagnosis in a neutered animal, will require other forms of therapy for the initiation of hair growth.

Growth hormone (bovine, porcine, or synthetic somatotrophin) may be tried (0.1 IU/kg; bovine somatotrophin in mg × 1.8 = IU), given 3 times a week for 6 weeks. Regrowth of hair is evident in 4–6 weeks, and a full coat is generally maintained for 2–3 years after which retreatment may be necessary. The treatment is very expensive and diabetes mellitus is a possible complication of growth hormone therapy. Because of this, weekly blood glucose determination should be made during therapy. If diabetes mellitus does develop it will generally resolve when growth hormone therapy is discontinued.

Methyltestosterone (1 mg/kg to a maximum dose of 30 mg/dog) every other day for a period of 3 months (or for a shorter duration if a clinical response is noted) may result in hair regrowth in some intact or neutered dogs. Liver enzymes should be monitored every 1–3 months in animals treated with methyltestosterone.

Therapy with mitotane (Lysodren (o'p'DDD)) may also be tried. It is administered at induction doses of 15–25 mg/kg q 24 h for 2–5 days with ACTH testing after 7 days. Cortisol concentrations should be in the range of 138–193 nmol/l (5–7 μg/dl) and may be followed by maintenance dosage of 15–25 mg/kg at biweekly intervals[1,2]. Favorable results should be seen within 3 months. Dogs should be monitored carefully for evidence of hypocortisolemia.

KEY POINT
- Theories on etiology, classification, and management of disease in this area are far from satisfactory.

Dermatoses Related to Adrenal Sex Hormones

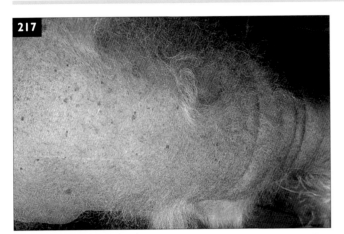

217, 218 Two cases of adult onset growth responsive dermatosis characterized by symmetrical alopecia.

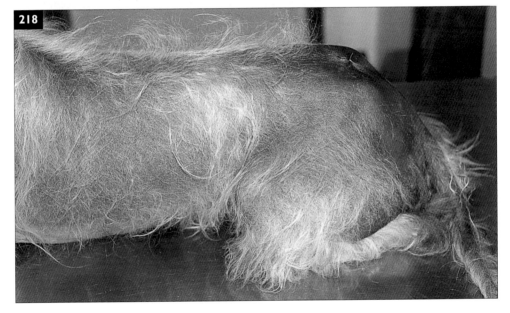

Telogen Effluvium and Anagen Defluxion

DEFINITION

These shedding abnormalities are a disruption of the normal mosaic hair replacement of the dog and cat. Normal replacement is affected primarily by photoperiod and, to a lesser extent, ambient temperature[1-3].

ETIOLOGY AND PATHOGENESIS

Anagen defluxion occurs when a condition, such as metabolic disease, endocrine disorders, infectious diseases, or treatment with antimitotic drugs, interferes with anagen, resulting in a sudden hair loss (occurring within days of the insult)[4].

Telogen defluxion occurs when a condition, such as whelping and lactation, pregnancy, high fever, severe illness, shock, surgery, or anaesthesia, results in the cessation of hair growth in many anagen follicles. This results in synchronization of these follicles to catagen and then telogen. When root activity begins again, typically after 1–3 months, large amounts of hair are shed[4].

The pathogenesis of wave shedding, diffuse shedding, and excessive continuous shedding has not been established.

CLINICAL FEATURES

Wave shedding concerns clients because they have noticed either a localized thinning of the coat, shedding of hair from a particular area, difference in coat color that is spreading, or differences in hair length between one region and another (**219**). It is characterized by a diffuse shedding that generally starts on the dorsum of the animal and descends ventrally on a horizontal plan. The coat is almost completely shed at the edge of the wave with new hair regrowth behind the wave. This often creates a contrast in coat length, coat color (new hair tends to be darker), coat density (new coat tends to be less dense), and texture (the new coat has a higher ratio of primary hairs).

Anagen defluxion is a diffuse shedding, especially of the trunk, that occurs within days of a systemic insult (**220**).

Telogen defluxion is a diffuse shedding, especially of the trunk, that occurs 1–3 months after a systemic insult.

Diffuse shedding occurs when an animal does not shed in a mosaic pattern but sheds the majority of its coat at one time, in the absence of a systemic insult, with normal regrowth.

Excessive continuous shedding is characterized by an animal who sheds excessive amounts of hair, but the coat never becomes thinned and no areas of alopecia develop.

DIFFERENTIAL DIAGNOSES

- Systemic disease, metabolic stress, long-standing pyrexia
- Post-clipping alopecia
- Endocrine diseases
- Toxicoses

DIAGNOSTIC TESTS

Diagnosis is based on history and clinical findings. Appropriate diagnostics to rule in or out a particular systemic insult should be performed as indicated. Histopathologic examination of biopsy samples is helpful in ruling in or out endocrinopathies.

MANAGEMENT

Wave and diffuse shedding will self-cure in 3–6 months. Anagen and telogen defluxion will self-cure 3–6 months after the systemic insult has been resolved. Removal of dead telogen hairs with a brush or comb so that they do not accumulate on household furnishings is the extent of management for excessive continuous shedding.

KEY POINT

- Another poorly defined group of diseases.

Telogen Effluvium and Anagen Defluxion

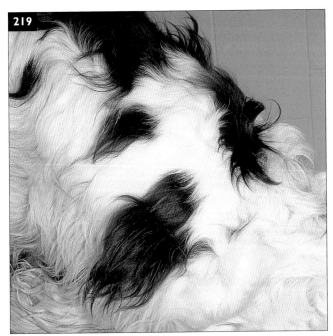

219, 220 Abnormal shedding with overlong regrowth of the black hairs (**219**) and patchy alopecia (**220**).

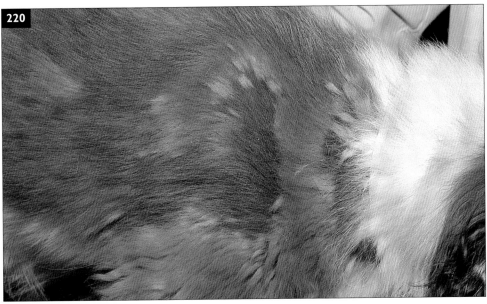

Post-clipping Alopecia

DEFINITION
Post-clipping alopecia is the failure of hair growth after the clipping of hair from a dog.

ETIOLOGY AND PATHOGENESIS
The exact mechanism for the arrest of hair growth in the clipped area is unknown. One theory is that decreased perfusion of hair follicles, secondary to vasoconstriction due to cooling of the skin by removal of the hair, may lead to premature termination of the growing phase[1]. Alternatively, it may simply reflect a very long anagen period.

CLINICAL FEATURES
Although post-clipping alopecia may occur in any breed, it occurs primarily in long-coated breeds, such as Siberian Huskies, Alaskan Malamutes, Samoyeds, Chow Chows and Keeshonds[1]. Clinically, the hair does not regrow after close clipping for venipuncture, surgery, wound management, or summer grooming (**221**). Occasionally, a few guard hairs will regrow in the affected area. Hair growth generally resumes 6–12 months after initial clipping.

DIFFERENTIAL DIAGNOSES
- Iatrogenic or endogenous hyperglucocorticoidism
- Growth hormone/castration responsive dermatosis
- Therapy with cytotoxic drugs
- Hypothyroidism

DIAGNOSTIC TESTS
The diagnosis is based on history and clinical findings as well as ruling out conditions in the differential diagnosis. Histopathologic findings on biopsy samples are supportive.

MANAGEMENT
There is no treatment that benefits this condition. With time hair will regrow in most animals.

KEY POINT
- A poorly understood condition.

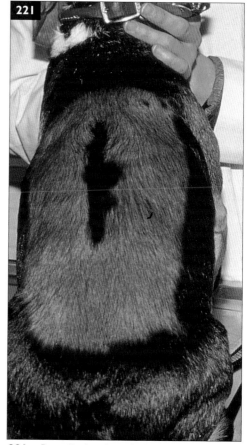

221 Post-clipping alopecia. (Illustration courtesy of S. Torres.)

Otitis Externa

GENERAL APPROACH
1 Always attempt to make a definitive diagnosis – do not rely on polypharmacy.
2 Remember that otitis commonly results from underlying disease.

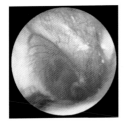
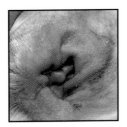
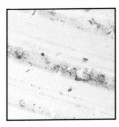
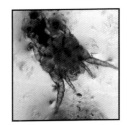

Otitis Externa

DEFINITION
Otitis externa results from inflammation of the epithelial lining of the external auditory canal. The inflammation may arise within the external ear canal following, for example, grass seed penetration, or result from conditions affecting the pinnae or middle ear.

ETIOLOGY AND PATHOGENESIS
Otitis externa may result from many causes and it has proven useful to classify these as primary, predisposing, and secondary[1].

Primary factors directly induce inflammation within the external ear canal:
- Ectoparasites
- Foreign bodies
- Hypersensitivities
- Disorders of keratinization
- Autoimmune conditions

Predisposing factors alter the environment within the eternal ear canal, which may result in quantitative and qualitative changes in otic microflora:
- Conformation
- Otic neoplasia or otopharyngeal polyp formation, which obstruct the ear canal
- Errors in otic pharmacy or errors in the management of ear disease
- Environmental temperature and humidity, lifestyle (particularly swimming)

Perpetuating factors arise within the external ear canal as a consequence of primary or predisposing conditions:
- Changes in microflora
- Otitis media
- Progressive changes in the otic epithelium and underlying cartilage

CLINICAL FEATURES
Clinical features will vary from individual to individual because of variation in primary cause, predisposing conditions, perpetuating factor, and individual expression[1,2]. In particular, the clinician should bear in mind a few key points:
- Acute, unilateral otitis externa is common in the dog and typically reflects a foreign body penetration. Acute, unilateral otitis externa is unusual in the cat.
- Chronic unilateral otitis externa in the cat is often associated with neoplasia or polyp formation, whereas bilateral otitis externa in the cat is considered to be otodectic mange until proven otherwise.

- Bilateral otitis externa in the dog, particularly if recurrent, is highly suggestive of hypersensitivity, such as atopy, dietary intolerance, or topical neomycin sensitivity.
- Chronic otitis externa results in a quantitative (more bacteria) and qualitative (initially more gram-positive and then more gram-negative bacteria) shift in microbial flora[3].
- Erythematous ulceration of the external ear canal suggests gram-negative infection.
- Pustules are rare on the concave aspect of the pinna and are often associated with pemphigus foliaceus rather than superficial pyoderma.

Foreign bodies
Foreign bodies, particularly grass seeds, are usually easily seen on otoscopic examination (**222**, **223**), although in some cases the ear canal needs to be cleaned before they can be visualized.

Otodectes cynotis
Infestation has a characteristic appearance and is associated with large amounts of dry, dark brown, waxy debris with variable amounts of inflammation (**224**). Careful otoscopic examination may allow for visualization of the mites as they move within the canal (**225**). Mites may also be seen on microscopic examination of scrapes from the external ear canal (**226**). Otodemodicosis (due to *Demodex canis*) is a rare cause of chronic otitis externa in the dog.

Bacterial infection
Infection with *Staphylococcus* spp., *Streptococcus* spp., and *Proteus* spp. is often, although not exclusively, associated with a light yellow exudate in most cases. The discharge becomes progressively darker if there is concomitant wax production.

Yeast infection
Infection, particularly *Malassezia* spp., may result in a chocolate brown waxy discharge (**227**). In cats, *Malassezia* spp. have been associated with chronic pruritic otitis externa characterized by minimal discharge. The status of *M. pachydermatis* as an otic pathogen is uncertain[4].

Pseudomonas spp.
Pseudomonas spp. are often found in ears that are very inflamed, eroded, or ulcerated and have copious amounts of bright yellow exudate (**228**). This organism is more likely to be present if the case is chronic.

Otitis Externa

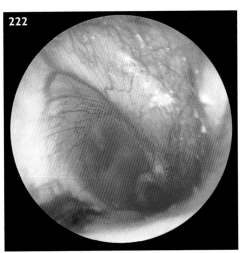 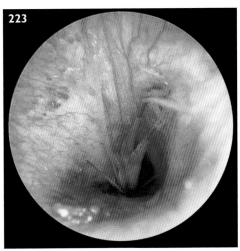

222–223   Otitis externa. Normal view of the tympanum (**222**) and of a foreign body (grass seed) adjacent to the tympanum (**223**).

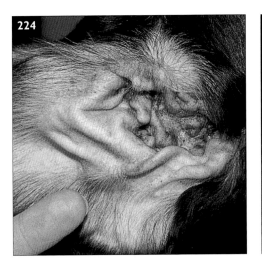 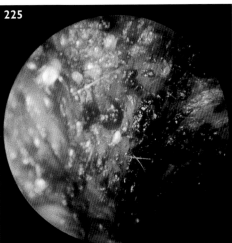

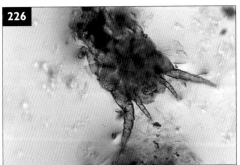

224–226   Otitis externa. Otic discharge secondary to *Otodectes cynotis* infection (**224**); the mites seen on otoscopic (**225**) and microscopic (**226**) examination.

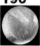

Otitis Externa

Hypersensitivities

Hypersensitivities are a common cause of chronic otitis externa, particularly in the dog (**229**). Early cases may exhibit erythema and lichenification of the concave aspect of the pinna and the vertical portion of the external ear canal. In these early cases the horizontal ear canal may appear quite normal. Most cases of atopy (or dietary intolerance) are associated with bilateral otitis externa, although unilateral ear disease may be seen occasionally. Furthermore, although most cases of atopy (in the dog) will be associated with pruritus (face, feet, and ventrum), a few atopic dogs will present with otitis externa alone.

Defects in keratinization

These are often associated with chronic otitis externa (**230**). Some breeds (notably Cocker Spaniels) are prone to both otitis externa and idiopathic defects in keratinization, possibly due to conformational problems such as narrow, hirsute ear canals[5].

Autoimmune diseases

These may be associated with pustules and crusts on the pinnae and otic epithelium. By far the most common of these rare diseases is pemphigus foliaceus, and the otic lesions may on rare occasions be confined to the pinnae and ear

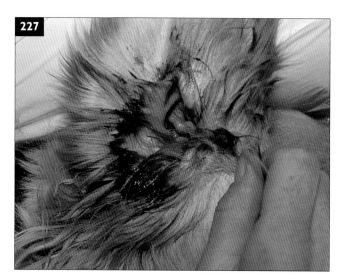

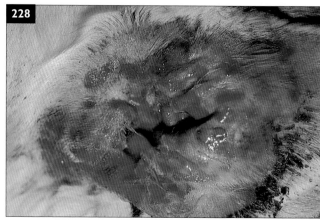

227, 228 Otitis externa. The typical brown discharge that is often associated with *Malassezia pachydermatis* infection (**227**); extensive ulceration associated with *Pseudomonas aeruginosa* infection (**228**).

Otitis Externa

canal. More usually there is extensive pustule and crust formation. The diseases which cause deeper lesions, such as pemphigus vulgaris and bullous pemphigoid, may cause ulceration in the ear canal, but will be associated with lesions elsewhere and systemic disease.

Whatever the cause of the otitis externa, the chronic changes to the external ear canal are associated with hyperplasia of the apocrine glands[6], thickening of the otic epithelium, a reduction in the effective diameter of the ear canal, and an increase in the humidity within the canal lumen[5,6]. Maceration of surface debris occurs and the potential for further microbial multiplication and continued inflammation is apparent. In severe, long-standing cases of otitis externa, ossification of the external ear canal and associated cartilage may occur.

DIFFERENTIAL DIAGNOSES

The differential diagnoses for otitis externa are formulated on the basis of history, clinical examination, and the observation of any association, or otherwise, with systemic or generalized disease. Broadly, all primary and most predisposing conditions should be considered.

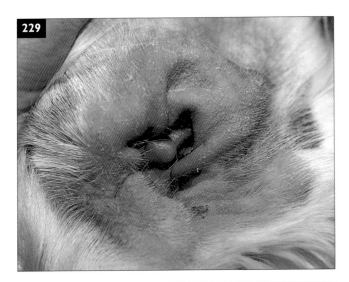

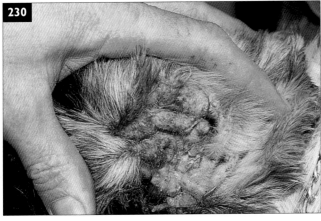

229, 230 Chronic otitis externa associated with atopic dermatitis (**229**); a defect in keratinization (**230**).

Otitis Externa

DIAGNOSTIC TESTS

Appropriate diagnostic and laboratory procedures should be performed to rule in or out the various predisposing conditions.

Cytologic evaluation of otic exudates or debris should be the initial diagnostic procedure. Smears should be stained with either Gram's stain or a modified Wright's stain (e.g. Diff-Quick) and examined for numbers and morphology of bacteria, yeast, leukocytes, and neoplastic cells (**231**, **232**). The presence of cocci on smears is indicative of *Staphylococcus* spp. or *Streptococcus* spp., while the presence of gram-negative rods may indicate either *Pseudomonas* spp. or *Proteus* spp. Peanut-shaped yeast are characteristic of *Malassezia* spp., which are the most commonly found yeast in the ear. In addition to stained smears, debris from the ear canal can be mixed with mineral oil and examined for ectoparasites and their eggs or larvae.

Samples of ear exudate should be submitted for culture and sensitivity when the presence of gram-negative rods is noted on cytology. This is because of the high likelihood of *Pseudomonas* spp., which can become resistant to a majority of systemic antibacterial agents. Samples for culture and sensitivity should also be submitted when there has not been significant response to initial treatment.

To diagnose a tumor or to differentiate neoplasia from proliferative tissue in the ear canal, a small pinch biopsy may be obtained with an endoscopic forceps passed through the otoscope cone.

MANAGEMENT

Predisposing conditions should receive appropriate treatment for the specific disease or factor.

In-hospital ear cleaning

To ensure that the ear canals are free of exudate and debris prior to topical treatment, it is recommended that the clinician, or an experienced technician, perform the initial cleaning. Ears with minimal secretions and patent canals may be cleaned without sedation. However, sedation is generally appropriate for the initial cleaning as it allows for a more through cleaning and better visualization of the ear canal and tympanic membrane. A combination of ketamine (1.36–2.2 mg/kg), diazepam (0.45 mg/kg), and acepromazine (0.23 mg/kg) mixed together and given IV has been used

satisfactorily for both examination and cleaning of the ears. The higher dose of ketamine (2.2 mg/kg) is preferred, and provides ample restraint for about 20 minutes.

The status of the tympanic membrane should be established before cleaning. If it cannot be visualized due to exudate or debris, or if it is known to be ruptured, saline can be used to rinse the ear. If an animal swallows, gags, or coughs when fluid is placed in the ear, it is a good indication that the tympanic membrane is ruptured. If saline is not able to rinse away the exudate or debris, then a solution containing propylene glycol, malic acid, benzoic acid, and salicylic acid (e.g. Oti-Clens (Pfizer), or Dermisol Multicleanse Solution (Pfizer)) is used[2,8]. This solution has been used for cleaning ears with ruptured tympanic membranes without any apparent signs of ototoxicity. However, the middle ear is always flushed after with saline. *It must be appreciated that there is no completely safe solution for cleaning the middle ear. Even water may cause a loss of cochlear and/or vestibular function*[7,8].

If the tympanic membrane is intact, the ear canal is filled with a solution containing dioctyl sodium sulfosuccinate, carbamide peroxide, and tetracaine (e.g. Clear-X Ear Cleansing Solution, DVM Pharmaceuticals). The ear canal is then massaged for 1 to 2 minutes to loosen and dissolve the debris, and the excess solution and debris that has floated to the surface is wiped away with a cotton ball. The ear canal is then flushed twice with lukewarm water using a bulb syringe. Failure to rinse this solution from the ear may result in irritation to the epithelium of the ear canal. If suction is available, it is attached to a No. 8 French urinary catheter cut to a length of 15 cm (6 in) and, while observing through a operating head otoscope, any remaining water and debris is suctioned from the canal and it is examined to verify that it is completely clean. If not, the process is repeated.

At-home ear cleaning

Periodic cleaning by the patient's owner is often necessary to remove secretions associated with continued inflammation or infection. The interval for this cleaning will vary from daily to weekly or longer, depending on the rate of accumulation of exudate or wax in the ear.

For removal of a waxy debris, a product containing docusate sodium (dioctyl sodium sulfosuccinate (DSS)), hexamethyltetracosane, or squalene

Otitis Externa

should be used. The following are examples of appropriate products:
- Epi-Otic, Allerderm/Virbac
- Otic Blue, Chesterfield
- Wax-O-Sol, Life Science Products
- Seb-O-Sol, Butler
- Cerumene, Evsco
- Leo Ear Cleaner, Leo Laboratories Ltd

Removal of a moist exudate from the ear can be accomplished by cleaning with one of the following:
- Oti-Clens, Pfizer
- Dermisol Multicleanse Solution, Pfizer
- Epi-Otic, Allerderm/Virbac
- Chlorhexiderm Flush, DVM Pharmaceuticals

A mixture of wax and exudate can be removed by cleaning with one of the following:
- Epi-Otic, Allerderm/Virbac
- Chlorhexiderm Flush, DVM Pharmaceuticals
- Leo Ear Cleaner, Leo Laboratories Ltd

Topical treatment
Topical antibacterial treatment
If doublets or packets of gram-positive cocci are present (most likely to be *Staphylococcus* spp.), topical preparations containing one of the following would be appropriate:
- Neomycin
- Gentamicin
- Chloramphenicol
- Fusidic acid

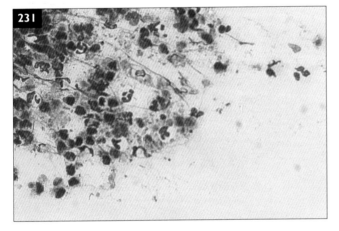

231   Otitis externa. Otic cytology may reveal many leukocytes.

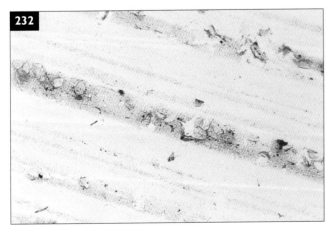

232   Otitis externa. Otic cytology may reveal masses of bacteria.

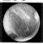

Otitis Externa

If chains of gram-positive cocci are present (most likely to be *Streptococcus* spp.), a topical preparation containing one of the penicillins would be appropriate.

If gram-negative rods are present (most likely to be *Pseudomonas* spp.), preparations containing one of the following would be appropriate pending the results of culture and sensitivity.

- Acetic acid based otic preparation, such as Oti Clens or Dermisol Multicleanse Solution, Pfizer
- Gentamicin
- Polymyxin B
- Amikacin
- Enrofloxacin
- Silver sulfadiazine suspension
- Ticarcillin

Neomycin, gentamicin, chloramphenicol, polymyxin B, and amikacin are ototoxic and should not be used if the tympanic membrane is ruptured[7, 8]. Antibacterials that would be appropriate for this situation include enrofloxacin, ticarcillin, penicillin, and silver sulfadiazine.

Topical antiyeast treatment
If yeast are present, topical preparations containing one of the following would be appropriate:
- Clotrimazole
- Miconazole
- Cuprimyxin
- Nystatin
- Amphotericin B

Topical anti-inflammatory treatment
Many otic preparations contain glucocorticoids, which will benefit most cases of otitis externa by reducing pruritus, swelling, exudation, and tissue hyperproliferation. Hyperplasia of tissues lining the ear canal benefits from the treatment of a solution containing flucinolone acetonide in 60% dimethylsulfoxide (Synotic, Syntex Animal Health). Long-term topical use of glucocorticoids in ears may result in systemic absorption, resulting in elevations of liver enzymes and suppression of the adrenal response to adrenocorticotrophic hormone (ACTH)[9].

Topical antiparasitic treatment
Ears with *O. cynotis* infestation should first be cleaned of excess wax and then treated daily for 20 days with a preparation containing one of the following:

- Rotenone
- Pyrethrin
- Carbaryl
- Monosulfiram

In addition, all contact animals – both dogs and cats – should be treated as asymptomatic carriers as they may be a source of reinfection. As *O. cynotis* can occasionally be found on other body areas, 3-weekly, whole-body treatments with pyrethrin sprays would be appropriate.

Systemic treatment
Prednisolone (0.1–0.2 mg/kg q 12 h PO) or methylprednisolone (0.05–0.1 mg/kg q 12 h PO) may be administered for 10–14 days to reduce severe inflammation and swelling due to hypersensitivity states or the foreign body reaction that occurs due to rupture of cystic apocrine glands.

Systemic antibacterial agents are indicated when the tympanic membrane is ruptured and infection is present in the middle ear, or when there is poor response to topical treatment. Choice should be made according to culture and sensitivity results.

Extra-label use of ivermectin is effective for the treatment of *O. cynotis*. Three treatments (0.3 mg/kg SC) are given at 10-day intervals to the affected animal as well as all contact animals[10]. Ivermectin is contraindicated in Collies, Shetland Sheepdogs, and certain other herding breeds.

Indications for surgery
Surgery is indicated when a tumor or polyp is present in the ear canal or when the hyperplasia of the ear canal is so great the resulting stenosis precludes appropriate cleaning and application of medications. A surgical text should be consulted for the exact procedures, as techniques will vary depending on the extent and location of lesions.

KEY POINTS
- Treat otitis externa seriously.
- Failure to treat underlying disease results in recurrent otitis and irreversible changes may occur.

Disorders of the Nails

GENERAL APPROACH
1 Diagnosis is difficult.
2 Treatment is often very prolonged and good communication is important.

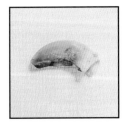 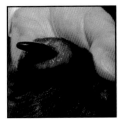 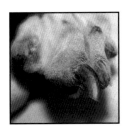

Disorders of the Nails

DEFINITION

Claw abnormalities are defined by certain terms. The following is a partial list of these terms and includes those that are used more frequently in association with conditions of the dog and cat[1]:

- Macronychia: unusually large claws
- Onychalgia: claw pain
- Onychia (onchitis): inflammation somewhere in the claw unit
- Onychoclasis: breaking of claws
- Onychocryptosis (onyxis): in-grown claws
- Onychodystrophy: abnormal claw formation
- Onychogryphosis: hypertrophy and abnormal curvature of claws
- Onychomadesis: sloughing of claws (**233**)
- Onychomalacia: softening of claws
- Onychomycosis: fungal infection of claws
- Onychorrhexis: longitudinal striations associated with brittleness and breaking of claws
- Onychoschizia: splitting and/or lamination of claws, usually beginning distally
- Onychopathy: disease abnormality of claws
- Paronychia: inflammation/infection of claw folds (**234, 235**)

ETIOLOGY AND PATHOGENESIS

Onycopathy may occur due to trauma, bacterial infection, neoplasia, dermatophytosis, pemphigus foliaceus, lupus erythematosus, other autoimmune diseases, deep mycotic infections, leishmaniasis, severe generalized systemic disease, severe nutritional deficiencies, and idiopathic changes[1-4].

CLINICAL FEATURES

Trauma

Trauma is the most common cause of damage to the claw of dogs and cats. This often occurs when a long claw is caught in a carpet or rug resulting in avulsion of the claw plate. Damage can also occur with bite wounds, or when a foot is run over by a motor vehicle or is stepped on. It may also occur in hunting dogs and racing Greyhounds due to the severe strain that is placed on the claws whilst the dogs are working. Onychalgia, onychoclasis, onychomadesis and, occasionally, onychorrexis are noted. Secondary bacterial infection with exudate formation is a frequent finding associated with trauma[1].

Bacterial infection

This is generally thought to be secondary to other conditions such as trauma, and it has been reported in association with systemic diseases such as hypothyroidism, hyperadrenocorticism, and atopic dermatitis[1]. However, it can occur as primary disease[4].

Onychoclasis

Onychoclasis may occur with or without onychorrhexis. The etiology is unknown but many of the animals respond to biotin therapy[4]. Small pieces of the claw break off, with or without longitudinal cracking. Generally, many but not all nails are affected.

Onychomycosis

Onychomycosis is a rare condition and is usually due to *Trichophyton mentagrophytes*[1,2]. Onychodystrophy is the predominant clinical finding with the nails appearing friable and misshapen. Generally, only one to two nails are affected, but many or all can suffer from the disease.

Autoimmune/immune-mediated diseases

Pemphigus vulgaris, pemphigus foliaceus, bullous pemphigoid, systemic lupus erythematosus, a lupus-like syndrome, cold agglutinin disease, drug eruption, and vasculitis have been associated with onychomadesis and onychodystrophy[2]. Often, most claws on many of the feet are affected[2]. Macronychia and onychomalacia were the only clinical signs in one dog with pemphigus foliaceus[4].

Lupoid onychodystrophy

Onychomadesis with exudate under the claw plate of one or a few claws is the most common clinical presentation. In some cases, infection will initially occur in only 1–3 nails, but slowly over a 4–8 month period many if not all the claws will become involved[4].

Recently, an immune-mediated tissue pattern has been described in the nail bed of dogs with idiopathic onychomadesis.

Neoplastic diseases

Squamous cell carcinoma, melanoma, mast cell tumor, keratoacanthoma, inverted papilloma, lymphosarcoma, eccrine adenocarcinoma, neurofibrosarcoma, hemangiopericytoma, fibrosarcoma, and osteosarcoma have all been reported to occur in the digit/claw and/or the claw fold[2]. Animals are presented for swelling of the claw or digit and variable degrees of paronychia, erosion, and ulceration. Squamous cell carcinoma arising from germinal claw epithelium is the most common

Disorders of the Nails

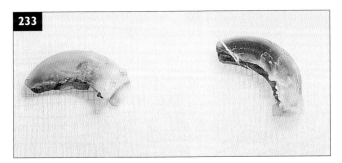

233–235   Shedding of nails (**233**) and paronychia (**234, 235**). **235** shows erythematous swelling around the base of a nail.

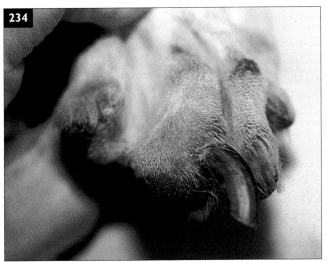

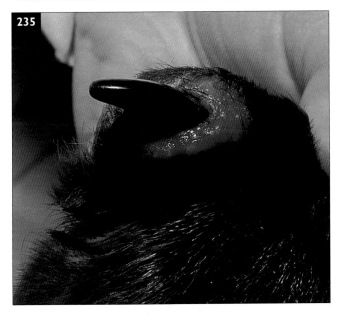

Disorders of the Nails

digital tumor of the dog[2]. It develops more frequently in black Standard Poodles and black Labrador Retrievers, and multiple digits may be involved over a course of 2–6 years[2,4].

DIFFERENTIAL DIAGNOSES
See the conditions listed under 'Etiology and Pathogenesis'.

DIAGNOSTIC TESTS
Bacterial culture and sensitivity of any exudates, after appropriate cleaning. Fungal culture of dystrophic claws. Biopsy is difficult since the nail bed is essential for a definitive diagnosis. This is achieved by amputating P3 and its associated claw, or a proximal transection of the claw, and there is often considerable owner resistance to this procedure. Appropriate diagnostic tests to rule in or out systemic diseases in the differential diagnosis would also be indicated.

MANAGEMENT
Trauma
Any loose fragments of the claw plate should be removed. If large amounts of the claw plate are missing, the area can be dressed with silver sulfadiazine and bandaged for 2–3 days. Systemic antibiotics (if possible based on culture and sensitivity) are appropriate for 4–6 weeks as secondary infection is common with trauma[1,2].

Bacterial infection
The animal should be anesthetized and all loose claw plates removed. Treatment as described for trauma should then be carried out.

Onychoclasis
The claws should be kept trimmed short. Clients should use an electric disc sanding tool designed for use on nails as it does not split or crack the nails. Biotin (0.05 mg/kg PO q 24 h) is beneficial in many cases[2,4]. Gelatin (10 grains PO q 12 h) has also been reported to be beneficial[1].

Autoimmune/immune-mediated diseases
These and other systemic diseases are treated as appropriate for the specific disease.

Neoplasitc diseases
Surgical removal of the affected digit or digits. The lung fields should be radiographed prior to surgery to demonstrate the presence, or otherwise, of metastases. The prescapular lymph node should be excised and submitted for histopathologic examination.

Lupoid onychodystrophy
Systemic glucocorticoids, at anti-inflammatory (0.5–0.7 mg/kg PO q 12 h) or moderate (1.0–1.2 mg/kg PO q 12 h) immunosuppressive doses are the most logical treatments for this pattern of tissue infiltrate (as with the lupoid diseases, for example). However, there are a few case reports suggesting that n:6 fatty acids, or mixtures of n:6 and n:3 fatty acids, may be helpful in the long-term management of lupoid onychodystrophy.

KEY POINTS
- Nail disorders are frustrating for owners and clinicians.

Dermatoses Characterized by Patchy Alopecia

GENERAL APPROACH
1 The differential diagnoses are dominated by demodicosis – scrape everything.
2 Dermatophytosis may be zoonotic.

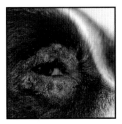
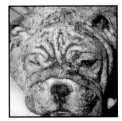
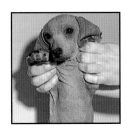
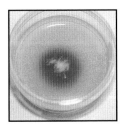

Canine Demodicosis

(Red Mange, Demodectic Mange, Demodicosis, Demodectic Acariasis, Follicular Mange)

DEFINITION

Demodicosis is a parasitic disease resulting from the presence of increased numbers of demodicid mites belonging to the genus *Demodex* in the skin.

ETIOLOGY AND PATHOGENESIS

Demodex canis is responsible for the majority of lesions in dogs[1]. The mites generally reside in the hair follicles but have been found in adjacent sebaceous and apocrine glands. Transmission from animal to animal is thought to be restricted to mother and offspring and is confined to the immediate post-natal period[1]. Completion of the entire life cycle requires from 20–35 days and consists of five stages: spindle-shaped eggs; small larvae which have three pairs of short legs; protonymphs which also have three pair of legs; nymphs which have four pair of legs; and adults which have a head, thorax, and four pair of legs[1].

Demodex canis are present in small numbers in the skin of a majority of healthy dogs and are asymptomatic. The mites feed primarily on follicular cells, follicular debris, and to a lesser extent sebum[1]. Adult mites survive for only a short period of time off the host[1].

The reason that some animals develop clinical disease is not completely understood. Studies have shown that there is a serum factor present in dogs with generalized demodectic mange that results in lymphocyte suppression[2–6]. However, lymphocyte suppression is also influenced by secondary bacterial infection[7]. Therefore, it appears that demodectic mites as well as a secondary bacterial pyoderma result in lymphocyte suppression, which may allow for excessive proliferation of the mite population. A hereditary factor also appears to play a role, as elimination of affected as well as carrier dogs (both parents and siblings) from a breeding programme greatly reduces or eliminates the incidence of clinical disease[8].

CLINICAL FEATURES

Localized demodicosis

The localized form of demodicosis is more common in younger dogs (3–11 months of age). Lesions consist of one or more focal areas of either scaling, thinning of the hair, alopecia, or erythema with alopecia (**236, 237**). They may be located on any area of the body, but are most frequently noted on the face and forelimbs.

Approximately 90% of these cases will self-cure, while 10% will progress and develop into generalized disease[1].

Generalized demodicosis

The generalized form of demodicosis occurs as a progression of localized lesions, and can be extremely varied with regard to clinical appearance. Widespread areas of alopecia develop with scaling, seborrhea, erythema, pustules, papules, crusts, and ulcers (**238, 239**). Furunculosis follows rupture of hair follicles and foreign body reactions to mites, keratin debris, and sebum. Follicular hyperkeratosis is a common feature, which appears clinically as dilated hair follicles containing keratin plugs. Animals with erythema, papules, and ulcers are often pruritic. Lesions can become secondarily infected with *Staphylococcus intermedius*, *Pseudomonas aeruginosa*, or *Proteus mirabilis*, which can facilitate ulceration and result in lesions that are exudative and crusting. Peripheral lymphadenopathy is marked. Dogs with generalized demodicosis often become debilitated, anorectic, lethargic, depressed, and febrile. Pododermatitis may occur and is characterized by swelling of the feet, with the development of interdigital cysts that ulcerate and drain a serosanguineous to exudative material. Pododemodicosis carries a poor prognosis since resolution of the mites is very difficult (**240**).

DIFFERENTIAL DIAGNOSES

- Dermatophytosis
- Color-dilute alopecia
- Sebaceous adenitis
- Superficial pyoderma
- Deep pyoderma
- Juvenile pyoderma
- Zinc responsive dermatitis
- Post-injection alopecia
- Alopecia areata
- Deep mycotic infection
- Pemphigus foliaceus
- Mycosis fungoides
- Drug eruption

DIAGNOSTIC TESTS

Microscopic examination of skin scrapings will usually reveal demodectic mites (**241**). The process is aided by squeezing the skin (which forces mites out of the follicles) before scraping.

Canine Demodicosis

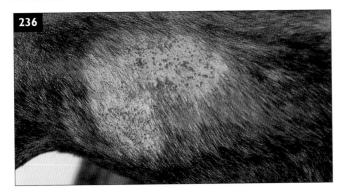

236, 237 Localized demodicosis on the forelimb of a Boxer (**236**); periorbital alopecia and crusting (**237**).

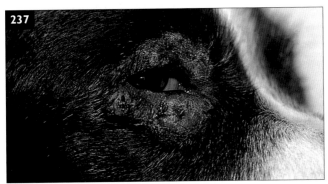

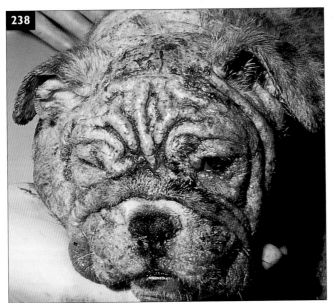

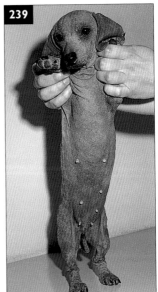

238, 239 Generalized demodicosis. Multiple erosions and furunculosis on the face of a 6-month-old English Bulldog (**238**); generalized alopecia and hyperpigmentation in a Dachshund (**239**).

Canine Demodicosis

Very thickened skin, chronic pedal lesions, and Chinese Shar-Peis may carry mites too deeply to be revealed by skin scrapings. In these cases, biopsy should be considered. Bacterial culture and sensitivity would be appropriate for those cases that have secondary infection.

MANAGEMENT

Localized demodicosis

The value of topical treatment of localized lesions with benzoyl peroxide gel or rotenone preparations on a daily basis remains in question as most cases resolve spontaneously. Such therapies may be dispensed to quell an owner's anxieties, but re-examinations should be scheduled at 2–3 week intervals to assess whether or not the case is resolving or becoming generalized.

Generalized demodicosis

Clipping medium- and long-haired dogs, bathing with benzoyl peroxide shampoo, and then saturating the total body either weekly or every 2 weeks with an amitraz solution is the most frequently used treatment protocol. Skin scrapings are taken prior to each treatment, and therapy is continued 4–6 weeks beyond the point where the scrapings become negative for mites. Reported cure rates for this treatment vary from 50–86%[9,10], although up to 12 weeks' treatment may be necessary.

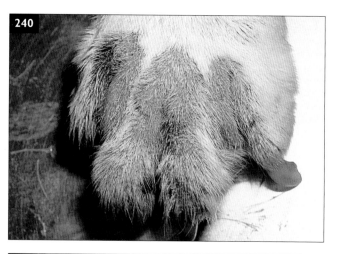

240 Generalized demodicosis. Pododemodicosis.

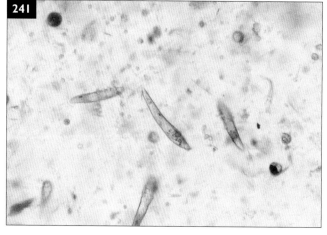

241 Photomicrograph of adult *Demodex canis* mites recovered in a skin scrape from a dog.

Canine Demodicosis

Animals not cured will be clinically improved, but yield a few mites on scrapings. Others will exhibit clinical relapse once treatment is stopped. Clinical disease can be controlled in many of these animals if treatments are continued at intervals of 4–6 weeks.

Transient sedation is the most common side-effect of amitraz and it may not occur with subsequent treatments. Severe pruritus, sedation, weakness, and ataxia are noted in some cases, but these side-effects are rare. Amitraz should not be used on Chihuahuas.

Other therapeutic strategies
Milbemycin
Milbemycin (0.5 mg/kg PO q 12 h) for 90 days[11]. If mites are still present, the dose can be increased (to 1.0–2.0 mg/kg PO q 12 h) with re-examinations to assess progress every 30 days. Expected cure rates for generalized demodectic mange using milbemycin are approximately 60%[11]. Most animals are negative for mites on skin scrapings at 60–90 days. Treatment should be continued 30 days beyond negative scrapings. Side-effects of milbemycin at the higher dose have included vomiting, stupor, trembling, and ataxia in small numbers of cases[11,12]. The neurologic signs disappeared within 24 hours of drug withdrawal, and did not recur when the lower dose was used. Vomiting did not recur even at the higher dose when the medication was given with meals. Another consideration for the use of milbemycin is the high cost of the medication.

Ivermectin
Ivermectin (0.6 mg/kg of the injectable solution q 24 h PO). Animals are re-examined and skin scrapings taken at 42-day intervals and treatment is continued 45 days beyond the time when skin scrapings become negative[13]. Collies, Collie cross-breeds, and some herding dogs and their crosses should not be treated with ivermectin due to CNS side-effects. Mydriasis, ataxia, disorientation, and lethargy are occasional side-effects in other breeds[13]. Relapses can occur in some animals (especially those with pododermatitis). The authors have found that if these animals are retreated until skin scrapings are negative and then maintained on ivermectin (0.6 mg/kg PO q 3 weeks), they will generally not relapse again. Expected cure rates for generalized demodectic mange using ivermectin are approximately 85%[13].

Adjunctive measures
Secondary bacterial infection should be treated with appropriate systemic antibacterial agents. Weekly baths with benzoyl peroxide shampoos are helpful for removing crusts, debris, and surface bacteria. Antihistamines may be used to ameliorate pruritus.

> *Note: Systemic steroids should never be used in the treatment of demodectic mange as their immunosuppressive effects exacerbate the infestation.*

As there appears to be a hereditary predisposition to the development of demodectic mange, it is recommended that generalized cases should not be used for breeding. The definition of generalized demodicosis is 'A dog who has five or more localized lesions, has involvement of an entire body region (e.g. facial area), or has complete involvement of two or more feet'[14].

KEY POINTS
- Possibly the most serious non-neoplastic dermatologic disease. Client education and good communication are essential.
- Do not be tempted to skip re-examination and do repeat skin scrapings.

Dermatophytosis

DEFINITION
Dermatophytosis is an infection (of the skin, hair, or nail) due to fungi of the genera *Microsporum*, *Trichophyton* , or *Epidermophyton*[1].

ETIOLOGY AND PATHOGENESIS
The most common cause of dermatophytosis in cats is *M. canis*[2,3]. In dogs the most common causes are *M. canis* and *M. gypseum*[2,3]. Other dermatophytes isolated less frequently include *T. mentagrophytes*, *M. persicolor*, *M. erinacei*, and *M. verrucosum*[2]. Dermatophytes can be isolated from the skin and hair of apparently normal cats, particularly those in colonies, show circles, and pounds, although healthy pet cats are unlikely to be infected[4–7].

Certain groups of animals appear to be predisposed to infection. Thus, dermatophytes can be recovered more frequently from animals less than 12 months of age, presumably because of a poorly developed immune response[2,3]. Dermatophytosis, in general, is more common in young animals[2], and dermatophytosis due to *M. canis* is more common in Persian cats[3]. Animals which are old, infirm, immunoincompetent, or severely stressed are also predisposed to dermatophytosis and exhibit more severe clinical signs[2,8]. Jack Russell Terriers appear predisposed to dermatophytosis due to *T. mentagrophytes* and *T. erinacei*[3].

Following infection with a dermatophyte, the animal responds with both a cell-mediated and humoral response[9,10]. The immune response, particularly the cell-mediated response, results in clearing of the infection[11]. The inflammatory reaction provoked by the dermatophyte also results in increased epidermal proliferation, which will tend to 'wash out' the dermatophyte in the epidermal tide. This state of immunity does not appear to confer complete resistance, although subsequent infection, in an immune host, results in a more rapid onset of clinical signs and a tendency to clear infections more quickly[9]. Experimental infection results in lesions reaching maximum size about 5 weeks after infection[12,13]. Self-cure of dermatophytosis has been reported, but the risk of zoonotic infection makes treatment mandatory.

Of major importance to other cats, and to people, within the same household or colony is the shedding of viable fungal spores into the immediate environment from the infected animal. These have the potential to remain viable for as long as 18 months[7]. Control of contamination from this source is of great importance in the management of dermatophytosis.

CLINICAL FEATURES
The clinical signs of *M canis* infection in cats can vary from an asymptomatic carrier to a crusting dermatitis[5–7]. Typical lesions consist of one or more 3-cm (1.2 in) diameter, discrete focal areas of fine scale and stubbled hair, typically on the face, head, or feet[2] (**242**, **243**). Pruritus and inflammation may occur but are usually minimal with focal lesions. Other manifestations of dermatophytosis due to *M. canis* include regional or generalized alopecia (**244**), papulocrustous dermatitis, localized subcutaneous granulomas, and onychomycosis.

Canine *M. canis* dermatophytosis is, in general, more inflammatory than that seen in the cat. The classical lesion is a slowly expanding zone of inflammation, crust, and alopecia with central healing, although multiple lesions may, occasionally, be seen. Surface scale is common and crusted papules within the zone of alopecia may be noted.

Dermatophytosis due to *T. mentagrophytes* (and *M. gypseum*) is much more inflammatory (**245**, **246**). Facial lesions may be strikingly symmetrical with erythema, crust, alopecia, and furunculosis. Large areas may be affected and it is not uncommon for the entire skin surface of a limb to be involved. The affected area has a well-demarcated border, often marked by a zone of inflammation and crusting. Pruritus is variable.

Dermatophytosis due to *M. persicolor* is rare. It is unusual in that the fungal hyphae are confined to the stratum corneum and do not invade the hair. Clinical lesions associated with *M. persicolor* dermatophytosis frequently are seen on the head, and are characterized by surface scale with minimal alopecia and inflammation[14].

DIFFERENTIAL DIAGNOSES
Cat
Focal lesions:
- Cat bite abscess
- Cheyletiellosis
- Demodicosis

Regional/generalized lesions:
- Flea bite hypersensitivity
- Telogen/anagen defluxion
- Psychogenic alopecia

Dog
Focal lesions:
- Superficial pyoderma
- Demodicosis
- Defects in keratinization
- Post-injection alopecia

Dermatophytosis

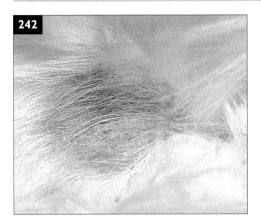

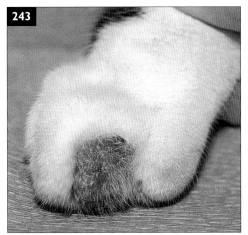

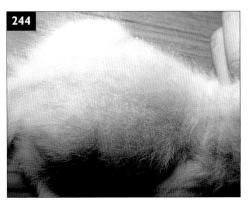

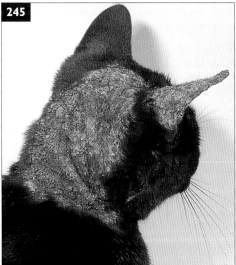

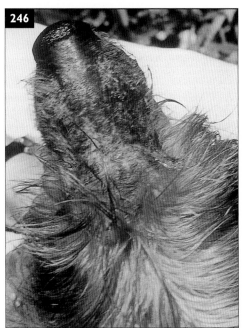

245, 246 Dermatophytosis. *Trychophyton mentagrophytes* infection usually results in well-demarcated inflammatory lesions in both cats (**245**) and dogs (**246**).

242–244 Dermatophytosis. *Microsporum canis* dermatophytosis usually results in focal alopecia (**242, 243**), although in some cases, particularly young animals, generalized lesions may occur (**244**).

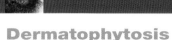

Dermatophytosis

Facial/regional lesions:
- Demodicosis
- Superficial pyoderma
- Immune-mediated diseases
- Deep mycotic lesions

DIAGNOSTIC TESTS

Clinical examination and, possibly, the presence of zoonotic lesions may be suggestive, but treatment should never be initiated without a definitive diagnosis. Microscopic examination of KOH preparations may reveal the presence of spores around the hair shaft (**247**), but the technique yields many false negatives. Examination of the cat in a darkened room with a Wood's light (that has been allowed properly to warm up) will reveal green fluorescence in some cases of *M. canis* dermatophytosis, but not in all cases. Culture of suspect material on Dermatophyte Test Medium or Sabouraud's medium (**248, 249**) is the only way to obtain a definitive diagnosis and the only reliable method of declaring a negative finding[15–17].

MANAGEMENT

Cats with minimal, well-demarcated isolated lesions probably do not need clipping[16]. However, all cases of generalized dermatophytosis and dermatophytosis in long-haired cats should be body clipped and the clippings burnt. This process may help to reduce some of the environmental contamination associated with dermatophytosis[16].

Topical therapeutics

It is inappropriate to use topical treatments alone. Specific, topical antifungal agents, such as miconazole and clotrimazole, may be useful adjuncts for focal lesions whereas enilconazole or lime sulfur (4–8 oz/ gallon) dips are preferred for more extensive conditions[16]. Chlorhexidine alone is ineffective in clearing dermatophytosis or inhibiting environmental contamination[12,16]. Infections in catteries require prolonged therapy and necessitate difficult management changes[12,17].

Systemic therapy

Systemic therapy is advocated for all cases of feline dermatophytosis[16]. The initial agent of choice is griseofulvin (50 mg/kg PO q 24 h), given with an oily meal[16,18]. Griseofulvin is a potent teratogen and should not be used for treatment of pregnant animals. Depression,

ataxia, and anemia are occasional side-effects. These side-effects generally resolve when griseofulvin therapy is discontinued. Bone marrow depression occurs more commonly in cats with FeLV infection. Alternative drugs, such as ketoconazole (5–10 mg/kg PO q 24 h) or, preferably, itraconazole (10 mg/kg PO q 24 h) may be used[3,16,18]. Treatment must be continued for at least 4–6 weeks and should not be suspended until fungal cultures are negative. This is particularly important as fungal cultures may continue to be positive long after apparent clinical resolution[12,16,19].

Environmental therapy

Areas in the house frequented by the animal should be vacuum cleaned daily to remove contaminated hair and spores. Cages and other surfaces which will tolerate bleach should be washed daily with a 1:10 solution of household bleach. Enilconazole spray may also be used as an environmental agent.

KEY POINTS
- There is great potential for misdiagnosis.
- Be aware of zoonotic risk.
- Good client communication is imperative.

Dermatophytosis

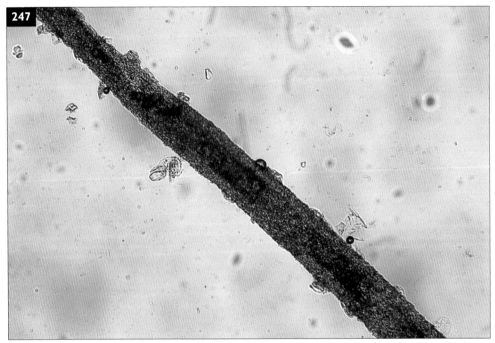

247 Photomicrograph of a hair shaft exhibiting spores and hyphae. Note that these impart a 'dirty', thickened appearance to the hair.

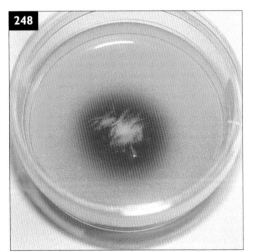

248 Positive culture on Dermatophyte Test Medium. The critical observation is the appearance of color change at the same time as colony growth becomes apparent.

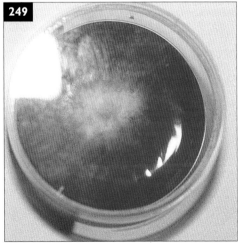

249 This is the same plate as in **248** but a week later. The uniform red color now makes it impossible to tell if the fungal growth appeared after the color change or before.

Follicular Dysplasia

DEFINITION
Non-color-linked follicular dysplasia is a rare, tardive disorder in which abnormal follicular function results in either a patchy loss of hair or generalized abnormality of hair structure.

ETIOLOGY AND PATHOGENESIS
The disorder is of unknown etiology, although the fact that individuals of certain breeds appear to exhibit similar signs suggests an inherited component. The abnormalities in follicle function result in failure to cycle properly, pigment clumping, shaft abnormalities, hypotrichosis or alopecia, and follicular hyperkeratosis.

CLINICAL FEATURES
Although any individual animal may be affected, a number of syndromes have been recognized in various breeds.

Siberian Husky
There is incomplete shedding of the juvenile coat, fracture and loss of guard hairs, and a reddish discoloration of remaining hair[1].

Doberman Pinscher
There is a slowly progressive, non-pruritic symmetrical loss of hair, usually starting on the dorsal lumbosacral region[2]. Hair loss begins at about 12 months of age and remains confined to the sublumbar fossae (**250**) and dorsal lumbosacral region. Animals are prone to secondary superficial pyoderma.

Airedale Terrier, Boxer, Staffordshire Bull Terrier
Tardive, non-cyclic, symmetrical, non-pruritic, often hyperpigmented alopecia confined to the sublumbar fossae (**251**). In some cases the alopecia is cyclic, often annual, in pattern[3,4].

Curly Coated Retriever, Irish Water Spaniel, Portuguese Water Dog
Affected individuals of these breeds exhibit loss of primary hairs and the remaining secondary hairs become dull and of a lighter shade[4].

DIFFERENTIAL DIAGNOSES
- Endocrinopathy
- Color-dilute alopecia
- Demodicosis
- Dermatophytosis

DIAGNOSTIC TESTS
Clinical history, physical examination, and basic investigatory tests will rule out infectious causes. Histopathologic examination of biopsy samples will reveal changes consistent with follicular dysplasia, although in some cases a definitive diagnosis is difficult.

MANAGEMENT
There is no treatment for these cases other than appropriate management of secondary folliculitis or local scaling as necessary. There are no systemic changes.

KEY POINT
- Breed-associated syndromes greatly facilitate recognition of these diseases, but do not forget the differential dignoses.

Follicular Dysplasia

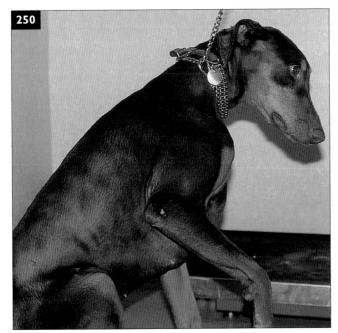

250, 251   Follicular dysplasia in a red Doberman Pinscher (251) and an Airedale Terrier (252).

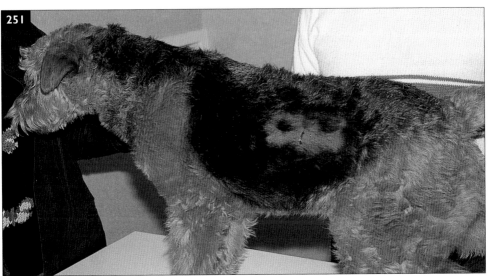

Injection Site Alopecia

DEFINITION
Injection site alopecia occurs at the site of subcutaneously administered drugs, including vaccines.

ETIOLOGY AND PATHOGENESIS
The etiology of this condition is not known, although a number of different mechanisms may be involved. Focal alopecia occurring after rabies vaccination is reported to affect particularly, though not exclusively, Poodles[1]. A vasculitis was noted in these cases and an immune-mediated etiology proposed[1]. Subcutaneous injections with progestagen suspensions may also result in focal alopecia. Inadvertent deep dermal injection may result in panniculitis and nodule formation[2]. Fibrosarcoma following feline leukemia (or rabies) vaccination has been reported in cats, although the exact mechanism of tumor induction is not known[3]. Extravascular injection of sodium thiopentone will cause a well-defined slough due to local necrosis of tissues.

CLINICAL SIGNS
Focal alopecia occurs 3–6 months after rabies injection[1]. Areas overlying the site of injection become hyperpigmented and alopecic, and may measure 2–5 cm (0.8–2 in) in diameter. Reactions following progestagen injection also occur at the site of injection, although this tends to be dorsal mid-line in the interscapular region (**252**).

DIFFERENTIAL DIAGNOSES
- Demodicosis
- Dermatophytosis
- Dermatomyositis
- Alopecia areata

DIAGNOSIS
Clinical history and examination is normally sufficient to suggest the diagnosis. Examination of skin scrapings and fungal culture will rule out infectious causes, and histopathologic examination of biopsy samples will confirm the diagnosis.

MANAGEMENT
There is no treatment. The atrophic changes following the injection are permanent.

KEY POINT
- It may be best to avoid the dorsal midline when injecting shorthaired show animals.

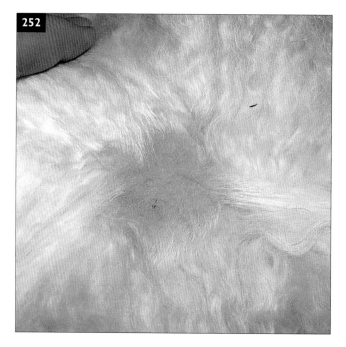

252 Focal alopecia and cutaneous atrophy following subcutaneous injection of progestagen.

Feline Demodicosis

DEFINITION

Feline demodicosis is a rare parasitic disease resulting from the presence of increased numbers of mites belonging to the genus *Demodex* in the skin.

ETIOLOGY AND PATHOGENESIS

Feline demodicosis is due to either *D. cati* or a species of demodectic mite that has not as yet been named[1]. Reasons as to why the mite populations increase and produce clinical signs in some cats has not been studied[2]. However, some cases have been associated with underlying systemic disease[2-4].

CLINICAL FEATURES

Demodicosis in cats can appear as a localized, generalized or otic condition. The disease has been diagnosed in both males and females, pure and mixed breeds, short- and long-haired, and young (1.5 years) and old (10 years) animals[5]. The localized form is characterized by single or multiple focal areas of alopecia and scaling, and occasional erythema and crusting of the eyelids (**253**), periocular area, chin, head, and neck. Infestation of the chin may result in the lesions of feline acne. Clinical signs of the generalized form can be seen as circumscribed areas of alopecia, scaling, erythema, hyperpigmentation, and crusting on areas of the head, trunk, and limbs. Some cases may be pruritic, especially if the infestation is due to the unnamed species of mite[1]. The otic form may be associated with ears of normal appearance with the mites being an incidental finding, or the ears may have a dark-brown ceruminous exudate[1].

DIFFERENTIAL DIAGNOSES

- Dermatophytosis
- Bacterial folliculitis-furunculosis
- Psychogenic alopecia
- Atopic dermatitis
- Adverse reaction to food
- Contact dermatitis
- Flea bite hypersensitivity
- Infestation with *Cheyletiella* spp.
- Infestation with *Notoedres cati*

DIAGNOSTIC TESTS

Skin scrapings. The unnamed adult mite is unusual as it has a broad, blunted abdomen and resides superficially in the stratum corneum[1].

MANAGEMENT

Because the mites are often superficial on the skin surface, many cases will respond to 2% lime sulfur dips weekly for 4–6 weeks. Alternatively, if this should fail, 0.015% amitraz may be used as a weekly dip and continued for 3 weeks beyond the presence of negative skin scrapings[2]. Amitraz is not approved for use in cats and the strength recommended is half that which the manufacturer recommends for dogs. Toxic side-effects of amitraz at this strength include mild sedation, pytalism anorexia, depression, and diarrhea[2,6].

KEY POINT

- Examination of skin scrapes is just as important in feline dermatology as it is in canine dermatology.

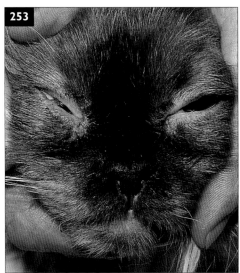

253 Focal alopecia and erythema due to feline demodicosis.

Alopecia Areata

DEFINITION
Alopecia areata is a rare condition characterized by focal areas of non-inflammatory hair loss.

ETIOLOGY AND PATHOGENESIS
Autoimmune mechanisms are believed to be responsible. Both a cellular and humoral immune response is directed against the inferior portion of the hair follicles[1].

CLINICAL FEATURES
Alopecia areata appears as focal or multifocal areas of well-circumscribed alopecia (**254**) in which the skin of the affected area appears normal, although hyperpigmentation may be present in chronic cases[2]. In some animals the disease may restrict itself to one hair color. Lesions are most frequently found about the head and neck[2]. A characteristic finding is 'exclamation-mark' hairs which are short and stubby with dystrophic proximal tapered portions and frayed, damaged distal portions[2,3].

DIFFERENTIAL DIAGNOSES
- Post-injection alopecia
- Demodicosis
- Dermatophytosis
- Follicular dysplasia
- Acquired pattern alopecia

DIAGNOSTIC TESTS
Histopathologic examination of biopsy samples may be diagnostic.

MANAGEMENT
There is no evidence that any therapy is beneficial. Many cases will undergo spontaneous resolution within 6 months to 2 years[3].

KEY POINT
- Definitive diagnosis is important as some of the differentials mandate specific treatment.

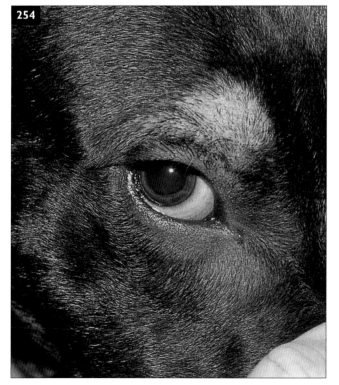

254

254 Focal alopecia due to alopecia areata. Note the complete absence of primary and secondary lesions apart from alopecia.

Black Hair Follicle Alopecia

DEFINITION
Black hair follicle dysplasia is a rare, tardive disorder affecting growth of black hairs, with sparing of white hairs[1].

ETIOLOGY AND PATHOGENESIS
The underlying etiology of the disorder is not understood. Abnormally large granules of melanin are present within the pigmented hair shafts, which may exhibit microscopic defects, and there are areas of epidermal pigment clumping, suggesting defects in pigment handling[1]. The dermatosis has been shown to be autosomally transmitted in one study in an affected cross-bred litter[2], although the mode of inheritance was not determined[1]. Other breeds reportedly affected include Bearded Collies[3] and Salukis[1].

CLINICAL FEATURES
Only pigmented hair is affected. There is a patchy hypotrichosis associated with pigmented regions of skin (**255**). Affected areas produce short, dry, lusterless hair, although severity varies both within and between individuals. Affected animals are normal at birth. Abnormalities may be detected both microscopically and grossly from as early as 3 weeks of age[2] and, rarely, are delayed later than 6 weeks[1].

DIFFERENTIAL DIAGNOSES
- Demodicosis
- Superficial pyoderma
- Color-dilute alopecia
- Endocrinopathy

DIAGNOSTIC TESTS
The history of normal pups developing lesions which are confined to the pigmented areas only is highly suggestive of black hair follicle dysplasia. Skin scrapes should be taken to rule out demodicosis. Histopathologic examination of biopsy samples is diagnostic.

MANAGEMENT
The dermatosis is not responsive to treatment. Only the pigmented areas of the skin are affected and there are no systemic signs. Management should be symptomatic; mild shampoos and systemic antibacterial therapy may be indicated if secondary superficial pyoderma develops.

KEY POINT
- Almost pathognomonic presentation.

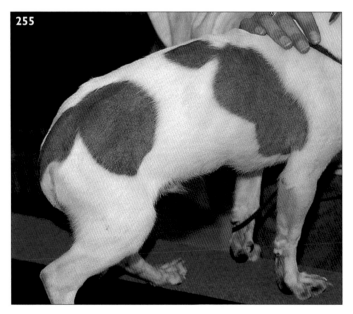

255 Black hair follicle alopecia in a Jack Russel Terrier. (Illustration courtesy of C.M. Knottenbelt.)

References

Section 1: Pruritic dermatoses
FLEA BITE HYPERSENSIVITY

1 Halliwell REW (1986) Flea bite hypersensitivity in dogs and cats – the current status. *Tijdschrift voor Diergeneeskunde*, **111**: 84S–87S.
2 Halliwell REW, Preston SF and Nesbitt JG (1987) Aspects of the immunopathogenesis of flea allergy dermatitis in dogs. *Vet. Immunol. and Immunopathol.*, **17**: 483–94.
3 Nesbitt GH (1978) Flea bite allergic dermatitis: a review and survey of 330 cases. *JAVMA*, **173**: 282–8.
4 Kristensen S, Haarlov N and Mourier H (1978) A study of skin disease in dogs and cats. IV. Patterns of flea infestation in dogs and cats in Denmark. *Nord. Vet.*, **30**: 401–13.
5 Kristensen S and Kieffer M (1978) A study of skin disease in dogs and cats. V. The intradermal test in the diagnosis of flea allergy in dogs and cats. *Nord. Vet.*, **30**: 414–23.
6 Dryden MW (1993) Biology of fleas of dogs and cats. *Comp. on Continuing Ed.*, **15**: 569–77.
7 Osbrink WLA, Rust MK and Reierson DA (1986) Distribution and control of cat fleas in homes in Southern California (Siphonaptera: Pulicidae). *J. of Med. Entomol.*, **79**: 135–40.
8 Melman SA and Hutton P (1985) Flea control on dogs and cats indoors and in the environment. *Comp. on Continuing Ed.*, **7**: 869–79.
9 Fisher MA, Hutchinson MJ, Jacobs DB and Dick IGC (1993) Efficacy of fenthion against the flea, *Ctenocephalides felis*, on the cat. *J. of Small Animal Practice*, **34**: 434–5.
10 Everett RE, Cunningham JR, Cox DD and Arther RG (1986) Efficacy of fenthion solution against repeated flea infestations of dogs. *Canine Practice*, **13**: 6–8.
11 Fisher MA, Hutchinson MJ, Jacobs DE and Dick IGC (1994) Comparative efficacy of fenthion, dichlorvos/fenitrothion and permethrin against the flea, *Ctenocephalides felis*, on the dog. *J. of Small Animal Practice*, **35**: 244–6.

12 Willemse T (1993) The effect of insect growth regulator lufenuron on flea reproduction. *Advances in Veterinary Dermatology* Vol. 2 (eds PJ Ihrke, IS Mason and SD White), Pergamon Press, Oxford, pp. 207–10.
13 Hink WF, Zakson M and Barnett S (1994) Evaluation of single oral dose of lufenuron to control flea infestations in dogs. *Am. J. of Vet. Research*, **55**: 822–4.
14 Fisher MA, Jacobs DE, Hutchinson MJ and Dick IGC (1996) Evaluation of flea control programmes for cats using fenthion and lufenuron. *Vet. Record*, **138**: 79–81.
15 Heath AW, Arfsten A, Yamanaka M et al. (1994) Vaccination against the cat flea *Ctenocephalides felis felis*. *Parasite Immunol.*, **16**: 187–91.
16 Halliwell REW (1993) Clinical and immunological response to alum-precipitated flea antigen in immunotherapy of flea-allergic dogs: results of a double blind study. *Advances in Veterinary Dermatology* Vol. 2 (eds PJ Ihrke, IS Mason and SD White), Pergamon Press, Oxford, pp. 41–50.

ATOPIC DERMATITIS

1 Rhodes KH, Kerdel F and Soter NA (1987) Comparative aspects of canine and human atopic dermatitis. *Seminars in Vet. Med. and Surg. (Small Animal)*, **2**: 166–72.
2 Cooper KD (1994) Atopic dermatitis: recent trends in pathogenesis and therapy. *J. of Invest. Dermatol.*, **102**: 128–37.
3 Griffin CE (1993) Canine atopic disease. *Current Veterinary Dermatology* (eds CE Griffin, KW Kwochka and JM McDonald), Mosby Year Book, St Louis, pp. 90–120.
4 Scott DW, Miller WM and Griffin CE (1995) Immunologic skin diseases. *Muller and Kirk's Small Animal Dermatology*, WB Saunders, Philadelphia, pp. 484–626.
5 Conder EC and Lessard P (1993) Comparison of intradermal allergy test and enzyme-linked immunosorbent assay in dogs with allergic skin disease. *JAVMA*, **202**: 739–43.
6 Bond R and Lloyd DH (1992) A double-blind compari-

son of olive oil and a combination of evening primrose oil and fish oil in the management of canine atopy. *Vet. Record,* **131**: 558–60.

7 Cambell KL (1993) Clinical use of fatty acid supplements in dogs. *Vet. Dermatol.,* **4**: 167–73.

8 Harvey RG (1993) Essential fatty acids and the cat. *Vet. Dermatol.,* **4**: 175–9.

9 Logas D and Kunkle GA (1994) Double-blinded crossover study with marine oil supplementation containing high-dose eicosapentanoic acid for the treatment of canine pruritic skin disease. *Vet. Dermatol.,* **5**: 99–104.

10 Scarff DH and Lloyd DH (1992) Double-blind, placebo-controlled, crossover study of evening primrose oil in the treatment of canine atopy. *Vet. Record,* **131**: 97–9.

11 Scott DW, Miller WH, Decker GA and Wellington JR (1992) Comparison of the clinical efficacy of two commercial fatty acid supplements (Efa Vet® and DVM Derm Caps®), evening primrose oil, and cold water marine fish oil in the management of allergic pruritus in dogs: a double-blinded study. *Cornell Vet.,* **82**: 319–29.

12 Scott DW and Miller WH (1990) Nonsteroidal management of canine pruritus: chlorpheniramine and a fatty acid supplement (DVM Derm Caps®) in combination, and the fatty acid supplement at twice the manufacturer's recommended dosage. *Cornell Vet.,* **80**: 381–7.

13 Miller WM, Scott DW, Wellington JR et al. (1993) Evaluation of the performance of a serologic allergy system in atopic dogs. *J. of the Am. Animal Hosp. Assoc.,* **29**: 545–50.

ADVERSE REACTIONS TO FOOD (DIETARY INTOLERANCE)

1 Metcalfe DD (1984) Food hypersensitivity. *J. Allergy and Clin. Immunol.,* **73**: 749–62.

2 Carlotti DN, Remy L and Prost C (1990) Food allergy in dogs and cats: a review and report of 43 cases. *Vet. Dermatol.,* **1**: 55–62.

3 Harvey RG (1993) Food allergy and dietary intolerance in dogs: a report of 25 cases. *J. of Small Animal Practice,* **34**: 175–9.

4 Reedy LM and Miller WH (1989) Food hypersensitivity. *Allergic Skin Diseases of Dogs and Cats,* WB Saunders, Philadelphia, pp. 147–58.

5 Walton GS (1967) Skin response in the dog and cat to ingested allergens: observations on one hundred confirmed cases. *Vet. Record,* **81**: 709–13.

6 White SD (1986) Food hypersensitivity in 30 dogs. *JAVMA,* **188**: 695–8.

7 White SD and Sequoia D (1989) Food hypersensitivity in cats: 14 cases (1982–1987). *JAVMA,* **194**: 692–5.

8 Wills JM (1992) Diagnosing and managing food sensitivity in cats. *Vet. Med./Small Animal Clin.,* **87**: 884–92.

9 Kunkle G and Horner S (1992) Validity of skin testing for diagnosis of food allergy in dogs. *JAVMA,* **200**: 677–80.

10 Rosser EJ (1990) Diagnosis of allergy in dogs. *JAVMA,* **203**: 259–62.

SARCOPTIC MANGE

1 Fain A (1978) Epidemiological problems of scabies. *Intl J. of Dermatol.,* **17**: 20–30.

2 Moriello KA (1987) Common ectoparasites of the dog. Part 2: *Sarcoptes scabiei* v. *canis* and *Demodex canis. Canine Practice,* **14**: 25–41.

3 Scott DW and Horn RT (1987) Zoonotic dermatoses of dogs and cats. *Vet. Clinics of N. Am.,* **17**: 117–44.

CHEYLETIELLA SPP. INFESTATION

1 Alexander MA and Ihrke PJ (1982) *Cheyletiella* dermatitis in small animal practice: a review. *Californian Vet.,* **36**: 9–12.

2 Cohen SR (1980) *Cheyletiella* dermatitis (in rabbit, cat, dog, man). *Archives of Dermatol.,* **116**: 435–7.

3 Scott DW and Horne RT (1987) Zoonotic dermatoses of dogs and cats. *Vet. Clinics of N. Am.,* **21**: 535–41.

4 McKeever PJ and Allen SK (1979) Dermatitis associated with *Cheyletiella* infestation in cats. *JAVMA,* **174**: 718–20.

5 Ottenschott TRF and Gil D (1978) Cheyletiellosis in long-haired cats. *Tijdschrift voor Diergeneeskunde,* **103**: 1104–8.

PYOTRAUMATIC DERMATITIS

1 Jennings S (1953) Some aspects of veterinary dermatology. *Vet. Record,* **46**: 809–16.

2 Reinke SI, Stannard AA, Ihrke PJ and Reinke JD (1987) Histopathological features of pyotraumatic dermatitis. *JAVMA,* **190**: 57–60.

MALASSEZIA PACHYDERMATIS DERMATITIS

1 Plant JD, Rosenkrantz WS and Griffin CE (1992) Factors associated with and prevalence of high *Malassezia pachydermatis* numbers on dog skin. *JAVMA,* **201**: 879–82.

2 Dufait R (1983) *Pityrosporon canis* as the cause of canine chronic dermatitis. *Vet. Med./Small Animal Clin.,* **78**: 1055–7.

3 Mason KV and Evans AG (1991) Dermatitis associated with *Malassezia pachydermatis* in 11 dogs. *J. of Am. Animal Hosp. Assoc.,* **27**: 14–20.

4 Bond R, Collin NS and Lloyd DH (1994) Use of contact plates for the quantitative culture of *Malassezia pachydermatis* from canine skin. *J. of Small Animal Practice,* **35**: 68–72.

PEDICULOSIS

1 Fadok FA (1980) Miscellaneous parasites of the skin (Part I). *Comp. on Continuing Ed.,* **2**: 707–12.

2 Shastra UV (1991) Efficacy of ivermectin against lice infestation in cattle, buffaloes, goats, and dogs. *Indian Vet. J.,* **68**: 191.

3 Cooper PR and Penaliggon EJ (1996) Use of fipronil to eliminate recurrent infestation by *Trichodectes canis* in a pack of bloodhounds. *Vet. Record,* **139**: 195.

PELODERA STRONGYLOIDES DERMATITIS

1 Nesbitt GH (1983) Parasitic diseases. *Canine and Feline*

Dermatology: A Systematic Approach, Lea & Febiger, Philadelphia, p. 77.

2   Willers WB (1970) *Pelodera strongyloides* in association with canine dermatitis in Wisconsin. *JAVMA*, **156**: 319–20.

HARVEST MITE INFESTATION

1   Greene RT, Scheidt VJ and Moncol DJ (1986) Trombiculiasis in a cat. *J. of the Am. Vet. Med. Assoc.*, **188**: 1054–5.
2   Folz SD, Ash KA, Conder GA and Rector DL (1986) Amitraz: a tick and flea repellent and tick detachment drug. *J. of Vet. Pharmacol. and Therapeut.*, **9**: 150–6.
3   Famose F (1995) Efficacy of fipronil (Frontline) spray in the prevention of natural infestation by *Trombicula autumnalis* in dogs. *Proc. of the Roy. Vet. Coll. Seminar – Ectoparasites and Their Control*, pp. 28–30.

ALLERGIC AND IRRITANT CONTACT DERMATITIS

1   Brasch J, Burgard J and Sterry W (1992) Common pathogenetic pathways in allergic and irritant contact dermatitis. *J. of Invest. Dermatol.*, **98**: 166–70.
2   Thomsen MK and Thomsen HK (1989) Histopathological changes in canine allergic contact dermatitis patch test reactions. A study on spontaneously hypersensitive dogs. *Acta Vet. Scand.*, **30**: 379–84.
3   Walton GW (1977) Allergic contact dermatitis. *Current Veterinary Therapy VI* (ed. RW Kirk), WB Saunders, Philadelphia, pp. 571–5.
4   Thomsen MK and Kristensen F (1986) Contact dermatitis in the dog. *Nord. Vet.*, **38**: 129–47.
5   Gaafar SM and Krawiec DR (1974) Chemical sensitisers and contact dermatitis. *J. of the Am. Animal Hosp. Assoc.*, **10**: 133–8.
6   Nesbitt GH and Schmitz JA (1977) Contact dermatitis in the dog: a review of 35 cases. *J. of the Am. Animal Hosp. Assoc.*, **13**: 155–63.

NOTOEDRIC MANGE

1   Scott DW and Horn RT (1987) Zoonotic dermatoses of dogs and cats. *Vet. Clinics of N. Am.*, **17**: 117–44.

EPITHELIOTROPIC LYMPHOMA (CUTANEOUS T CELL LYMPHOMA, MYCOSIS FUNGOIDES)

1   Baker JL and Scott DW (1989) Mycosis fungoides in two cats. *J. of the Am. Animal Hosp. Assoc.*, **25**: 97–101.
2   DeBoer DJ, Turrel JM and Moore PF (1990) Mycosis fungoides in a dog: demonstration of T-cell specificity and response to radiotherapy. *J. of the Am. Animal Hosp. Assoc.*, **26**: 566–72.
3   Walton DK (1986) Canine epidermotropic lymphoma. *Current Veterinary Therapy IX* (ed. RW Kirk), WB Saunders, Philadelphia, pp. 609–14.
4   Wilcock BP and Yager JA (1989) The behavior of epidermotropic lymphoma in twenty-five dogs. *Can. Vet. J.*, **30**: 754–6.
5   Beale KM, Dill-Macky E, Meyer DJ and Calderwood-Mays M (1990) An unusual presentation of cutaneous lymphoma in two dogs. *J. of the Am. Animal Hosp. Assoc.*, **26**: 429–32.

6   Kwochka KW (1989) Retinoids in dermatology. *Current Veterinary Therapy X* (ed. RW Kirk), WB Saunders, Philadelphia, pp. 553–63.

PSYCHOGENIC DERMATOSES

1   Scott DW, Miller WH and Griffin CE (1995) Psychogenic skin diseases. *Muller and Kirk's Small Animal Dermatology*, WB Saunders, Philadelphia, pp. 846–58.
2   Van Ness JJ (1986) Electrophysiological evidence of a sensory nerve dysfunction in 10 dogs with acral lick dermatitis. *J. of the Am. Animal Hosp. Assoc.*, **22**: 157–60.
3   Walton DK (1986) Psychodermatoses. *Current Veterinary Therapy IX* (ed. RW Kirk), WB Saunders, Philadelphia, pp. 557–9.
4   Shanley K and Overall K (1992) Psychogenic dermatoses. *Current Veterinary Therapy XI* (eds RW Kirk and JD Bonagura), WB Saunders, Philadelphia, pp. 552–8.
5   Dodman NH, Shuster L, White SD *et al.* (1988) Use of narcotic antagonists to modify stereotypic self-licking, self-chewing, and scratching behaviour in dogs. *JAVMA*, **193**: 815–19.
6   White SD (1990) Naltrexone for treatment of acral lick dermatitis in dogs. *JAVMA*, **196**: 1073–6.
7   Willemse T, Spruijt BM and Osterwyck A. van (1989) Feline psychogenic alopecia and the role of the opioid system. *Advances in Veterinary Dermatology* Vol. 1 (eds C von Tscharner and REW Halliwell), Baillière Tindall, London, pp. 195–8.

ANCYLOSTOMIASIS (HOOKWORM DERMATITIS)

1   Bowman DD (1992) Hookworm parasites of dogs and cats. *Comp. on Continuing Ed.*, **14**: 585–93.
2   Scott DW, Miller WM and Griffin CE (1995) Parasitic skin diseases. *Muller and Kirk's Small Animal Dermatology*, WB Saunders, Philadelphia, pp. 393–5.
3   Buelke DL (1971) Hookworm dermatitis. *JAVMA*, **158**: 735–9.
4   Baker KP (1979) Clinical aspects of hookworm dermatitis. *Vet. Dermatol. Newsletter*, **6**: 69–74.

SCHNAUZER COMEDO SYNDROME

1   Morriello KA and Mason IS (1995) Scaling and crusting. *Handbook of Small Animal Dermatology*, Elsevier Science Ltd, Oxford, pp. 75–91.
2   Kwochka KW (1993) Primary keratinization disorders of dogs. *Current Veterinary Dermatology* (eds CE Griffin, KW Kwochka and JM McDonald), Mosby Year Book, St Louis, pp. 176–90.
3   Scott DW, Miller WM and Griffin CE (1995) Congenital and hereditary disorders. *Muller and Kirk's Small Animal Dermatology*, WB Saunders, Philadelphia, pp. 136–805.

Section 2: Nodular dermatoses
EPIDERMAL AND FOLLICULAR INCLUSION CYSTS

1 Goldschmidt MH and Shofer FS (1992) *Skin Tumors of the Dog and Cat*, Pergamon Press, Oxford.

PAPILLOMATOSIS

1 Goldschmidt MH and Shofer FS (1992) Cutaneous papillomas. *Skin Tumors of the Dog and Cat*, Pergamon Press, New York, pp. 11–15.

2 Gross TL, Ihrke PJ and Walder EJ (1992) Epidermal tumors. *Veterinary Dermatopathology*, Mosby Year Book, St. Louis, pp. 334–6.

3 Scott DW, Miller WM and Griffin CE (1995) Neoplastic and non–neoplastic tumors. *Small Animal Dermatology*, WB Saunders, Philadelphia, pp. 994–7.

4 Sansom J, Barnett KC, Blunden AS et al. (1996) Canine conjunctival papilloma: a review of five cases. *J. of Small Animal Practice*, **37**: 84–6.

5 Watrach AM, Small E and Case MT (1970) Canine papillomas: progression of oral papilloma to carcinoma. *J. of the National Cancer Inst.*, **45**: 915–20.

6 Bergman CL, Hirth RS, Sundberg JP and Christensen EF (1987) Cutaneous neoplasia in dogs associated with canine papillomavirus vaccine. *Vet. Pathol.*, **24**: 477–87.

MAST CELL NEOPLASIA

1 Tamms TR and Macy DW (1981) Canine mast cell tumors. *Comp. on Continuing Ed.*, **3**: 869–82.

2 Bevier DE and Goldschmidt MH (1981) Skin tumors in the dog. Part 2. Tumors of the soft (mesenchymal) tissues. *Comp. on Continuing Ed.*, **3**: 506–16.

3 Rothwell TLW, Howlett CR, Middleton DJ et al. (1987) Skin neoplasms in Sydney. *Austr. Vet. J.*, **64**: 161–4.

4 Holzinger EA (1973) Feline cutaneous mastocytomas. *Cornell Vet.*, **63**: 87–93.

5 Brown CA and Chalmer SA (1990) Diffuse cutaneous mastocytosis in a cat. *Vet. Pathol.*, **27**: 360–6.

6 Chastain CB, Turk MAM and O'Brian D (1988) Benign cutaneous mastocytomas in two litters of Siamese kittens. *JAVMA*, **193**: 959–60.

7 Barton CL (1987) Cytologic diagnosis of cutaneous neoplasia: an algorithmic approach. *Comp. on Continuing Ed.*, **9**: 20–33.

8 Dobson, JM and Gorman, NT (1988) A clinical approach to the management of skin tumours in the dog and cat. *In Practice*, **March 1988**: 55–68.

9 Al-Sarraf, R, Maudlin, N, Patnaik, AK and Meleo, KA (1996) A prospective study of radiation therapy for the treatment of Grade 2 mast cell tumors in dogs. *J. of Vet. Int. Med.*, 10: 376–8.

10 Dean, PW (1988). Mast cell tumors in dogs: diagnosis, treatment, and prognosis. *Pet Practice*, **February 1988**: 185–92.

11 Grier, RL, Guardo, GD, Schaffer, CB et al. (1990) Mast cell destruction by deionized water. *Am. J. of Vet. Res.*, **51**: 1116–20.

BASAL CELL TUMOR

1 Miller SJ (1991) Biology of basal cell carcinoma. *J. of the Am. Acad. of Dermatol.*, **24**: 161–75.

2 Miller MA, Nelson SL, Turk JR et al. (1991) Cutaneous neoplasia in 340 cats. *Vet. Pathol.*, **28**: 389–95.

3 Macy DW and Reynolds HA (1981) The incidence, characteristics and clinical management of skin tumors of cats. *J. of the Am. Animal Hosp. Assoc.*, **17**: 1026–34.

4 Rothwell TLW, Howlett CR, Middleton DJ et al. (1987) Skin neoplasms of dogs in Sydney. *Austr. Vet. J.*, **64**: 161–4.

5 Bevier DE and Goldschmidt MH (1981) Skin tumors in the dog. Part 1. Epithelial tumors and tumor-like lesions. *Comp. on Continuing Ed.*, **3**: 389–400.

6 Barton CL (1987) Cytological diagnosis of cutaneous neoplasia: an algorithmic approach. *Comp. on Continuing Ed.*, **9**: 20–33.

COLLAGENOUS NEVI

1 Scott DW, Yager-Johnson JA, Manning TO et al. (1984) Nevi in the dog. *J. of the Am. Animal Hosp. Assoc.*, **20**: 505–12.

2 Calderwood-Mays MB, Bellah JR and Pohlenz-Zertuche HO (1993) Regional collagenous nevi in three dogs: nevus nodular dermatofibrosis or something new? *Advances in Veterinary Dermatology* Vol. 2 (eds PJ Ihrke, IS Mason and SD White), Pergamon Press, New York, pp. 315–21.

MELANOCYTIC NEOPLASIA

1 Sober AJ (1991) Biology of malignant melanoma. *Pathophysiology of Dermatologic Diseases* (eds NA Soter and HP Baden), McGraw-Hill, New York, pp. 515–28.

2 Bostock DE (1979) Prognosis after surgical excision of canine melanomas. *Vet. Pathol.*, **16**: 32–40.

3 Aronsohn MG and Carpenter JL (1990) Distal extremity melanocytic nevi and malignant melanoma in dogs. *J. of the Am. Animal Hosp. Assoc.*, **26**: 605–12.

4 Goldschmidt MH, Liu SMS and Shofer FS (1993) Feline dermal melanoma. *Advances in Veterinary Dermatology* (eds PJ Ihrke, IS Mason and SD White), Pergamon Press, Oxford, pp. 285–91.

5 Rothwell TLW, Howlett CR, Middleton DJ et al. (1987) Skin neoplasms of dogs in Sydney. *Austr. Vet. J.*, **64**: 161–4.

6 Richardson RC, Rebar AH and Elliott GS (1984) Common skin tumors of the dog: a clinical approach to diagnosis and treatment. *Comp. on Continuing Ed.*, **6**: 1080–5.

7 Marino DJ, Mattieson DT, Stefanacci JD and Morroff SD (1995) Evaluation of dogs with digital masses: 117 cases (1981–1991). *JAVMA*, **207**: 726–8.

HYPERANDROGENISM

1 Aronsohn M (1979) Canine testicular hyperplasia. *Comp. on Continuing Ed.*, **1**: 925–8.

2 Schmeitzel LP and Lothrop CD (1990) Sex hormones and skin disease. *Vet. Med. Report*, **2**: 28–41.

3 Scott DW and Reimers TJ (1986) Tail gland and perianal gland hyperplasia associated with testicular neoplasia and

hypertestosteronemia in a dog. *Canine Practice*, **13**: 15–17.

4   Wilson GP and Hayes HM (1979) Castration for treatment of perianal gland neoplasms in the dog. *JAVMA*, **174**: 1301–3.

PANNICULITIS

1   Scott DW and Anderson WI (1988) Panniculitis in dogs and cats: a retrospective analysis of 78 cases. *J. of the Am. Animal Hosp. Assoc.*, **24**: 551–9.

2   Shanley KJ and Miller WH (1985) Panniculitis in the dog: a report of five cases. *J. of the Am. Animal Hosp. Assoc.*, **21**: 545–50.

3   Hendrick MJ and Dunagan CA (1991) Focal necrotizing granulomatous panniculitis associated with subcutaneous injection of rabies vaccine in cats and dogs: 10 cases (1988–1989). *JAVMA*, **198**: 304–5.

4   Gross TL, Ihrke PJ and Walder EJ (1992) Diseases of the panniculus. *Veterinary Dermatopathology*, Mosby Year Book, St. Louis, pp. 316–26.

5   Hagiwara MK, Guerra JL and Maeoka MRM (1986) Pansteatitis (yellow fat disease) in a cat. *Feline Practice*, **16**: 25–7.

6   Edgar TP and Furrow RD (1984) Idiopathic nodular panniculitis in a German Shepherd Dog. *J. of the Am. Animal Hosp. Assoc.*, **20**: 603–6.

7   Kunkle GA, White SD, Calderwood-Mays M and Pohlenz-Zerruche HO (1993) Focal metatarsal fistulas in five dogs. *JAVMA*, **202**: 756–7.

8   Paterson S (1995) Sterile idiopathic pedal panniculitis in the German Shepherd Dog – clinical presentation and response to treatment of four cases. *J. of Small Animal Practice*, **36**: 498–501.

CRYPTOCOCCOSIS

1   Wolf AM and Troy GC (1995) Deep mycotic diseases. *Textbook of Veterinary Internal Medicine* (eds SJ Ettinger and EC Feldman), WB Saunders, Philadelphia, pp. 439–62.

2   Ackerman L (1988) Feline cryptococcosis. *Comp. on Continuing Ed.*, **10**: 1049–55.

3   Medleau L and Barsanti JA (1990) Cryptococcosis. *Infectious Diseases of Dogs and Cats* (ed. CE Green), WB Saunders, Philadelphia, pp. 687–95.

4   Medleau L, Hall EJ, Goldschmidt MH and Irby N (1995) Cutaneous cryptococcosis in three cats. *JAVMA*, **187**: 169–70.

5   Legendre AM (1995) Antimycotic drug therapy. *Current Veterinary Therapy XII* (ed. JD Bonagura), WB Saunders, Philadelphia, pp. 327–31.

6   Medleau L, Jacobs GJ and Marks MA (1995) Itraconazole for the treatment of cryptococcosis in cats. *J. of Vet. Int. Med.*, **9**: 39–42.

INFUNDIBULAR KERATINIZING ACANTHOMA

1   Scott DW, Miller WM and Griffin CE (1995) Neoplastic and non-neoplastic tumors. *Muller and Kirk's Small Animal*

Dermatology, WB Saunders, Philadelphia, pp. 999–1001.

2   Goldschmidt MH and Shofer FS (1992) Intracutaneous cornifying epithelioma. *Skin Tumors of the Dog and Cat*, Pergamon Press, New York, pp. 109–14.

3   Gross TL, Ihrke PJ and Walder EJ (1992) Follicular tumors. *Vet. Dermatopathol.*, Mosby Year Book, St. Louis, pp. 361–3.

4   White SD (1991) Isotretinoin and etretinate in the treatment of benign and malignant cutaneous neoplasia and sebaceous adenitis in longhaired dogs. *Proc. of the 7th Ann. Members' Meeting, AAVD, ACVD*, pp. 101–2.

5   Henfrey JI (1991) Treatment of multiple intra-cutaneous cornifying epitheliomata using isotretinoin. *J. of Small Animal Practice*, **32**: 363–5.

6   Scott DW, Miller WM and Griffin CE (1995) Dermatologic therapy. *Muller and Kirk's Small Animal Dermatology*, WB Saunders, Philadelphia, pp. 238–40.

SYSTEMIC HISTIOCYTOSIS AND OTHER HISTIOCYTOSES

1   Moore PF (1984) Systemic histiocytosis in Bernese Mountain Dogs. *Vet. Pathol.*, **21**: 544–63.

2   Scott DW and Angorano DK (1987) Systemic histiocytosis in two dogs. *Canine Practice*, **14**: 7–12.

3   Padgett GA, Madewell BR, Kellert ET et al. (1995) Inheritance of histiocytosis in Bernese Mountain Dogs. *J. of Small Animal Practice*, **36**: 93–8.

4   Calderwood-Mays MB and Bergeron JA (1986) Cutaneous histiocytosis in dogs. *JAVMA*, **188**: 377–81.

5   Wellman ML, Davenport DJ, Morton D and Jacobs RM (1985) Malignant histiocytosis in four dogs. *JAVMA*, **187**: 919–21.

CUTEREBRA SPP. INFESTATION

1   Bowman DD and Lynn RC (1995) Arthropods. *Georgis' Parasitology for Veterinarians*, WB Saunders, Philadelphia, pp. 29–31.

2   Hatziolos BC (1966) *Cuterebra* larva in the brain of a cat. *JAVMA*, **148**: 787–92.

3   Hendrix CM, Cox NR, Clemans-Chevis CL et al. (1989) Aberrant intracranial myiasis caused by larval *Cuterebra* infection. *Comp. on Continuing Ed.*, **11**: 550–62.

4   Kazocos KR, Bright RM, Johnson KE et al. (1980) *Cuterebra* species as a cause of pharyngeal myiasis in cats. *J. of the Am. Animal Hosp. Assoc.*, **16** 773–6.

DRACUNCULIASIS

1   Giovengo SL (1993) Canine dracunculiasis. *Comp. on Continuing Ed.*, **15**: 726–9.

2   Scott DW, Miller WM and Griffin CE (1995) Parasitic skin diseases. *Muller and Kirk's Small Animal Dermatology*, WB Saunders, Philadelphia, pp. 400–1.

BLASTOMYCOSIS

1   Attleberger MH (1980) Subcutaneous and opportunistic mycoses. *Current Veterinary Therapy VII* (ed. REW Kirk), WB Saunders, Philadelphia, pp. 1177–80.

2 Fadok VA (1987) Granulomatous dermatitis in dogs and cats. *Seminars in Vet. Med. and Surg. (Small Animal)*, **2**: 186–94.
3 Rudmann DG, Coolman BR, Perez CM and Glickman LT (1992) Evaluation of risk factors for blastomycosis in dogs: 857 cases (1980–1990). *JAVMA*, **201**: 1754–9.
4 Legendre AM (1995) Antimycotic drug therapy. *Current Veterinary Therapy XII* (ed. JD Bonagura), WB Saunders, Philadelphia, pp. 327–31.

PHAEOHYPHOMYCOSIS

1 Odds FC, Arai T, Disalvo AF et al. (1992) Nomenclature of fungal diseases: a report and recommendations from a sub-committee of the International Society for Human and Animal Mycology (ISHAM). *J. of Med. and Vet. Mycology*, **30**: 1–10.
2 Dhein CR, Leathers CW, Padhye AA and Ajello L (1988) Phaeomycosis caused by *Alternaria alternata* in a cat. *JAVMA*, **193**: 1101–3.
3 Beale KM and Pinson D (1990) Phaeomycosis caused by two different species of *Curvularia* in two animals from the same household. *J. of the Am. Animal Hosp. Assoc.*, **26**: 67–70.
4 Attleburger MH (1980) Mycoses and mycosis-like diseases. *Current Veterinary Therapy VII* (ed. RW Kirk), WB Saunders, Philadelphia, pp. 1177–80.
5 Fadok VA (1987) Granulomatous dermatitis in dogs and cats. *Seminars in Vet. Med. and Surg. (Small Animal)*, **2**: 186–94.
6 Kettlewell P, McGinnis MR and Wilkinson GT (1989) Phaeomycosis caused by *Exophiala spinifera* in two cats. *J. of Med. and Vet. Mycology*, **27**: 257–64.

Section 3: Ulcerative dermatoses
FELINE EOSINOPHILIC GRANULOMA COMPLEX

1 Leiferman KM (1991) A current perspective on the role of eosinophils in dermatologic diseases. *J. of the Am. Acad. of Dermatol.*, **24**: 1101–12.
2 Mason KV and Evans AG (1991) Mosquito bite-caused eosinophilic dermatitis in cats. *JAVMA*, **198**: 2086–8.
3 Rosenkrantz WS (1993) Feline eosinophilic granuloma complex. *Current Veterinary Dermatology* (eds CE Griffin, KW Kwochka and JM McDonald), Mosby Year Book, St Louis, pp. 319–24.
4 Power HT (1990) Eosinophilic granuloma in a family of specific pathogen-free cats. *Proc. of the Ann. Members' Meeting of the Am. Assoc. of Vet. Dermatol. and Am. Acad. of Vet. Dermatol.*, p. 45.
5 Wilkinson GT and Bate MJ (1984) A possible further manifestation of the feline eosinophilic granuloma complex. *J. of the Am. Animal Hosp. Assoc.*, **20**: 325–31.
6 MacEwan EG and Hess PW (1987) Evaluation of effect of immunomodulation on the feline eosinophilic granuloma complex. *J. of the Am. Animal Hosp. Assoc.*, **23**: 519–26.

GERMAN SHEPHERD DOG PYODERMA

1 Bell A (1995) Prophylaxis of German Shepherd recurrent furunculosis (German Shepherd pyoderma) using cephalexin pulse therapy. *Austr. Vet. Prac.*, **25**: 30–6.
2 Wisselink MA, Bernadina WE, Willemse A and Noordzij A (1988) Immunologic aspects of German Shepherd Dog pyoderma (GSP), *Vet. Immunol. and Immunopathol.*, **19**: 67–77.
3 Wisselink MA, Koeman JP, van den Ingh TSGAM and Willemse A (1990) Investigations on the role of staphylococci in the pathogenesis of German Shepherd Dog pyoderma (GSP), *Vet. Q.*, **12**: 29–34.
4 Chabanne L, Marchal T, Denerolle P et al. (1995) Lymphocyte subset abnormalities in German Shepherd Dog pyoderma (GSP), *Vet. Immunol. and Immunopathol.*, **49**: 189–98.

CALCINOSIS CUTIS

1 Scott DW (1982) Histopathological findings in endocrine skin disorders. *J. of the Am. Animal Hosp. Assoc.*, **18**: 173–83.
2 Zerbe CA and MacDonald JM (1994) Canine and feline Cushing's syndrome. *Current Veterinary Dermatology* (eds CE Griffin, KW Kwochka and JM McDonald), Mosby Year Book, St Louis, pp. 273–87.
3 White SD, Ceragioli KL, Bullock LP and Mason GD (1989) Cutaneous markers of canine hyperadrenocorticism. *Comp. on Continuing Ed.*, **11**: 446–64.
4 Scott DW (1979) Hyperadrenocorticism. *Vet. Clinics of N. Am.*, **9**: 3–28.

DECUBITAL ULCERS

1 Fadok VA (1983) Necrotizing skin diseases. *Current Veterinary Therapy VIII* (ed. RW Kirk), WB Saunders, Philadelphia, pp. 473–80.
2 Waldron DR and Trevor P (1993) Management of superficial skin wounds. *Textbook of Small Animal Surgery* (ed. D Slatter), WB Saunders, Philadelphia, pp. 276–9.

SQUAMOUS CELL CARCINOMA

1 Kwa RE, Campana K and Moy RL (1992) Biology of cutaneous squamous cell carcinoma. *J. of the Am. Acad. of Dermatol.*, **26**: 1–26.
2 Hargis AM, Thomassen RW and Rheimister RD (1977) Chronic dermatosis and cutaneous squamous cell carcinoma in the beagle dog. *Vet. Pathol.*, **14**: 218–88.
3 Taylor CR, Stern RS, Leyden JJ and Gilchrest BA (1990) Photoaging/photodamage and photoprotection. *J. of the Am. Acad. of Dermatol.*, **22**: 1–15.
4 Bevier DE and Goldschmidt MH (1981) Skin tumors in the dog. Part 1. Epithelial tumors and tumor-like lesions. *Comp. on Continuing Ed.*, **3**: 389–400.
5 Rothwell TLW, Howlett CR, Middleton DJ et al. (1987) Skin neoplasms of dogs in Sydney. *Austr. Vet. J.*, **64**: 161–4.
6 Miller MA, Nelson SL, Turk JR et al. (1991) Cutaneous neoplasia in 340 cats. *Vet. Pathol.*, **28**: 389–95.
7 Macy DW and Reynolds HA (1981) The incidence, char-

acteristics, and clinical management of skin tumors of cats. *J. of the Am. Animal Hosp. Assoc.,* **17**: 1026–34.

8   Barton CL (1987) Cytological diagnosis of cutaneous neoplasia: an algorithmic approach. *Comp. on Continuing Ed.,* **9**: 20–33.

9   Peaston AE, Leach MW and Higgins J (1993) Photodynamic therapy for nasal and aural squamous cell carcinoma in cats. *JAVMA,* **202**: 1261–5.

EPIDERMAL METABOLIC NECROSIS (DIABETIC DERMATOPATHY, HEPATOCUTANEOUS SYNDROME, NECROLYTIC MIGRATORY ERYTHEMA, SUPERFICIAL NECROLYTIC DERMATITIS)

1   Gross TL, Song MD, Havel PJ and Ihrke PJ (1993) Superficial necrolytic dermatitis (necrolytic migratory erythema) in dogs. *Vet. Pathol.,* **30**: 75–81.

2   Miller WH, Scott DW, Buerger RG et al. (1990) Necrolytic migratory erythema in dogs: a hepatocutaneous syndrome. *J. of the Am. Animal Hosp. Assoc.,* **26**: 573–81.

3   Scott DW, Miller WM and Griffin CE (1995) Endocrine and metabolic diseases. *Small Animal Dermatology,* WB Saunders, Philadelphia, pp. 706–11.

4   Gross TL, Ihrke PJ and Walder EJ (1992) Necrotizing diseases of the epidermis. *Veterinary Dermatopathology,* Mosby Year Book, St. Louis, pp. 46–8.

DISCOID LUPUS ERYTHEMATOSUS

1   Norris DA (1993) Pathomechanisms of photosensitive lupus erythematosus. *J. of Invest. Dermatol.,* **100**: 58S–68S.

2   Walton DK, Scott DW, Smith CS and Lewis RM (1981) Canine discoid lupus erythematosus. *J. of the Am. Animal Hosp. Assoc.,* **17**: 851–8.

3   Scott DW, Walton DK, Manning TO et al. (1983) Canine lupus erythematosus. Part 2. Discoid lupus erythematosus. *J. of the Am. Animal Hosp. Assoc.,* **19**: 481–6.

4   Scott DW, Walton DK, Slater MR et al. (1987) Immune-mediated dermatoses in domestic animals: ten years after. Part 2. *Comp. on Continuing Ed.,* **9**: 539–51.

5   Willemse T and Koeman JP (1989) Discoid lupus erythematosus in cats. *Vet. Dermatol.,* **1**: 19–24.

6   White SD, Rosychuk RAW, Reinke SI and Paradis M (1992) Use of tetracycline and niacinamide for treatment of autoimmune skin disease in 32 dogs. *JAVMA,* **200**: 1497–500.

FELINE COWPOX INFECTION

1   Bennett M, Gaskell CJ, Gaskell RM et al. (1986) Poxvirus infection in the domestic cat: some clinical and epidemiological observations. *Vet. Record,* **118**: 387–90.

2   Gaskell RM, Gaskell CJ, Evans RJ et al. (1983) Natural and experimental poxvirus infection in the domestic cat. *Vet. Record,* **112**: 164–70.

3   Thomsett LR (1989) Cowpox in cats. *J. of Small Animal Practice,* **30**: 236–41.

4   Brown A, Bennett M and Gaskell CJ (1989) Fatal poxvirus infection in association with FIV infection. *Vet. Record,* **124**: 19–20.

5   Bennett M, Blaxby D, Gaskell RM et al. (1985) Laboratory diagnosis of orthopoxvirus infection in the domestic cat. *J. of Small Animal Practice,* **26**: 653–62.

DRUG ERUPTION

1   Mason KV (1990) Cutaneous drug eruptions. *Vet. Clinics of N. Am.,* **20**: 1633–53.

2   Mason KV (1988) Fixed drug eruption in two dogs caused by diethylcarbamazine. *J. of the Am. Animal Hosp. Assoc.,* **24**: 301–3.

3   Medleau L, Shanley KJ, Rakich PM and Goldschmidt MH (1990) Trimethoprim-sulfonamide-associated drug eruptions in dogs. *J. of the Am. Animal Hosp. Assoc.,* **26**: 305–11.

4   Cribb AE (1989) Idiosyncratic reactions to sulfonamides in dogs. *JAVMA,* **195**: 1612–14.

5   Delmage DA and Payne-Johnson CE (1991) Erythema multiforme in a Dobermann on trimethoprim-sulphamethoxazole therapy. *J. of Small Animal Practice,* **32**: 635–9.

6   McEwan NA, McNeil PA, Kirkham D and Sullivan M (1987) Drug eruption in a cat resembling pemphigus foliaceus. *J. of Small Animal Practice,* **28**: 713–20.

7   Daniel GB and Patterson JS (1985) Toxic epidermal necrosis. *J. of the Am. Animal Hosp. Assoc.,* **21**: 631–5.

NOCARDIOSIS

1   Hardie EM (1990) Actinomycosis and nocardiosis. *Infectious Diseases of Dogs and Cats* (ed. CE Green), WB Saunders, Philadelphia, pp. 585–91.

2   Kirpensteijn J and Fingland RB (1992) Cutaneous actinomycosis and nocardiosis in dogs: 48 cases (1980–1990), *JAVMA,* **201**: 917–20.

PLASMA CELL PODODERMATITIS OF CATS

1   Gruffyd-Jones TJ, Orr CM and Lucke VM (1980) Foot pad swelling and ulceration in cats: a report of five cases. *J. of Small Animal Practice,* **21**: 381–9.

2   Taylor JE and Schmeitzel LP (1990) Plasma cell pododermatitis with chronic footpad ulceration in two cats. *JAVMA,* **197**: 375–7.

3   Medleau L, Kaswan RL, Lorenz MD and Dawe DL (1982) Ulcerative pododermatitis in a cat: immunofluorescent findings and response to chrysotherapy. *J. of the Am. Animal Hosp. Assoc.,* **18**: 449–51.

PEMPHIGUS VULGARIS

1   Burge SM, Wilson CL, Dean D and Wojnarowska F (1993) An immunohistological study of desmosomal components on pemphigus. *Br. J. of Dermatol.,* **128**: 163–70.

2   Suter MM, Wilkinson JE, Dougherty EP and Lewis RM (1990) Ultrastructural localization of pemphigus vulgaris antigen on canine keratinocytes *in vivo* and *in vitro*. *Am. J. of Vet. Res.,* **51**: 507–11.

3 Scott DW, Walton DK, Slater MR *et al.* (1987) Immune-mediated dermatoses in domestic animals: ten years after. Part 1. *Comp. on Continuing Ed.*, **9**: 424–35.
4 Gorman NT and Werner LL (1986) Immune-mediated diseases of the dog and cat III. Immune-mediated diseases of the integument, urogenital, endocrine and vascular systems. *BVJ*, **142**: 491–7.
5 Werner LL, Brown KA and Halliwell REW (1983) Diagnosis of autoimmune skin disease in the dog: correlation between histopathologic, direct immunofluorescent and clinical findings. *Vet. Immunol. and Immunopathol.*, **5**: 57–64.
6 Scott DW, Manning TO, Smith CA and Lewis RM (1982) Observations on the immunopathology and therapy of canine pemphigus and pemphigoid. *JAVMA*, **180**: 48–52.
7 Beale KM (1988) Azathioprine for treatment of immune-mediated diseases of dogs and cats. *JAVMA*, **192**: 1316–18.
8 Serra DA and White SD (1989) Oral chrysotherapy with auranofin in dogs. JAVMA, **194**: 1327–30.

FELINE CUTANEOUS HERPESVIRUS AND FELINE CUTANEOUS CALICIVIRUS INFECTION
1 Flecknell PA, Orr CM, Wright AI *et al.* (1979) Skin ulceration associated with herpesvirus infection in cats. *Vet. Record*, **104**: 313–15.
2 Johnson RP and Sabine M (1971) The isolation of herpesviruses from skin ulcers in domestic cats. *Vet. Record*, **89**: 360–3.
3 Cooper LM and Sabine M (1972) Paw and mouth disease in a cat. *Austr. Vet. J.*, **48**: 644.

SYSTEMIC LUPUS ERYTHEMATOSUS
1 Lewis RM and Picut CA (1989) Multisystem disorders. *Veterinary Clinical Immunology*, Lea & Febiger, Philadelphia, pp. 167–91.
2 Tizard J (1992) The systemic autoimmune diseases. *Veterinary Immunology: An Introduction*, WB Saunders, Philadelphia, pp. 405–10.
3 Thompson JP (1995) Immunologic diseases. *Textbook of Veterinary Internal Medicine* (eds SJ Ettinger and EC Feldman), WB Saunders, Philadelphia, pp. 2017–20.
4 Gross TL, Ihrke PJ and Walder EJ (1992) Bullous and vesicular diseases of the epidermis and dermal–epidermal junction. *Veterinary Dermatopathology*, Mosby Year Book, St. Louis, pp. 24–6.
5 Halliwell REW and Gorman NT (1989) Autoimmune blood diseases. *Veterinary Clinical Immunology*, WB Saunders, Philadelphia, pp. 308–34.

BULLOUS PEMPHIGOID
1 Guidice GJ, Emery DJ and Diaz LA (1992) Cloning and primary structural analysis of the bullous pemphigoid autoantigen BP180. *J. of Invest. Dermatol.*, **99**: 243–50.
2 Ackerman LJ (1985) Canine and feline pemphigus and pemphigoid. Part II. Pemphigoid. *Comp. on Continuing Ed.*, **7**: 281–5.
3 Gorman NT and Werner LL (1986) Immune–mediated

diseases of the dog and cat III. Immune–mediated diseases of the integument, urogenital, endocrine and vascular systems. *BVJ*, **142**: 491–7.
4 Scott DW, Walton DK, Slater MR *et al.* (1987) Immune–mediated dermatoses in domestic animals: ten years after – Part I. *Comp. on Continuing Ed.*, **9**: 424–35.
5 Scott DW, Manning TO, Smith CA and Lewis RM (1982) Observations on the immunopathology and therapy of canine pemphigus and pemphigoid. *JAVMA*, **180**: 48–52.
6 Werner LL, Brown KA and Halliwell REW (1983) Diagnosis of autoimmune skin disease in the dog: correlation between histopathologic, direct immunofluorescent and clinical findings. *Vet. Immunol. and Immunopathol.*, **5**: 57–64.
7 Beale KM (1988) Azathioprine for treatment of immune–mediated diseases of dogs and cats. *JAVMA*, **192**: 1316–18.
8 Serra DA and White SD (1989) Oral chrysotherapy with auranofin in dogs. *JAVMA*, **194**: 1327–30.

SPOROTRICHOSIS
1 Wolf AM and Troy GC (1995) Deep mycotic diseases. *Textbook of Veterinary Internal Medicine* (eds SJ Ettinger and EC Feldman), WB Saunders, Philadelphia, pp. 453–5.
2 Gross TL, Ihrke PJ and Walder EJ (1992) Infectious nodular and diffuse granulomatous and pyogranulomatous diseases of the dermis. *Veterinary Dermatopathology*, Mosby Year Book, St. Louis, pp. 181–4.
3 Dunston, R., Lanham, RF, Reimann, KA and Wakemell, PS (1996) Feline sporotrichosis. A report of five cases with transmission to humans. *J. of the Am. Acad. of Derm.*, 15: 37–45.

IDIOPATHIC EAR MARGIN VASCULITIS
1 Gross TL, Ihrke PJ and Walder EJ (1992) Vascular diseases of the dermis. *Veterinary Dermatopathology*, Mosby Year Book, St. Louis, pp. 135–40.
2 Griffin CE (1985) Pinnal diseases. *The Complete Manual of Ear Care*, Solvay Animal Health Inc., Veterinary Learning Systems Co. Inc., Trenton, pp. 21–35.
3 Manning TO and Scott DW (1980) Cutaneous vasculitis in a dog. *J. of the Am. Animal Hosp. Assoc.*, **16**: 61–7.

Section 4: Papular and pustular dermatoses
SUPERFICIAL PYODERMA
1 Berg JN, Wendell DE, Vogelweid C and Fales WH (1984) Identification of the major coagulase-positive *Staphylococcus* sp. of dogs as *Staphylococcus intermedius*. *Am. J. of Vet. Res.*, **45**: 1307–9.
2 Cox HU, Newman SS, Roy AF and Hoskins JD (1984) Species of *Staphylococcus* isolated from animal infections. *Cornell Vet.*, **74**: 124–35.
3 Lloyd DH (1992) Therapy for canine pyoderma. *Current Veterinary Therapy XI* (eds RW Kirk and JD Bonagura), WB Saunders, Philadelphia, pp. 539–44.
4 Ihrke PJ (1987) An overview of bacterial skin disease in the dog. *BVJ*, **143**: 112–18.
5 Mason IS (1991) Canine pyoderma. *J. of Small Animal*

Practice, **32**: 381–6.

6 Mason IS and Lloyd DH (1992) The role of allergy in the development of canine pyoderma. *J. of Small Animal Practice,* **30**: 216–18.

7 Medleau L, Long RE, Brown J and Miller WH (1986) Frequency and antimicrobial susceptibility of *Staphylococcus* species isolated from canine pyodermas. *Am. J. of Vet. Res.,* **47**: 229–31.

PEMPHIGUS FOLIACEUS

1 Angarano DW (1987) Autoimmune dermatoses. *Contemporary Issues in Small Animal Practice 8* (ed. GH Nesbitt), Churchill Livingstone, New York, pp. 79–94.

2 August JR and Chickering WR (1985) Pemphigus foliaceus causing lameness in four dogs. *Comp. on Continuing Ed.,* **7**: 894–902.

3 Beale KM (1988) Azathioprine for treatment of immune-mediated disease of dogs and cats. *JAVMA,* **192**: 1316–18.

4 Halliwell REW and Gorman NT (1989) (eds) *Veterinary Clinical Immunology,* WB Saunders, Philadelphia, pp. 285–307.

5 Kristensen F and Mehl NB (1989) The use of gold in the treatment of auto-immune disease in the dog and cat. *Dansk Veterinär Tidsskrift,* **15**: 883–7.

6 Manning TO, Scott DW, Smith CA and Lewis RM (1982) Pemphigus diseases in the feline: seven case reports. *J. of the Am. Animal Hosp. Assoc.,* **18**: 433–43.

7 McEwan NA, McNeil PE and Kirkham D (1986) Pemphigus foliaceus: a report of two cases in the dog. *J. of Small Animal Practice,* **27**: 567–75.

8 Norman NJ (1990) Pemphigus. *Dermatol. Clinics,* **84**: 689–700.

9 Scott DW, Walton DK, Slater MR et al. (1987) Immune-mediated dermatoses in domestic animals: ten years after. Part I. *Comp. on Continuing Ed.,* **9**: 424–35.

10 Serra DA and White SD (1989) Oral chrysotherapy with auranofin in dogs. *JAVMA,* **194**: 1327–30.

ZINC RESPONSIVE DERMATOSIS

1 Jezyk PF, Haskins ME, Mackay-Smith WE and Patterson DF (1986) Lethal acrodermatitis in bull terriers. *JAVMA,* **188**: 833.

2 Lewis LD (1981) Cutaneous manifestations of nutritional imbalances. *Proc. of the 48th Ann. Meeting of the Am. Animal Hosp. Assoc.,* p. 263.

3 Thoday KL (1989) Diet-related zinc-responsive skin disease in dogs: a dying dermatosis? *J. of Small Animal Practice,* **30**: 213.

4 Willemse T (1992) Zinc-related cutaneous disorders. *Current Veterinary Therapy XI* (eds RW Kirk and JD Bonagura), WB Saunders, Philadelphia, pp. 532–34.

CANINE JUVENILE CELLULITIS (JUVENILE PYODERMA, PUPPY STRANGLES)

1 Mason IS and Jones J (1989) Juvenile cellulitis in Gordon Setters. *Vet. Record,* **124**: 642.

2 White SD, Rosychuk RAW, Stewart LJ et al. (1989) Juvenile cellulitis in dogs: 15 cases (1979–1988). *JAVMA,* **195**: 1609–11.

3 Moriello KA and Mason IS (1995) Nodular lesions, non-healing wounds and common skin tumours. *Handbook of Small Animal Dermatology,* Elsevier Science Ltd, Oxford, p. 146.

4 Scott DW, Miller WM and Griffin CE (1995) Miscellaneous skin diseases. *Small Animal Dermatology,* WB Saunders, Philadelphia, pp. 938–41.

Section 5: Diseases characterized by sinus formation
BITE WOUNDS

1 Kelly PJ, Mason PR, Els J and Matthewman LA (1992) Pathogens in dog bite wounds in dogs in Harare, Zimbabwe. *Vet. Record,* **131**: 464–6.

2 Carro T, Pederson NC, Beaman BL and Munn R (1989) Subcutaneous abscesses and arthritis caused by a probable bacterial L-form in cats. *JAVMA,* **194**: 1583–8.

3 Cowell AC and Penwick RC (1989) Dog bite wounds: a study of 93 cases. *Comp. on Continuing Ed.,* **11**: 313–18.

ANAL FURUNCULOSIS (PERIANAL FISTULAS)

1 Harvey, CE (1972) Perianal fistula in the dog. *Vet. Record,* **91**: 25–32.

2 Day, MJ (1993) Immunopathology of anal furunculosis in the dog. *J. of Small Animal Practice,* 34: 381–9.

3 Christie, TR (1975) Perianal fistulas in the dog. *Vet. Clinics of N. Am.,* **5**: 353–62.

4 Van E RT (1993) Perianal fistulas. *Disease Mechanisms in Small Animal Surgery* (ed. MJ Bojrab), Lea & Febiger, Philadelphia, pp. 285–6.

5 Vasseur, .B (1981). Perianal fistulae in dogs: a retrospective analysis of surgical techniques. *J. of the Am. Animal Hosp. Assoc.,* **17**: 177–180.

6 Van E RT and Palminteri, A (1987) Tail amputation for treatment of perianal fistulas in dogs. *J. of the Am. Animal Hosp. Assoc.,* **23**: 95–100.

FOREIGN BODY SINUS

1 Fadok VA (1987) Granulomatous dermatitis in dogs and cats. *Seminars in Vet. Med. and Surg. (Small Animal),* **2**: 186–94.

ATYPICAL MYCOBACTERIAL INFECTIONS

1 Chapman JS (1971) The ecology of the atypical mycobacteria. *Arch. of Environ. Health,* **22**: 41–6.

2 Kunkle GA, Gulbas NK, Fadok V et al. (1983) Rapidly growing mycobacteria as a cause of cutaneous granulomas: report of five cases. *J. of the Am. Animal Hosp. Assoc.,* **19**: 513–21.

3 Mason KV and Wilkinson GT (1989) Results of treatment of atypical mycobacteriosis. *Advances in Veterinary Dermatology* (eds C von Tscharner and REW Halliwell), Baillière Tindall, London, p. 452.

4 Monroe WE and Chickering WR (1988) Atypical my-

cobacterial infections in cats. *Comp. on Continuing Ed.*, **10**: 1044–8.

5 Studdert VP and Hughes KL (1992) Treatment of opportunistic mycobacterial infections with enrofloxacin in cats. *JAVMA*, **201**: 1388–90.

FELINE LEPROSY

1 Schieffer HB and Middleton DM (1983) Experimental transmission of a feline mycobacterial skin disease (feline leprosy). *Vet. Pathol.*, **20**: 460–71.

2 McIntosh DW (1982) Feline leprosy: a review of forty-four cases from Western Canada. *Can. Vet. J.*, **23**: 291–5.

3 Mundell AC (1989) The use of clofazimine in the treatment of three cases of feline leprosy. *Advances in Veterinary Dermatology* Vol. 1 (eds C von Tscharner and REW Halliwell), Baillière Tindall, London, p. 451.

DERMOID SINUS

1 Lord LH, Cawley AJ and Gilray J (1957) Mid-dorsal dermoid sinus in Rhodesian Ridgeback dogs – a case report. *JAVMA*, **149**: 515–18.

2 Fatone G, Brunetti A, Lamagus F and Potena A (1995) Dermoid sinus and spinal malformations in a Yorkshire Terrier: diagnosis and follow-up. *J. of Small Animal Practice*, **36**: 176–80.

3 Mann GE and Stratton J (1966) Dermoid sinus in the Rhodesian Ridgeback. *J. of Small Animal Practice*, **7**: 631–42.

4 Selcer EA, Helman RG and Selcer RR (1984) Dermoid sinus in a Shi-Tzu and a Boxer. *J. of the Am. Animal Hosp. Assoc.*, **20**: 634–6.

BLASTOMYCOSIS

1 Legendre AM (1990) Blastomycosis. *Infectious Diseases of Dogs and Cats* (ed. CE Green), WB Saunders, Philadelphia, pp. 669–78.

2 Wolf AM and Troy G. C. (1995) Deep mycotic diseases. *Textbook of Veterinary Internal Medicine* (eds SJ Ettinger and EC Feldman), WB Saunders, Philadelphia, pp. 453–5.

3 Archer JR, Trainer DO and Schell RF (1987) Epidemiologic study of canine blastomycosis in Wisconsin. *JAVMA*, **190**: 1292–5.

4 Rudmann DG, Coolman BR, Perez CM and Glickman LT (1992) Evaluation or risk factors for blastomycosis in dogs: 857 cases (1980–1990). *JAVMA*, **201**: 1754–9.

5 Legendre AM (1995) Antimycotic drug therapy. *Current Veterinary Therapy XII* (ed. JD Bonagura), WB Saunders, Philadelphia, pp. 327–31.

SUBCUTANEOUS MYCOSES

1 Attleberger MH (1980) Subcutaneous and opportunistic mycoses. *Current Veterinary Therapy VII* (ed. RW Kirk), WB Saunders, Philadelphia, pp. 1177–80.

2 Beale KM and Pinson D (1990) Phaeohyphomycosis caused by two different species of *Curvularia* in two animals from the same household. *J. of the Am. Animal Hosp.*

Assoc., **26**: 67–70.

3 Fadok VA (1987) Granulomatous dermatitis in dogs and cats. *Seminars in Vet. Med. and Surg. (Small Animal)*, **2**: 186–94.

4 Kettlewell P, McGinnis MR and Wilkinson GT (1989) Phaeohyphomycosis caused by *Exophiala spinifera* in two cats. *J. of Med. and Vet. Mycol.*, **27**: 257–64.

5 Macartney L, Rycroft AN and Hammil J (1988) Cutaneous protothecosis in the dog: first confirmed case in Britain. *Vet. Record*, **123**: 494–6.

Section 6: Diseases characterized by crust and scale
SEBACEOUS ADENITIS

1 Dunstan RW and Hargis AM (1995) The diagnosis of sebaceous adenitis in Standard Poodle dogs. *Current Veterinary Therapy XII* (ed. JD Bonagura), WB Saunders, Philadelphia, pp. 619–22.

2 Gross TL, Ihrke PJ and Walder EJ (1992) Hyperkeratotic diseases of the epidermis. *Veterinary Dermatopathology*, Mosby Year Book, St Louis, pp. 100–2.

3 Stewart LJ (1990) Newly reported skin disease syndromes in the dog. *Vet. Clinics of N. Am.*, **20**: 1603–13.

4 Power HT and Ihrke PJ (1990) *Vet. Clinics of N. Am.*, **20**: 1525–39.

5 Carothers MA, Kwochka KW and Rojko JL (1991) Cyclosporine-responsive granulomatous sebaceous adenitis in a dog. *JAVMA*, **198**: 1645–8.

FELINE ACNE

1 Rosenkrantz WS (1991) The pathogenesis, diagnosis, and management of feline acne. *Vet. Med.*, **86**: 504–12.

2 Gross TL, Ihrke PJ and Walder EJ (1992) Pustular and nodular diseases with follicular destruction. *Veterinary Dermatopathology*, Mosby Year Book, St. Louis, pp. 258–9.

IDIOPATHIC SEBORRHEA OF COCKER SPANIELS

1 Kwochka KW and Rademakers AM (1989) Cell proliferation of epidermis, hair follicles, and sebaceous glands of Beagles and Cocker Spaniels with healthy skin. *Am. J. of Vet. Res.*, **50**: 587–91.

2 Kwochka KW and Rademakers AM (1989) Cell proliferation of epidermis, hair follicles, and sebaceous glands of Cocker Spaniels with idiopathic seborrhea. *Am. J. of Vet. Res.*, **50**: 1918–22.

3 Kwochka KW (1990) Cell proliferation kinetics in the hair root matrix of dogs with healthy skin and dogs with idiopathic seborrhea. *Am. J. of Vet. Res.*, **51**: 1570–3.

4 Kunkle GA (1983) Managing canine seborrhea. *Current Veterinary Therapy VIII* (ed. RW Kirk), WB Saunders, Philadelphia, pp. 518–23.

5 Austin VH (1983) A clinical approach to abnormal keratinization disease of the dog. *Comp. on Continuing Ed.*, **5**: 890–7.

6 Campbell KA, Uhland CF and Dorn GP (1992) Effects of oral sunflower oil on serum and cutaneous fatty acid

concentration profiles in seborrheic dogs. *Vet. Dermatol.*, **3**: 29–35.

7 Power HT, Ihrke PJ, Stannard AA and Backus KQ (1992) Use of etretinate for treatment of primary keratinization disorders (idiopathic seborrhoea) in Cocker Spaniels, West Highland White Terriers, and Basset Hounds. *JAVMA*, **201**: 419–29.

ACTINIC DERMATOSES

1 Hruza LH and Pentland AP (1993) Mechanisms of UV-induced inflammation. *J. of Invest. Dermatol.*, **100**: 35S–41S.

2 Streilen JW, Taylor JR, Vincek V et al. (1994) Immune surveillance and sunlight-induced skin cancer. *Immunol. Today*, **15**: 174–9.

3 Frank LA and Calderwood-Mays MB (1994) Solar dermatitis in dogs. *Comp. on Continuing Ed.*, **16**: 465–72.

4 Frank LA, Calderwood-Mays MB and Kunkle GA (1996) Distribution and appearance of elastic fibers in the dermis of clinically normal dogs and dogs with solar dermatitis and other dermatoses. *Am. J. of Vet. Res.*, **57**: 178–81.

LEISHMANIASIS

1 Bravo LA, Frank LA and Brenneman KA (1993) Canine leishmaniasis in the United States. *Comp. on Continuing Ed.*, **15**: 699–705.

2 Slappendel RJ and Green CE (1990) Leishmaniasis. *Infectious Diseases of Dogs and Cats* (ed. CE Green), WB Saunders, Philadelphia, pp. 769–77.

3 Koutinas AF, Scott DW, Kantos V and Lekkas S (1992) Skin lesions in canine leismaniasis (Kala-Azar): a clinical and histopathological study on 22 spontaneous cases in Greece. *Vet. Dermatol.*, **3**: 121–30.

4 Ferrer L (1992) Leishmaniasis. *Current Veterinary Therapy XI* (eds RW Kirk and JD Bonagura), WB Saunders, Philadelphia, pp. 266–70.

5 Slappendel RJ (1988) Canine leishmaniasis: a review based on 95 cases in the Netherlands. *Vet. Q.*, **10**: 1–16.

CUTANEOUS HORN

1 Scott DW (1984) Feline dermatology, 1079–1982. *J. of the Am. Animal Hosp. Assoc.*, **20**: 537.

NASAL AND DIGITAL HYPERKERATOSIS

1 Paradis M (1992) Footpad hyperkeratosis in a family of Dogues de Bordeaux. *Vet. Dermatol.*, **3**: 75–8.

2 August JR and Chickering WR (1985) Pemphigus foliaceus causing lameness in four dogs. *Comp. on Continuing Ed.*, **11**: 894–902.

3 Ihrke PJ (1980) Topical therapy – uses, principles, and vehicles in dermatologic therapy (Part 1) *Comp. on Continuing Ed.*, **11**: 28–35.

4 Kwochka KW (1993) Primary keratinization disorders of dogs. *Current Veterinary Dermatology* (eds CE Griffin, KW Kwochka and JM McDonald), Mosby Year Book, St Louis, pp. 176–90.

VITAMIN A RESPONSIVE DERMATOSIS

1 Blumenberg M, Connelly DM and Freedberg IM (1992) Regulation of keratin gene expression: the role of the nuclear receptors of retinoic acid, thyroid hormone, and vitamin D_3. *J. of Invest. Dermatol.*, **98**: 42S–49S.

2 Ihrke PJ and Goldschmidt MH (1983) Vitamin A responsive dermatosis in the dog. *J. of the Am. Animal Hosp. Assoc.*, **182**: 687–90.

ERYTHEMA MULTIFORME

1 Mason KV (1990) Cutaneous drug eruption. *Vet. Clinics of N. Am.*, **20**: 633–53.

2 Medleau L, Chalmers S, Kirpensteijn J et al. (1990) Erythema multiforme and disseminated intravascular coagulation in a dog. *J. of the Am. Animal Hosp. Assoc.*, **26**: 643–6.

3 Delmage DA and Payne-Johnson CE (1991) Erythema multiforme in a Dobermann on trimethoprim-sulphamethoxazole therapy. *J. of Small Animal Practice*, **32**: 635–9.

4 McMurdy MA (1990) A case resembling erythema multiforme major (Stevens–Johnson syndrome) in a dog. *J. of the Am. Animal Hosp. Assoc.*, **26**: 297–300.

Section 7: Pigmentary abnormalities
COLOR-DILUTION ALOPECIA (COLOR-MUTANT ALOPECIA, BLUE DOBERMAN SYNDROME)

1 Miller WH (1990) Color dilution alopecia in Doberman Pinschers with blue or fawn coat colours: a study on the incidence and histopathology of this disorder. *Vet. Dermatol.*, **1**: 113–21.

2 Miller WH (1991) Alopecia associated with coat color dilution in two Yorkshire Terriers, one Saluki, and one mix-breed. *J. of the Am. Animal Hosp. Assoc.*, **27**: 39–43.

3 Brignac MM, Foil CS, Al-Bagdadi FAK and Kreeger J (1990) Microscopy of color mutant alopecia. *Advances in Veterinary Dermatology* Vol. 1 (eds C von Tscharner and REW Halliwell), Baillière Tindall, London, p. 448.

4 Gross TL, Ihrke PJ and Walder EJ (1992) Color-mutant alopecia. *Veterinary Dermatopathology*, Mosby Year Book, St Louis, pp. 298–301.

VITILIGO

1 Naughton GK, Mahaffey M and Bystryn JC (1986) Antibodies to surface antigens of pigmented cells in animals with vitiligo. *Proc. of the Soc. for Exp. Biol. and Med.*, **181**: 423–6.

2 Mosher DB, Fitzpatrick TB, Ortonne JP and Hori Y (1987) Disorders of pigmentation. *Dermatology in General Medicine* (eds TB Fitzpatrick, AZ Eisen, K Wolff, I Freedberg and KF Austen), McGraw-Hill Inc., New York, pp. 794–876.

3 Gross TL, Ihrke PJ and Walder EJ (1992) Vitiligo. *Veterinary Dermatopathology*, Mosby Year Book, St Louis, pp. 150–3.

4 Guagure E and Alhaidari Z (1989) Disorders of melanin pigmentation in the skin of dogs and cats. *Current Veterinary Therapy X* (ed. RW Kirk), WB Saunders, Philadelphia, pp. 628–32.

CANINE UVEODERMATOLOGIC SYNDROME (VOGT–KOYANAGI– HARADA–LIKE (VKH) SYNDROME)

1 Gross TL, Ihrke PJ and Walder EJ (1992) Vogt–Koyanagi–Harada-like syndrome. *Veterinary Dermatopathology*, Mosby Year Book, St Louis, pp. 148–50.
2 Kern TJ, Walton DK, Riis RC et al. (1985) Uveitis associated with poliosis and vitiligo in six dogs. *JAVMA*, **187**: 408–14.
3 Morgan RV (1989) Vogt–Koyanagi–Harada syndrome in humans and dogs. *Comp. on Continuing Ed.*, **11**: 1211–49.
4 Vercelli A and Taraglio S (1990) Canine Vogt–Koyanagi–Harada-like syndrome in two Siberian Husky dogs. *Vet. Dermatol.*, **1**: 151–8.

LENTIGO AND LENTIGINOSIS PROFUSA

1 Mackie RM (1992) Melanocytic naevi and malignant melanomas. *Textbook of Dermatology* (eds RH Champion, JL Burton and FJG Ebling), OUP, Oxford. pp. 1525–60.
2 Nagata M, Nanko H, Moriyama A et al. (1996) Pigmented plaques associated with papillomavirus infection in dogs: is this epidermodysplasia verruciformis? *Vet. Dermatol.*, **6**: 179–86.
3 Prunieras M (1986) Melanocytes, melanogenesis and inflammation. *Intl J. of Dermatol.*, **25**: 624–8.
4 Briggs OM (1985) Lentiginosis profusa in the pug: three case reports. *J. of Small Animal Practice*, **26**: 675–80.
5 Scott DW (1987) Lentigo simplex in orange cats. *Companion Animal Practice*, **1**: 23–5.
6 Van Rensburg IBJ and Briggs OM (1986) Pathology of canine lenitigosis profusa. *J. of the S. Afr. Vet. Assoc.*, **56**: 159–61.
7 Nash S and Paulsen D (1990) Generalized lentigines in a silver cat. *JAVMA*, **196**: 1500–1.
8 Selmanowitz VJ, Orentreiach N and Felsenstein JM (1971) Lentiginosis profusa syndrome (multiple lentigines syndrome). *Arch. of Dermatol.*, **104**: 393–401.

Section 8: Environmental dermatoses
TICK INFESTATION

1 Hoskins JD and Cupp EW (1988) Ticks of veterinary importance. Part I. The Ixodes family: identification, behavior, and associated diseases. *Comp. on Continuing Ed.*, **10**: 564–80.
2 Hoskins JD and Cupp EW (1988) Ticks of veterinary importance. Part II. The Argasidae family: identification, behavior, and associated diseases. *Comp. on Continuing Ed.*, **10**: 699–708.
3 Appel MJ and Jacobson RH (1995) CVT update: canine Lyme disease. *Current Veterinary Therapy XII* (ed. JD Bonagura), WB Saunders, Philadelphia, pp. 303–9.
4 Fadok VA (1980) Miscellaneous parasites of the skin (Part I). *Comp. on Continuing Ed.*, **11**: 707–12.

BEE STINGS AND SPIDER BITES

1 Elgart GW (1990) Ant, bee and wasp stings. *Dermatol. Clinics*, **8**: 229–36.
2 Wilson DC and King LE (1990) Spiders and spider bites. *Dermatol. Clinics*, **8**: 277–86.
3 Meerdink GI (1983) Bites and stings of venomous animals. *Current Veterinary Therapy VIII* (ed. RW Kirk), WB Saunders, Philadelphia, pp. 155–9.
4 Cowell AK, Cowell RL, Tyler RD and Nieves MA (1991) Severe systemic reactions to *Hymenoptera* stings in dogs. *JAVMA*, **198**: 1014–16.
5 Curtis CF, Bond R, Blunden AS et al. (1995) Canine eosinophilic folliculitis and furunculosis in three cases. *J. of Small Animal Practice*, **36**: 119–23.
6 Gross TL, Ihrke PJ and Walder EJ (1992) *Veterinary Dermatopathology*, Mosby Year Book, St Louis, pp. 269–70.
7 Walder EJ and Howard EB (1991) Persistent insect bite granuloma in a dog. *Vet. Pathol.*, **19**: 839–41.

FLY AND MOSQUITO BITE DERMATOSES

1 Mason KV and Evans AG (1991) Mosquito bite-caused eosinophilic dermatitis in cats. *JAVMA*, **198**: 2086–8.
2 Wilkinson GT and Bates MJ (1984) A possible further clinical manifestation of the feline eosinophilic granuloma complex. *J. of the Am. Animal Hosp. Assoc.*, **20**: 325–31.

BURNS

1 McKeever PJ (1980) Thermal injury. *Current Veterinary Therapy VII* (ed. RW Kirk), WB Saunders, Philadelphia, pp. 191–4.
2 Saxon WD and Kirby R (1992) Treatment of acute burn injury and smoke inhalation. *Current Veterinary Therapy XI* (eds RW Kirk and JD Bonagura), WB Saunders, Philadelphia, pp. 146–52.
3 Rudowski W, Nasitowski W, Zietkiewiez W and Ziemkiewiez K (1976) *Burn Therapy and Research*. Johns Hopkins University Press, Baltimore.
4 Stamp GL and Crow DT (1992) Triage and resuscitation of the catastrophic trauma patient. *Current Veterinary Therapy XI* (eds RW Kirk and JD Bonagura), WB Saunders, Philadelphia, pp. 75–82.
5 Ofeigsson OJ (1995) Water cooling: first aid treatment for scalds and burns. *Surgery*, **57**: 391–400.

MYIASIS

1 Hendrix CM (1991) Facultative myiasis in dogs and cats. *Comp. on Continuing Ed.*, **13**: 86–93.

FROSTBITE

1 Dietrich RA (1983) Cold injury (hypothermia, frostbite, freezing). *Current Veterinary Therapy VIII* (ed. RW Kirk), WB Saunders, Philadelphia, pp. 187–9.

Section 9: Endocrine dermatoses
HYPOTHYROIDISM

1 Gill GN, Bardin CW and Thau RB (1985) The hypothalamic–pituitary control system. *Best and Taylor's Physiological Basis of Medical Practice* (ed. JB West), Williams & Wilkins, Baltimore, pp. 856–71.
2 Kaptein EM and Hayes MT (1994) Thyroid hormone me-

tabolism – a comparative evaluation. *Vet. Clinics of N. Am.*, **24**: 431–61.

3 Scott DW, Miller WM and Griffin CE (1995) Endocrine and metabolic diseases. *Small Animal Dermatology*, WB Saunders, Philadelphia, pp. 628–719.

4 Ferguson DC (1995) Update on diagnosis of canine hypothyroidism. *Vet. Clinics of N. Am.*, **24**: 515–39.

5 Kemppainen RJ and MacDonald JM (1993) Canine hypothyroidism. *Current Veterinary Dermatology* (eds CE Griffin, KW Kwochka and JM Macdonald), Mosby Year Book, St Louis, pp. 265–72.

6 Feldman EC and Nelson RW (1987) Hypothyroidism. *Canine and Feline Endocrinology and Reproduction*, WB Saunders, Philadelphia, pp. 55–90.

7 Kemppainen RJ and Clark TP (1995) Etiopathogenesis of canine hypothyroidism. *Vet. Clinics of N. Am.*, **24**: 467–76.

8 Moriello KA and Mason IS (1995) Alopecia. *Handbook of Small Animal Dermatology*, Elsevier Science Ltd, Oxford, pp. 75–91.

HYPERADRENOCORTICISM

1 Willeberg P and Priester WA (1982) Epidemiological aspects of clinical hyperadrenocorticism in dogs (canine Cushing's syndrome). *J. of the Am. Animal Hosp. Assoc.*, **18**: 717–24.

2 Nelson RW, Feldman EC and Smith MC (1988) Hyperadrenocorticism in cats: seven cases (1978–1987). *JAVMA*, **193**: 245–61.

3 Chastain CB and Graham CL (1979) Adrenocortical suppression in dogs on daily and alternate day prednisone administration. *Am. J. of Vet. Res.*, **40**: 936–41.

4 Zenoble RD and Kemppainen RJ (1987) Adrenocortical suppression by topically applied corticosteroids in healthy dogs. *JAVMA*, **191**: 685–8.

5 Murphy CJ, Feldman E and Bellhorn R (1990) Iatrogenic Cushing's syndrome in a dog caused by topical ophthalmic medications. *J. of the Am. Animal Hosp. Assoc.*, **26**: 640–2.

6 Peterson ME (1986) Canine hyperadrenocorticism. *Current Veterinary Therapy IX* (ed. RW Kirk), WB Saunders, Philadelphia, pp. 963–72.

7 Ling GV, Stabenfeldt GH, Comer KM et al. (1979) Canine hyperadrenocorticism: pretreatment clinical and laboratory evaluation of 117 cases. *JAVMA*, **174**: 1211–15.

8 White SD, Ceragioli KL, Bullock LP and Mason GD (1989) Cutaneous markers of canine hyperadrenocorticism. *Comp. on Continuing Ed.*, **11**: 446–64.

9 Scott DW (1982) Histopathological findings in endocrine skin disorders. *J. of the Am. Animal Hosp. Assoc.*, **18**: 173–83.

10 Hansen BL, Kamppainen RJ and MacDonald JM (1994) Synthetic ACTH (cosyntropin) stimulation tests in normal dogs: comparison of intravenous and intramuscular administration. *J. of the Am. Animal Hosp. Assoc.*, **30**: 38–40.

11 Huntley K, Frazer J, Gibbs C and Gaskell CJ (1982) The radiological features of canine Cushing's syndrome: a review of forty eight cases. *J. of Small Animal Practice*, **23**: 369–80.

12 Reusch C and Feldman EC (1991) Canine hyperadrenocorticism due to adrenocortical neoplasia: pretreatment evaluation of 41 dogs. *J. of Vet. Int. Med.*, **5**: 3–10.

13 Widmer WR and Guptill L (1995) Imaging techniques for facilitating the diagnosis of hyperadrenocorticism in dogs and cats. *JAVMA*, **206**: 1857–64.

14 Scavelli TD, Peterson ME and Matthieson DT (1986) Results of surgical treatment for hyperadrenocorticism caused by adrenocortical neoplasia in the dog: 25 cases (1980–1984). *JAVMA*, **189**: 1360–4.

15 Kintzer PP and Peterson ME (1994) Mitotane treatment of 32 dogs with cortisol-secreting adrenocortical neoplasms. *JAVMA*, **205**: 54–61.

16 Emms SG, Johnston DE, Eigenmann JE and Goldschmidt MH (1997) Adrenalectomy in the management of canine hyperadrenocorticism. *J. of the Am. Animal Hosp. Assoc.*, **23**: 557–64.

17 Bruyette DS, Ruehl WW, Entriken T, Darling LA and Griffin DW (1997) Treating canine pituitary-dependent hyperadrenocorticism with L-deprenyl. *Veterinary Medicine*, **August 1997**: 711–27.

PITUITARY DWARFISM

1 Scott DW, Miller WM and Griffin CE (1995) Endocrine and metabolic diseases. *Small Animal Dermatology*, WB Saunders, Philadelphia, pp. 628–719.

2 Lund-Larson TR and Grondalen J (1976) Aetiolitic dwarfism in the German Shepherd Dog. Low somatomedin activity associated with apparently normal pituitary function (two cases) and with panadenopituitary dysfunction (one case). *Acta Vet. Scand.*, **17**: 293–306.

3 Chastain CB and Ganjam VK (1986) The endocrine brain. *Clinical Endocrinology of Companion Animals*, Lea & Febiger, Philadelphia, pp. 37–96.

4 Eigenmann JE (1986) Growth hormone-deficient disorders associated with alopecia in the dog. *Current Veterinary Therapy IX* (ed. RW Kirk), WB Saunders, Philadelphia, pp. 1006–14.

5 DeBowes LJ (1987) Pituitary dwarfism in a German Shepherd puppy. *Comp. on Continuing Ed.*: **9**: 931–7.

6 Feldman EC and Nelson RW (1987) Growth hormone. *Canine and Feline Endocrinology and Reproduction*, WB Saunders, Philadelphia, pp. 29–54.

7 Bell AG (1993) Growth hormone responsive dermatosis in three dogs. *NZ Vet. J.*, **41**: 195–9.

CANINE FAMILIAL DERMATOMYOSITIS

1 Hargis AM and Haupt KH (1990) Review of familial canine dermatomyositis. *Vet. Ann.*, **30**: 227–82.

2 Hargis AM and Mundell AC (1992) Familial canine dermatomyositis. *Comp. on Continuing Ed.*, **14**: 855–64.

3 Haupt KH, Prieur DJ, Moore MP et al. (1985) Familial canine dermatomyositis: clinical, electrodiagnostic, and genetic studies. *Am. J. of Vet. Res.*, **46**: 1861–9.

4 Gross TL, Ihrke PJ and Walder EJ (1992) Necrotizing dis-

eases of the epidermis. *Veterinary Dermatopathology*, Mosby Year Book, St Louis, pp. 34–6.

SERTOLI CELL AND OTHER TESTICULAR NEOPLASIA

1 Aronsohn M (1979) Canine testicular neoplasia. *Comp. on Continuing Ed.*, **1**: 925–8.
2 Lipowitz AJ, Schwartz A, Wilson GP and Ebert JW (1973) Testicular neoplasms and concomitant clinical changes in the dog. *JAVMA*, **163**: 1364–8.
3 Scott DW and Reimers T (1986) Tail gland and perianal gland hyperplasia associated with testicular neoplasia and hypertestosteronemia in a dog. *Canine Practice*, **13**: 15–17.
4 Sherding RG, Wilson GP and Kociba GJ (1981) Bone marrow hypoplasia in eight dogs with Sertoli cell tumour. *JAVMA*, **175**: 197–501.
5 Suess RP, Barr SC, Sacre BJ and French TW (1992) Bone marrow hypoplasia in a feminized dog with an interstitial cell tumour. *JAVMA*, **200**: 1346–8.
6 Weaver AD (1983) Survey with follow-up of 67 dogs with testicular Sertoli cell tumours. *Vet. Record*, **113**: 105–7.
7 Wilson GP and Hayes HM (1979) Castration for treatment of perianal gland neoplasms in the dog. *JAVMA*, **174**: 1301–3.

DERMATOSES RESPONSIVE TO NEUTERING

1 Rosser EJ (1989) Castration responsive dermatosis in the dog. *Advances in Veterinary Dermatology* Vol. 1 (eds C von Tscharner and REW Halliwell), Baillière Tindall, London, pp. 34–42.
2 Gross TL, Ihrke PJ and Walder EJ (1992) *Veterinary Dermatopathology*, Mosby Year Book, St Louis, pp. 280–4.
3 Fiorito DA (1992) Hyperestrogenism in bitches. *Comp. on Continuing Ed.*, **14**: 727–9.
4 Medleau L (1989) Sex hormone-associated endocrine alopecias in dogs. *J. of the Am. Animal Hosp. Assoc.*, **25**: 689–94.
5 Nemzek JA, Homco LD, Wheaton LG and Gorman GL (1992) Cystic ovaries and hyperestrogenism in a canine female pseudohermaphrodite. *J. of the Am. Animal Hosp. Assoc.*, **28**: 402–6.

DERMATOSES RELATED TO ADRENAL SEX HORMONES (GROWTH HORMONE RESPONSIVE DERMATOSIS)

1 Rosenkrantz WS (1995) Alopecia associated with adrenal sex hormone abnormalities. *Proc. 19th Waltham/OSU Symp. for the Treatment of Animal Dis.*, Columbus, pp. 59–62.
2 Rosenkrantz WS and Griffin CE (1992) Lysodren therapy in suspect adrenal sex hormone dermatoses. *Advances in Veterinary Dermatology* Vol. 2 (eds PJ Ihrke, IS Mason and SD White), Pergamon Press, Oxford, pp. 451–4.
3 Schmeitzel LP and Lothrop CD (1990) Hormonal ab-

normalities in Pomeranians with normal coat and in Pomeranians with growth hormone-responsive dermatosis. *JAVMA*, **107**: 1333–41.

TELOGEN EFFLUVIUM AND ANAGEN DEFLUXION

1 Baker KP (1974) Hair growth and replacement in the cat. *BVJ*, **130**: 327–34.
2 Hale PA (1982) Periodic hair shedding by a normal bitch. *J. of Small Animal Practice*, **23**: 345–50.
3 Gunaratnam P and Wilkinson GT (1983) A study of normal hair growth in the dog. *J. of Small Animal Practice*, **24**: 445–53.
4 Scott DW, Miller WM and Griffin CE (1995) Acquired alopecias. *Small Animal Dermatology*, WB Saunders, Philadelphia, pp. 720–35.

POST-CLIPPING ALOPECIA

1 Gross TL, Ihrke PJ and Walder EJ (1992) Post-clipping alopecia. *Veterinary Dermatopathology*, Mosby Year Book, St Louis, pp. 285–6.

Section 10: Otitis externa

1 August, JR (1988) Otitis externa: a disease of multifactorial etiology. *Vet. Clinics of N. Am.*, 18: 731–42.
2 McKeever, PJ (1995) Canine otitis externa. *Kirk's Current Veterinary Therapy XII* (ed. JD Bonagura), WB Saunders, Philadelphia, pp. 647–55.
3 McArthy, G and Kelly, WR (1982) Microbial species associated with canine ear disease and their antibacterial sensitivity patterns. *Irish Vet. J.*, **36**: 53–6.
4 Mansfield PD, Boosinger TR and Attleburger MH (1990) Infectivity of *Malassezia pachydermatis* in the external ear canal of dogs. *J. of the Am. Animal Hosp. Assoc.*, **26**: 97–100.
5 Stout-Graham, MS, Kainer, RA, Whalen, LR and Macey, DW (1990). Morphological measurements of the horizontal ear canal of dogs. *Am. J. of Vet. Research*, **51**: 990–4.
6 Van der Gaag, I (1986) The pathology of the external ear canal in dogs and cats. *Vet. Quarterly*, **8**: 307–17.
7 Neer, MT and Howard, PE (1982) Otitis media. *Comp. on Continuing Ed.*, 4: 410–17.
8 Mansfield, PD (1990). Ototoxicity in dogs and cats. *Comp. on Continuing Ed.*, 12: 331–7.
9 Morrielo, KA, Fehrer-Sawyer, SL, Meyer, DJ and Feder, B (1988) Adrenocortical suppression associated with topical otic administration of glucocorticoids in dogs. *J. of the Am. Vet. Med. Assoc.*, **193**: 329–31.
10 Paradis, M (1989) Ivermectin in small animal dermatology. *Current Veterinary Therapy X* (ed. RW Kirk), WB Saunders, Philadelphia, pp. 560–3.

Section 11: Disorders of the nails

1 Scott DW and Miller WH (1992) Disorders of the claw and clawbed in dogs. *Comp. on Continuing Ed.*, **14**: 1448–58.
2 Rosychuck RAW (1995) Diseases of the claw and claw fold. *Current Veterinary Therapy XII* (ed. JD Bonagura), WB

Saunders, Philadelphia, pp. 641–7.

3 Foil CS (1987) Disorders of the feet and claws. *Proc. of Ann. Kal Kan Symposium*, **11**: 23–32.

4 McKeever PJ (1972–96) Unpublished observations.

Section 12: Dermatoses characterized by patchy alopecia
CANINE DEMODICOSIS (RED MANGE, DEMODECTIC MANGE, DEMODICOSIS, DEMODECTIC ACARIASIS, FOLLICULAR MANGE)

1 Folz SD (1983) Demodicosis (*Demodex canis*). *Comp. on Continuing Ed.*, **5**: 116–24.

2 Barrage O, Al-Child NW, Martin S and Whyman M (1992) Evidence of immunosuppression by *Demodex canis*. *Vet. Immunol. and Immunopathol.*, **32**: 37–46.

3 Corbett R, Banks K, Hinrichs D and Bell T (1975) Cellular immune responsiveness in dogs with demodectic mange. *Transplant. Proc.*, **7**: 557–9.

4 Hirsh DC, Baker B, Wigner N et al. (1975) Suppression of *in vitro* lymphocyte transformation by serum from dogs with generalized demodicosis. *Am. J. of Vet. Res.*, **36**: 1591–5.

5 Krawiec DR and Gaafar SM (1980) Studies on the immunology of canine demodicosis. *J. of the Am. Animal Hosp. Assoc.*, **16**: 669–76.

6 Scott DW, Schultz RD and Baker E (1976) Further studies on the therapeutic and immunologic aspects of generalized demodectic mange in the dog. *J. of the Am. Animal Hosp. Assoc.*, **12**: 203–13.

7 Barta O, Waltman C, Oyekan PP et al. (1983) Lymphocyte transformation suppression caused by pyoderma – failure to demonstrate it in uncomplicated demodectic mange. *Comp. Immunol., Microbiol. and Inf. Dis.*, **6**: 9–18.

8 Scott DW, Farrow BRH and Schultz RD (1974) Studies on the therapeutic and immunologic aspects of generalized demodectic mange in the dog. *J. of the Am. Animal Hosp. Assoc.*, **10**: 233–44.

9 Kwochka KW, Kunkle GA and O'Neill Foil CO (1985) The efficacy of amitraz for generalized demodicosis in dogs: a study of two concentrations and frequencies of application. *Comp. on Continuing Ed.*, **7**: 8–18.

10 Muller GH (1983) Amitraz treatment of demodicosis. *J. of the Am. Animal Hosp. Assoc.*, **19**: 435–41.

11 Garfield RA and Reedy LM (1992) The use of oral milbemycin oxime (Interceptor) in the treatment of chronic generalized canine demodicosis. *Vet. Dermatol.*, **3**: 231–325.

12 Miller HW, Scott DW, Wellington JR and Panic R (1993) Clinical efficacy of milbemycin oxime in the treatment of generalized demodicosis in adult dogs. *JAVMA*, **203**: 1426–9.

13 Ristic A, Medleau L, Paradis M and White-Weithers NE (1995) Ivermectin for treatment of generalized demodicosis in dogs. *JAVMA*, **207**: 1308–10.

14 Scott DW, Miller WM and Griffin CE (1995) Parasitic skin diseases. *Small Animal Dermatology*, WB Saunders,

Philadelphia, pp. 392–467.

DERMATOPHYTOSIS

1 Odds FC, Araf T, Disolvo AF et al. (1992) Nomenclature of fungal diseases: a report and recommendation from a sub-committee of the International Society for Human and Animal Mycology. *J. of Med. and Vet. Mycol.*, **30**: 1–10.

2 Wright AI (1989) Ringworm in dogs and cats. *J. of Small Animal Practice*, **30**: 242–9.

3 Lewis DT, Foil CS and Hopgood G (1991) Epidemiology and clinical features of dermatophytosis in dogs and cats at Louisiana State University: 1981–1990. *Vet. Dermatol.*, **2**: 53–8.

4 Quaife RA and Womar SM (1982) *Microsporum canis* isolations from show cats. *Vet. Record*, **110**: 333–4.

5 Moriello KA, Kunkle G and DeBoer DJ (1994) Isolation of dermatophytes from the haircoats of stray cats from selected animal shelters in two different geographic regions in the United States. *Vet. Dermatol.*, **5**: 57–62.

6 Moriello KA and DeBoer DJ (1991) Fungal flora of the coat of pet cats. *Am. J. of Vet. Res.*, **52**: 602–6.

7 Sparkes AH, Werrett G, Stokes CR and Gruffydd-Jones TJ (1994) *Microsporum canis*: inapparent carriage by cats and the viability of arthropsores. *J. of Small Animal Practice*, **35**: 397–401.

8 Moriello KA (1990) Management of dermatophyte infections in catteries and multiple-cat households. *Vet. Clinics of N. Am.*, **20**: 1457–74.

9 DeBoer DJ and Moriello KA (1994) The immune response to *Microsporum canis* induced by a fungal cell wall vaccine. *Vet. Dermatol.*, **5**: 47–55.

10 Sparkes AH, Stokes CR and Gruffydd-Jones TJ (1993) Humoral immune responses in cats with dermatophytosis. *Am. J. of Vet. Res.*, **54**: 1869–73.

11 Jones HE (1993) Immune response and host resistance of humans to dermatophyte infection. *J. of the Am. Acad. of Dermatol.*, **28**: 12S–18S.

12 DeBoer DJ and Moriello KA (1995) Inability of two topical treatments to influence the course of experimental feline dermatophytosis. *JAVMA*, **207**: 52–7.

13 Moriello KA and DeBoer DJ (1994) Efficacy of griseofulvin and itraconazole in the treatment of experimental feline dermatophytosis. *JAVMA*, **207**: 439–44.

14 Bond R, Middleton DJ, Scarff DH and Lamport AI (1992) Chronic dermatophytosis due to *Microsporum persicolor* infection in three dogs. *J. of Small Animal Practice*, **33**: 571–6.

15 Harvey RG (1990) Fungal culture in small animal practice. *In Practice (Journal of Veterinary Postgraduate Clinical Study)*, **12**: 11–16.

16 Moriello KA and DeBoer DJ (1995) Feline dermatophytosis: recent advances and recommendations for therapy. *Vet. Clinics of N. Am.*, **25**: 901–21.

17 Carney HC and Moriello KA (1993) Dermatophytosis: cattery management plan. *Current Veterinary Dermatology* (eds CE Griffin, KW Kwochka and JM Macdonald), Mosby Year Book, St Louis, pp. 34–43.

18 Hill PB, Moriello KA and Shaw SE (1995) A review of systemic antifungal agents. *Vet. Dermatol.*, **6**: 59–66.

19 Sparkes AH, Werrett G, Stokes CR and Gruffydd-Jones TJ (1994) *Microsporum canis:* inapparent carriage by cats and the viability of arthrospores. *J. of Small Animal Practice*, **35**: 397–401.

FOLLICULAR DYSPLASIA

1 Post K, Dignean MA and Clark E (1988) Hair follicle dysplasia of Siberian Huskies. *J. of the Am. Animal Hosp. Assoc.*, **24**: 659–62.

2 Miller WH (1990) Follicular dysplasia in adult black and red Doberman Pinschers. *Vet. Dermatol.*, **1**: 181–7.

3 Miller MA and Dunstan RW (1993) Seasonal flank alopecia in Boxers and Airedale Terriers: 24 cases (1985–1992). *JAVMA*, **203**: 1567–72.

4 Gross TL, Ihrke PJ and Walder EJ (1992) *Veterinary Dermatopathology*, Mosby Year Book, St Louis, pp. 302–6.

INJECTION SITE ALOPECIA

1 Wilcock BP and Yager JA (1986) Focal cutaneous vasculitis and alopecia at sites of rabies vaccination in dogs. *JAVMA*, **188**: 1174–7.

2 Gross TL, Ihrke PJ and Walder EJ (1992) Atrophic diseases of the hair follicle. *Veterinary Dermatopathology*, Mosby Yearbook, St Louis, pp. 287–98.

3 Lester S, Clemett T and Burt A (1996) Vaccine site-associated sarcomas in cats: clinical experience and a laboratory review (1982–1993). *J. of the Am. Animal Hosp. Assoc.*, **32**: 91–5.

FELINE DEMODICOSIS

1 Conroy JD, Healey MC and Bane AG (1982) New *Demodex* sporotrichosis infesting a cat: a case report. *J. of the Am. Animal Hosp. Assoc.*, **18**: 405–7.

2 Cowan LA and Campbell K (1988) Generalized demodicosis in a cat responsive to amitraz. *JAVMA*, **192**: 1442–4.

3 Chalmers S, Schick RO and Jeffers J (1989) Demodicosis in two cats seropositive for feline immunodeficiency virus. *JAVMA*, **194**: 256–7.

4 White SD, Carpenter JL, Moore FM and Ogilvie G (1987) Generalized demodicosis associated with diabetes mellitus in two cats. *JAVMA*, **191**: 448–9.

5 Stogdale L and Moore DJ (1982) Feline demodicosis. *J. of the Am. Animal Hosp. Assoc.*, **18**: 427–32.

6 Gunaratnam, P, Wilkinson GT and Seawright AA (1983) A study of amitraz toxicity in cats. *Austr. Vet. J.*, **60**: 278–9.

ALOPECIA AREATA

1 Olivery T, Moore PF, Naydan SK *et al.* (1996) Antifollicular cell-mediated and humoral immunity in canine alopecia areata. *Vet. Dermatol.*, **7**: 67–77.

2 Gross TL, Ihrke PJ and Walder EJ (1992) Alopecia areata. *Veterinary Dermatopathology*, Mosby Year Book, St Louis, pp. 291–2.

3 Scott DW, Miller WM and Griffin CE (1995) Immunologic skin disease. *Small Animal Dermatology*, WB Saunders, Philadelphia, pp. 611–13.

BLACK HAIR FOLLICLE ALOPECIA

1 Hargis AM, Brignac MM, Al-Bagdadi FAK *et al.* (1991) Black hair follicular dysplasia in black and white Saluki dogs: differentiation from color mutant alopecia in the Doberman Pinscher by microscopic examination of hairs. *Vet. Dermatol.*, **2**: 69–83.

2 Selmanowitz VJ, Markofsky F and Orentreich N (1977) *JAVMA*, **171**: 1079–81.

3 Harper RC (1978) Congenital black hair follicle dysplasia in Bearded Collie pups. *Vet. Record*, **102**: 87.

Index